Community mental health nursing and dementia care

Community mental health nursing and dementia care

Practice perspectives

Edited by John Keady, Charlotte L. Clarke and Trevor Adams

Open University Press
Maidenhead · Philadelphia

Open University Press
McGraw-Hill Education
McGraw-Hill House
Shoppenhangers Road
Maidenhead
Berkshire
England
SL6 2QL

email: enquiries@openup.co.uk
world wide web: www.openup.co.uk

and
325 Chestnut Street
Philadelphia, PA 19106, USA

First published 2003

A catalogue record of this book is available from the British Library

ISBN 0 335 21142 9 (pb) 0 335 21143 7 (hb)

Library of Congress Cataloging-in-Publication Data
CIP data applied for

Typeset by RefineCatch Limited, Bungay, Suffolk
Printed in Great Britain by Biddles Ltd, *www.biddles.co.uk*

Contents

Contributors   viii
Acknowledgements   xiii
Editorial note   xiv
Foreword by Professor Mike Nolan   xv
Introduction   xvii

PART ONE
Setting the scene   1
The landscape of contemporary community mental health nursing practice in
dementia care

1 **Voices from the past**   3
   The historical alignment of dementia care to nursing
   Peter Nolan

2 **Integrating practice and knowledge in a clinical context**   17
   Charlotte L. Clarke, John Keady and Trevor Adams

3 **Multi-disciplinary teamworking**   33
   Trevor Adams, Mark Holman and Gordon Mitchell

4 **'We put our heads together'**   45
   Negotiating support with the community mental health nurse
   Anne Mason, Heather Wilkinson, Elinor Moore and Anne McKinley

5 **Risk and dementia**   63
   Models for community mental health nursing practice
   Jill Manthorpe

PART TWO
Dementia care nursing in the community   75
Assessment and practice approaches

6 **Assessment and therapeutic approaches for community mental health
   nursing dementia care practice**   77
   An overview
   Linda Miller

7   Cognitive-behavioural interventions in dementia   88
Practical and practice issues for community mental health nurses
Peter Ashton

8   Turning rhetoric into reality   104
Person-centred approaches for community mental health nursing
Tracy Packer

9   From screening to intervention   120
The community mental health nurse in a memory clinic setting
Sean Page

**10   The community mental health nurse role in sharing a diagnosis
of dementia**   134
Practice approaches from an early intervention study
Chris Clark

11   Group therapy   148
The double bonus effect of intervention for people with dementia and
their carers
Kath Lowery and Michelle Murray

12   Psychosocial interventions with family carers of people with dementia   160
Helen Pusey

13   Admiral Nurses   171
A model of family assessment and intervention
Alison Soliman

14   Normalization as a philosophy of dementia care   186
Experiences and practice illustrations from a dedicated community
mental health nursing team
Dot Weaks and Gill Boardman

15   Assessing and responding to challenging behaviour in dementia   199
A focus for community mental health nursing practice
Marilla Pugh and John Keady

PART THREE
Leading and developing community mental health nursing in dementia   213

16   Clinical supervision and dementia care
Issues for community mental health nursing practice   215
Angela Carradice, John Keady and Sue Hahn

17 Multi-agency and inter-agency working
Issues in managing a community mental health nursing service
in dementia   236
Cathy Mawhinney, Paul McCloskey and Assumpta Ryan

18 Higher-level practice   250
Addressing the learning needs for community mental health nursing
practice in dementia care
Jan Dewing and Vicki Traynor

Index   265

Contributors

Trevor Adams is a lecturer in mental health at the European Institute of Health and Medical Sciences, University of Surrey. Prior to teaching, Trevor worked as a community psychiatric nurse in Oldham. Trevor later completed an MSc Nursing Studies (Brunel University) and a PhD in Community Mental Health Nursing to People with Dementia (University of Surrey). Trevor has written widely on community mental health nursing to people with dementia, and with Dr Charlotte L. Clarke edited *Dementia Care: Developing Partnerships in Practice* (Baillière Tindall 1999).

Peter Ashton is a senior lecturer/course director in the School of Nursing, Midwifery and Health Studies at the University of Wales, Bangor. Previously, he practised for several years as a community mental health nurse with older adults. More recently he has qualified and become registered as a cognitive behaviour therapist, and provides an undergraduate level module on cognitive behaviour therapy for nurses.

Gill Boardman is a community mental health nurse based with the community mental health nursing team for people with dementia at Murray Royal Hospital, Perth, Scotland. Gill is both a general and mental health nurse and has worked in her current role since 1988. Gill is a long-standing council member of Alzheimer Scotland – Action on Dementia, and has previously served on the executive of this organization. Gill has a particular interest in ethics and dementia care.

Angela Carradice graduated from Hull University with a BSc (Hons) in Psychology in 1994. She then worked in a psychiatric institution with people with severe and enduring mental health problems, cognitive impairments and challenging behaviour. In 1996 Angela began a three-year doctorate training in clinical psychology at Sheffield University. The doctorate research project focused on how community mental health nurses think when they assess carers for people with dementia. This influenced her growing interest in clinical supervision and nursing. Angela now works half time in inpatient services and a community mental health team.

Chris Clark qualified as a registered mental nurse in 1981 and is currently working as a community mental health nurse with older people for Doncaster and South Humber Trust. Her completed research study *Early Interventions in Dementia* has led to developing the role of community mental health nursing in promoting early referral and diagnosis of people with dementia in primary care.

Charlotte L. Clarke has worked in dementia care practice and research since the mid-1980s. She is currently working at Northumbria University as Professor of Nursing Practice Development Research and as Head of the Nursing, Midwifery and Allied Health Professions Research and Development Unit.

Jan Dewing works as a consultant nurse with Milton Keynes Primary Care Trust and General NHS Trusts. She is also an associate fellow in practice development with the Royal College of Nursing. Her specialist practice interests are in dementia care and she is exploring the meaning and purpose of 'wandering' for a doctoral degree.

Sue Hahn is currently a senior lecturer at the University of Hertfordshire and is the Book Review Editor for *Dementia: The International Journal of Social Research and Practice*. Prior to this she worked as a research and training officer and a community mental health nurse for people with dementia and their carers.

Mark Holman works as a community mental health nurse in Derwentside, County Durham. He has been involved in supervisory relationships as both supervisee and supervisor for more than 12 years, eight of which he has spent working in older people's services.

John Keady worked as a community mental health nurse in a community dementia team in north west Wales before moving into teaching and research at the University of Wales, Bangor, in July 1993. John has maintained an active research and teaching interest in dementia care and his PhD was awarded on the basis of an in-depth study exploring the social construction of dementia.

Kath Lowery trained as an RMN and worked predominately with older people in the mental health services in a variety of settings. Following several years as a community mental health nurse located in a community mental health centre, she became a visiting worker at the Medical Research Centre as a project coordinator on studies relating to dementia. Currently she is involved in a number of research studies with a focus on service user involvement.

Jill Manthorpe is Reader in Community Care at the University of Hull. Her research interests lie in older people's services and she has recently completed projects on risk, dementia care, older nurses and care management. She is Chair of the Hull and East Yorkshire Adult Protection Committee and Vice Chair of the Social Services Research Group.

Anne Mason is a lecturer within the Faculty of Human Science Nursing and Midwifery Department based at the Highland Campus, University of Stirling. Anne's research interests centre on identifying ways of empowering people with dementia and their families, and understanding the experiences of living with dementia, particularly in rural areas.

Cathy Mawhinney is employed by Craigavon and Banbridge Community Health and Social Services Trust, Northern Ireland as a community psychiatric nurse team leader in a specialist dementia team. She was the principal catalyst and pioneering influence in the initiation, evolution and establishment of the Northern Ireland Dementia Forum and has held the post of chairperson.

Paul McCloskey is currently employed by North and West Belfast Health and Social Services Trust. He holds the position of community mental health nurse/team coordinator for mental health services for older people in north Belfast. He currently holds the position of secretary for the Northern Ireland Dementia Forum.

Anne McKinley has been working as a community psychiatric nurse for older adults since 1990 in Inverness city and the surrounding rural areas. She works within a small team, working mainly with people of varying degrees of cognitive impairment, their carers and families.

Linda Miller is a lecturer in nursing in the Department of Nursing and Midwifery at Keele University with the responsibility of teaching in the areas of gerontology, mental health and illness, and complementary therapies. She is particularly interested in dementia care mapping. Linda's clinical background is in community mental health and she works with students in pre- and post-registration education and training. She has strong links with North Staffordshire Carers and has been involved in the Royal College of Nursing special interest group on older people.

Gordon Mitchell is a senior lecturer in mental health nursing at the University of Teeside. Gordon started mental health nurse training in 1980 and has held a variety of positions in acute mental health units before moving into nurse education in 1992. In his present post, Gordon developed the module 'Care of the older person with mental health problems' and has worked with a department of old age psychiatry which has been accredited as a practice development unit.

Elinor Moore has been a community psychiatric nurse for 12 years and has a special interest in dementia care. Her interests centre round supporting carers, and advocating on behalf of people with dementia. She lives and works in Inverness and is a member of the local dementia network.

Michelle Murray is a specialist nurse for people under the age of 65 with a diagnosis of dementia in the city of Manchester. Michelle has been instrumental in the development of a specialist young onset dementia service for the city with the inception of a community-based service in March 1996. Michelle is the lead clinician for the multi-disciplinary service, which provides age appropriate day and community care. The service aims to provide support for both the younger person with dementia and for their carers.

Mike Nolan is Professor of Gerontological Nursing in the School of Nursing and Midwifery, University of Sheffield. For the past 20 years Mike has worked with older people and their carers as a practitioner, educator and researcher. He has particular interests in the design and evaluation of services for older people and in the assessment of family carers. Carer assessment instruments that he has developed with colleagues have been translated into several languages and are currently used for both research and practice in a variety of countries.

Peter Nolan has a long-standing interest in the history of mental health services in the UK. He has explored the various ideological shifts that have taken place and the impact that these have had on the work of nurses. He was for many years Professor of Mental Health Nursing at the University of Birmingham and is now Professor at Staffordshire University and the South Staffordshire Healthcare Trust.

Tracy Packer is a nurse consultant in dementia care working across a range of acute hospitals in Bristol. She has a particular interest in working with unqualified staff to develop training and extended practice opportunities in dementia care. Tracy has an extensive publication history in the field.

Sean Page is a clinical nurse specialist in the Manchester memory clinic. He has experience of managing drug treatments for dementia since 1994 and currently has responsibility for developing the role of mental health nursing in relation to memory clinic activity across the city of Manchester.

Marilla Pugh is a community mental health nurse specializing in the care of people with dementia and their families. Marilla is based in Bangor, North Wales, and has extensive experience of working with people with dementia in a variety of clinical setting and community settings. Marilla has recently completed a full-time BSc course at the University of Wales, Bangor, that included a specialist practice award of community mental health nursing.

Helen Pusey spent her early career working with vulnerable people before training as a mental health nurse in Oxford. Her clinical background is in older people's mental health, particularly dementia care. She is now a lecturer at the University of Manchester and undertakes research and educational development in the field.

Assumpta Ryan is a lecturer in nursing at the University of Ulster, Coleraine, Northern Ireland. Her clinical, teaching and research interest is in the care of older people. She has published in a range of journals and is currently undertaking research on the experiences of family carers following the nursing home placement of an older relative.

Alison Soliman is Operational Support Manager/Head of Education – Admiral Nurse Service at the Dementia Relief Trust. Since nurse training, Alison has worked in the NHS, in social housing and the voluntary sector. Her interest has always been in older people and she completed an MSc in Gerontology in 1998.

Vicki Traynor is a lecturer in the School of Nursing at the University of Nottingham and worked on the Admiral Nurses' Competency Project whilst with the Gerontological Nursing Programme at the Royal College of Nursing. Her interests are gerontological nursing and qualitative research methods. She completed her PhD at the University of Edinburgh and has worked with the Oxford Dementia Centre at Oxford Brookes University.

Dot Weaks has worked with people with dementia and their families both in hospital and community settings for over 20 years. Over that time she has enjoyed the challenge of innovative practice. She is co-author of *The Right to Know* (with Kate Fearnley and Jane McLennan, Alzheimer Scotland 1997) and was awarded the OBE for services to nursing in 1998. Dot has recently completed an MSc in Counselling Studies at the University of Abertay Dundee.

Heather Wilkinson currently holds a Royal Society of Edinburgh Personal Research Fellowship and is based at the Centre for Research on Families and Relationships in the Faculty of Medicine, University of Edinburgh. Heather's research interests centre on issues of inclusion and quality of life for people with dementia and for people with learning disabilities and dementia. A significant part of her work involves developing methods for including people with dementia in research and policy.

Acknowledgements

We would like to acknowledge the contribution of each of the authors represented in the book who gave their time to the project. The book would not exist without their enthusiasm and input, and for these qualities and more we are extremely grateful. The editors would also like to acknowledge the support of their respective universities in helping to facilitate this project and to the Open University Press for commissioning the book; in this latter instance, we would particularly like to thank Jacinta Evans for her support throughout the completion of the text. We would also like to thank the original reviewers of the book proposal who provided us with some very helpful feedback on the (eventual) shape and scope of the work. Last, and by no means least, we would like to extend a special thank you to Ms Nyree Hulme at the Research Office, School of Nursing, Midwifery and Health Studies, University of Wales, Bangor, for her invaluable administrative help, word processing skills and patience in helping us to pull this book together.

John Keady
Charlotte L. Clarke
Trevor Adams

Editorial note

To promote uniformity, and in response to recommendation 10 of the mental health nursing review (Department of Health 1994), the authors have used 'community mental health nurse' (CMHN) throughout the book as opposed to 'community psychiatric nurse' (CPN) unless individual authors have explicitly requested otherwise, or the text is referring to an original source/historical document.

Reference

 Department of Health (1994) *Working in Partnership: A Collaborative Approach to Care.* London: The Stationery Office.

Foreword
Professor Mike Nolan

> An understanding of illness that reunites the psychological with the experiential will, it has been suggested, require a far richer and more varied conception of evidence than that currently at stake in evidence-based medicine . . .
>
> (Evans 1999)

Anyone who has worked in the field of health and social care soon becomes accustomed to change being a fact of life. And yet in recent times the scale and pace of change has been more frenetic than ever. It seems that before one set of policies or recommendations have been introduced, they are replaced by another. Such an environment provides few opportunities for considered reflection nor is it possible to judge the impact or effectiveness of the currently popular 'policy of the month'.

The rhetoric of course is persuasive, who would argue against notions such as independence and autonomy, which have become watchwords for how we currently live. However, from an ethical perspective, Evans (1999) raises several objections about not only the ways in which evidence and knowledge are construed but also what this says about the values that underpin policy development and service delivery.

It is now widely acknowledged that improving the quality of health and social care requires a 'change in thinking' (Department of Health 1998), and recently a more person-centred approach has been advocated. Paradoxically, such a model with its focus on 'individuals and their needs' (Department of Health 2001) potentially ignores the 'communitarian' values that Evans (1999) asserts are essential if the needs of the most vulnerable and disadvantaged members of society are to receive the attention that they deserve.

That is what is so appealing and so important about this book. Not only does it recognize the need for a change of thinking but it also explicitly promotes the adoption of a broader, less individualistic set of values. As the editors point out in their introduction, the community mental health nurse (CMHN) interacts with several differing 'communities' and in so doing has to address disparate types of need whilst not simultaneously ignoring their own. In order to achieve this difficult balance the editors promote a vision of a 'triadic' partnership in which the person with dementia, their family carer (where one exists) and the CMHN each brings differing types of experience, expertise and evidence, which in combination far exceed the sum of their individual parts.

This is the 'richer and more varied conception of evidence' to which Evans (1999) refers and in providing such evidence the contributors to this book have done much to further debate in this important, but hitherto relatively neglected, area of practice.

I believe that this book marks a watershed in the evolution not just of the role of the CMHN, but also of a more holistic and inclusive form of partnership in which no one voice is privileged above another. Read this book, reflect upon the messages it contains and play your own part in shaping a new order of things.

Mike Nolan
Professor of Gerontological Nursing
University of Sheffield

References

Department of Health (1998) *A First Class Service: Quality in the New NHS*. London: Department of Health.

Department of Health (2001) *The National Service Framework for Older People*. London: The Stationery Office.

Evans, M. (1999) *Ethics: Reconciling Conflicting Values in Health Policy*, Policy Futures for the UK, no. 9. London: Nuffield Trust.

Introduction

Trevor Adams, John Keady and Charlotte L. Clarke

> . . . we found evidence of under-investment in training, support and super-vision for nursing staff in relation to the very complex and demanding needs of those suffering from dementia.
>
> (Department of Health 1994a: 34)

The above quotation is taken from the most recent mental health nursing review (Department of Health 1994a) and it is a statement that should send a shudder of disquiet throughout the profession. In 2003 it is salutary that these few words continue to pose key challenges to the mental health profession, and nursing as a whole, as we wrestle with the opportunities and challenges set by people with dementia and their families.

As editors and nurses who have worked with people with dementia and their families in a variety of settings and in the capacity of both clinicians and researchers, we know that nursing has, by and large, poorly prepared its students for a proactive role in dementia care and failed to seize therapeutic opportunities that exist in the field (see also Nolan *et al.* 2001). The fact that this is the first book of its type for a role that has its roots in the early 1960s says a lot about the under-investment in dementia care as observed by the mental health review team (Department of Health 1994a). However, it also says something about the lack of a cohesive identity for community mental health nurses (CMHNs) in dementia care, and an inadequacy of role preparation and role transparency.

That said, this book cannot hope to do justice to all community mental health nursing practice in dementia care, or adequately define its practice epistemology. However, the text can act as a springboard for understanding by bringing together the contribution of practitioners and/or research commentators with an interest in the field. The book can also highlight areas where further work is necessary in order to construct this shared identity and put in place foundations for future practice development. As you make your way through the book, you will see that CMHNs in dementia care are building a bridge towards a goal of commonality of purpose. Indeed, we have attempted to facilitate this process by including in the text contributions from CMHNs in each of the four countries of the UK. However, in order to make sure that the community mental health nursing role is both purposeful and transparent, the profession will need to reassure itself that its foundations are securely grounded and its objectives of care well defined, measured and evaluated. It is, perhaps, a lack of emphasis on these last three elements that has held back the community mental health nursing profession in recent years and caused uncertainty for other commentators as they try to interpret the evidence base for practice (see, for example, Carradice *et al.* 2002).

Echoing this dilemma, one of the major surprises we encountered in our preparation of this text was the fact that, at present, the quinquennial surveys of community mental health nursing practice in England and Wales (see White 1999a) are unable to define the precise number of CMHNs working with people with dementia and their families (Brooker 2001). What is known, however, is that the reported number of CMHNs in these two regions has increased from 4000 in 1990 to nearly 7000 in 1996 (White 1999a), but by 1996 it was reported that CMHNs were less likely to specialize in the care of older people. This fate was also shared with CMHNs working with children and adolescents, substance abusers and those with HIV and AIDS. Arguably, the most significant reason behind this diminished emphasis on mental health nursing and older people/dementia care centred on the UK government's policy push and, it must be said, some influential mental health nurse commentators, to define the community mental health nursing role in relation to those with a 'serious mental illness' – a label that was all but used to represent working-age adults with schizophrenia. This more targeted (and consequently selective) focus allowed CMHNs in adult psychiatry to specialize in case management, psychosocial interventions and brief intervention approaches (Gournay and Birley 1998; White 1999a). However, a product of this realignment was the displacement of 'dementia' within the community mental health nursing profession despite the value attached to the role in influential policy documents (see, for example, Department of Health 1995; Audit Commission 2000).

A further explanation for this dichotomy is that the CMHN role has, to date, been largely articulated through individual and isolated accounts of practice efficacy (Adams 1998; Gunstone 1999; Keady and Adams 2001a,b). Indeed, each of these sources indicate that community mental health nursing must be able to define its contribution to the care of people with dementia in a succinct and accessible way if it is to fully understand the contribution that can be made within a multi-disciplinary and inter-agency context. Furthermore, without a firm awareness of the position of contemporary practice, even with a clear idea of what the profession wishes to be, it becomes impossible to navigate a course towards that destination.

To begin to plot a path through the maze of possibilities, our intention in this book is to share existing community mental health nursing work in dementia care, demonstrate the extent of CMHNs' decision making and stretch practice boundaries by providing evidence of role efficacy. This Introduction also provides an initial marker for this journey by locating community mental health nursing practice within contemporary health policy in dementia care. After this discussion, a one-line synopsis of each chapter will be shared in order to provide readers with an overview of the book, its primary objectives and some of the major challenges facing the community mental health nursing profession at the dawning of a new millennium.

Health policy and dementia care

Community mental health nursing or, as it was then called, community psychiatric nursing, began in the UK in the mid-1950s (White 1999b). Its evolution was one of a number of initiatives aimed at relocating mental hospital patients to community settings. Initially, community psychiatric nurses (CPNs) were 'generic' and worked with a range of people with mental health problems. Their main role was to administer and monitor long-term intramuscular drugs to people with long-term conditions such as schizophrenia. This maintained the long-standing dependency of mental health nursing upon psychiatrists, as it was to them that CPNs reported patients' progress or deterioration.

In the 1960s, community psychiatric nursing to older people began to develop as a distinct speciality within community psychiatric nursing. Early accounts of their work are given by Greene (1968), Barker and Black (1971), Leopaldt *et al.* (1975) and Ainsworth and Jolley (1978). These accounts describe the work of CPNs with people with dementia and their family networks. For example, Greene (1968) argued that 'psychogeriatric' and 'partially confused' patients required a different approach to services than other client groups. Picking up on the practice examples provided in Greene's (1968) innovative paper, Keady and Adams (2001a: 37) suggested that for the CPN working with people with dementia and their families this early role description encompassed:

- the value of experience in working with people with dementia and their families;
- a knowledge of dementia and its likely course;
- attention to the personal care needs of people with dementia;
- information-sharing with families;
- promotion of autonomy for people with dementia;
- maintaining regular visits and contact;
- establishing trust with both the person with dementia and their family;
- service coordination.

Undoubtedly, the provision of care to people with dementia has changed considerably over the past 30 years and the institutional approach to care pre-1970 lent itself to two fundamental criticisms. First, to 'warehousing' where patients remained in the hospital for long periods with little hope of cure; and secondly, to the subordination of such individuals to the needs of the staff and the institution. These practices were reported in influential publications such as *Sans Everything* (Robb 1967) and research studies by Townsend (1962) and Meacher (1972). These works supported the general view that institutional care was dehumanizing and detrimental to people's welfare, and that at worse led to the physical and emotional abuse of residents and patients (Goffman 1961; Barton 1966). Later, Kitwood (1997) described this environment, and legacy, as 'the old culture of dementia care', although it would be unwise to believe that all continuing care facilities for people with dementia are currently run on person-centred values. Indeed, as reported in a recent extensive survey by Nolan *et al.* (2001), it was the poor environment of care encountered by student nurses on placement that militated against their positive view of gerontological nursing as a future practice specialism. Clearly, much work still needs to be done if the situation is to improve.

Since the early 1980s, institutional care has fallen out of favour and has been replaced by community care and person-centred values, as recently demonstrated in England by the production of the *National Service Framework for Older People* (Department of Health 2001). Multi-disciplinary and inter-agency working in health care is now the continuing goal of UK government policy with several recent reports advocating this as the way forward for a modern health and social care service (see, for example, National Health Service Executive 1993a,b; Department of Health 1994b, 1996, 1997a,b). This drive towards closer professional and agency collaboration has continued with the UK government White Paper *The New NHS* (Department of Health 1997b), with its emphasis on organizational partnership and shared responsibility, and initiatives such as health action zones and health improvement programmes.

The National Service Frameworks (NSFs) for Mental Health (Department of Health 1999a) and for Older People (Department of Health 2001) build on this foundation of health care and social services working in partnership, and reiterate that care planning, service delivery and review should be a multi-agency endeavour. The mental health system is therefore required to provide the range of interventions and integration across all specialist services. The growing belief that effective care in any setting relies on strong, inter-collaborative working (Miller *et al.* 2001) is supported by the National Health Service Executive (1993a) which examines nursing in primary care and states:

> The best and most effective outcomes for patients and clients are achieved when professionals work together, learn together, engage in clinical audit of outcomes together and generate innovation to ensure progress in practice and service.
>
> (paragraph 3)

As the main location of care for people with dementia and their families is within their own homes, two main approaches have developed to tackle this need. The first approach is the 'care for the carer approach' which focuses on the needs of carers, such as family, friends and neighbours as they provide care to people with dementia. The approach is advocated by numerous health and social policy documents, notably the Carers (Recognition and Services) Act 1995 and *Caring about Carers* (Department of Health 1999b). As a result, in dementia care, various approaches have developed that primarily support family carers. These include specific assessment and intervention strategies that centre on augmenting the carer's coping efforts and sources of well-being (for a review see Ferguson and Keady 2001), and specific community services that exist to solely support the carer in their caregiving role, for example the Admiral Nurses service (Greenwood and Walsh 1995). Both these perspectives are represented in Chapters 12 and 13, respectively, of this book.

However, an alternative approach to understanding the experience of dementia developed in the early 1990s. This approach focused on the person with dementia rather than their family carers. The approach began in the United States through the writings of people with the early stages of dementia, such as Davis (1989) and Hamilton (1994), and was developed in the UK in the work of Froggatt (1988), Goldsmith (1996), Downs (1997), Keady and Gilliard (1999) and Killick and Allan (2001). This work raised the profile of the person with dementia and their ability to make choices about the services they wished to receive. Promoting the personhood of people with dementia was also a feature of 'the new culture of dementia care' developed by Professor Tom Kitwood and his colleagues at the Bradford Dementia Group in the UK (see, for example, Kitwood and Bredin 1992; Kitwood and Benson 1995; Kitwood 1997), and such values have received an enduring legacy in social policy through their integration into the NSF for Older People (Department of Health 2001).

The existence of these two, seemingly contradictory, approaches to dementia care, one focusing on the needs of the carer and the other on the needs of the person with dementia, could be considered problematic for policy and practice in dementia care. More precisely, who should be the priority in the focus of nursing care? To address this potential conflict it might be useful to build upon the writings of Rolland (1988), Clarke (1997, 1999), Silliman (2000), Fortinsky (2001), Nolan *et al.* (2001) and Adams (2002), who have all suggested that making sense of perceptions and relationships are crucial variables in helping to work out the multiple constructions of reality that are present in any situation involving a chronic disease, dementia being no exception. In essence, this approach suggests that there are three parties associated with dementia care: the person with the dementia; the family carer; and the health and social care providers embracing, in the context of this book, the CMHN. Each of these parties is viewed as having their own perspectives and interests in what is happening, coupled to their own account of such realities. The importance of this triadic approach is that it moves dementia care away from static, dichotomous and polarizing ways of thinking about either 'the person with dementia' or 'the carer' and reconstructs dementia care in terms of a network of reciprocating, interpersonal relationships between people who are affected in different ways.

To a significant extent, CMHNs in dementia care have attempted to conceptualize their practice through a family-orientated approach that takes full account of the person with dementia and the family. Right from the start, CMHNs have highlighted the need to work not only with people who have dementia, but also with their family (Greene 1968). However, the triadic approach also recognizes that it is not just people with dementia and their families who have needs, but CMHNs too. Arguably, it can be comforting for CMHNs to imagine themselves as 'experts' in care provision and that the altruistic nature of the work causes relatively little or no upset to the worker. However, nothing could be further from the truth, and numerous studies have shown that this way of thinking needs to be challenged and that CMHNs frequently experience considerable stress as they work with people with mental health needs, including those with dementia (Hannigan *et al.* 2000).

From our practice and research experience, working alongside people who have a dementia can be emotionally challenging with the stress involved in some home care situations, such as supporting a person with dementia who lives alone or working with a younger person with dementia, can leave the CMHN exposed in their decision making and approaches to risk management. Moreover, as relationships with people with dementia and their families can be lengthy, close contact with people with dementia may give rise to CMHNs feeling emotional attachment and discomfort as they too take on board the families' changing sense of loss and reality. Additionally, CMHNs may feel emotional discomfort and are threatened about the possibility that one day they, or a member of their family, may have a dementia. Consequently, various writers have advocated that CMHNs in dementia care should have access to clinical supervision on a regular basis in order to keep such emotions 'in check' and allow a forum for reflection and practice evaluation (see, for example, Kitwood and Benson 1995; Adams 2001). Unfortunately, there remains a paucity of literature on the efficacy and approaches to supervision in dementia care. CMHNs, and health and social care professionals in general, there-fore, constitute a third area of need within dementia care. In our opinion, it is a distinctive feature of community mental health nursing practice in dementia care that it is underpinned by a triadic partnership relationship that seeks the well-being of each party, namely: the person with dementia, the family carer(s) and the CMHN. It is this triadic partnership that forms the cornerstone of the book, its philosophy and its structure.

The structure of the book

To provide an initial framework for articulating community mental health nursing practice in dementia care, this book is divided into three parts:

1. Setting the scene: the landscape of contemporary community mental health nursing practice in dementia care
2. Dementia care nursing in the community: Assessment and practice approaches
3. Leading and developing community mental health nursing in dementia.

As mentioned above, the book attempts to underscore its structure through cognisance of the triadic partnership, i.e. the person with dementia; the family carer(s); and the CMHN and the relationships that weave and flow between these partners. Accordingly, as editors, we had to take a pragmatic approach between balancing research commentary, evidence-based care and practice reality. Not all community mental health nursing practice is based on research evidence and the reliance, particularly in Parts Two and Three on the use of case studies to explain community mental health nursing decision making, reflects this point. However, such openness and honesty are necessary qualities if the community mental health nursing profession in dementia care is to reflect on its current practices and move forward as a result.

Before outlining the book's contents, it is also necessary to acknowledge its limitations. It would have been useful to include a chapter on palliative care and the role of the CMHN, as some people with dementia are cared for at home by family members until the time of their death. However, this specialist area of practice could not be located in the preparation of this text. Similarly, more emphasis on activities and the CMHN role in residential and nursing home settings would have aided understanding and enhanced the role dimension. These limitations are the responsi-bility of the editors and we would hope that an additional volume, and/or published works, would help to further develop the CMHN role.

What we have put together, however, is a book of 18 chapters split into three parts. The first part, 'Setting the scene: the landscape of contemporary community mental health nursing practice in dementia care' contains five chapters. The opening chapter by Peter Nolan describes the historical association of nursing to dementia care. Next, led by Charlotte L. Clarke, the editors provide an epistemology for community mental health nursing practice by exploring a range of sources of knowledge that inform professional practice. In the third chapter, Trevor Adams, Gordon Mitchell and Mark Holman set community mental health nursing practice within the context of multi-disciplinary teamwork. In the penultimate chapter of this part, Anne Mason and her colleagues draw on the results of a large-scale survey in Scotland to emphasize the users perspective on the value of community mental health nursing practice in dementia care. Finally, Jill Manthorpe debates the issues that face CMHNs as they seek to assess and manage the risks associated with dementia care.

Part Two of the book is the largest and comprises ten chapters that constitute 'Dementia care nursing in the community: Assessment and practice approaches'. Linda Miller begins the part by examining how various assessment and intervention strategies can be used by CMHNs. Continuing with this therapeutic focus, Peter Ashton explores the practice implications and use of cognitive behaviour therapy for CMHNs in dementia care. This is followed by Tracy Packer who examines how the personhood approach may be incorporated within routine community mental health nursing practice. The fourth chapter in this part sees the contribution of Sean Page who develops a framework for mental health nurses working with people in the early stages of dementia who are taking one of a variety of pharmacological treatments designed to enhance quality of life. Next, Chris Clark provides a further reminder of the necessity of early community mental health nursing intervention by describing the results of her study conducted in primary care. Building a bridge between interventions with people with dementia and their carers, Kath Lowery and Michelle Murray combine their extensive practice expertise by reviewing the community mental health nursing role in providing support groups for family carers and, separately, for people with dementia. The following chapter by Helen Pusey provides a systematic account of the research evidence that can be used by CMHNs in conducting psychosocial interventions with carers of people with dementia. This is developed in the next chapter when Alison Soliman describes the role of Admiral Nurses and their assessment and intervention profiles for carers of people with dementia. In the penultimate chapter in this part, Dot Weaks and Gill Boardman describe their dedicated community mental health nursing team in Perth, Scotland, and the emphasis they place on normalization as a guiding philosophy for practice. Finally, Marilla Pugh and John Keady explore the meaning of challenging behaviour in community mental health nursing practice and review three case illustrations where interventions are described and compared for their practice efficacy.

The last part of the book is entitled 'Leading and developing community mental health nursing in dementia'. This part comprises three chapters and starts with Angela Carradice, John Keady and Sue Hahn describing models of clinical supervision and the use of ecomaps in the structuring of such sessions. Next, Cathy Mawhinney, Paul McCloskey and Assumpta Ryan look at the management issues in providing a community mental health nursing service in Northern Ireland. The third and final chapter, by Jan Dewing and Vicki Traynor, outlines a competency framework for community mental health nursing practice that was inductively generated from the practice of Admiral Nurses.

What can be learnt from the community mental health nursing role?

By writing a book about community mental health nursing in dementia care it could be assumed that there is such a distinct area of practice to write about. What we have found is that this is not necessarily the case, although chapters in this book describe in some detail the work of Admiral Nurses (Chapter 13) and one team of CMHNs in Scotland (Chapter 14). These examples, however, are probably the exception rather than the rule. Most people with dementia are cared for by a more generic team of practitioners who are either more broad-based in the disciplinary composition (perhaps including social workers and therapists), or have a wider caseload of older people with other mental health needs. However, as Mawhinney, McCloskey and Ryan suggest in Chapter 17, it is necessary to have a commitment to the community mental health nursing service and a goal of combining social and health care needs within a practice domain. Perhaps it is this combination that will help the community mental health nursing profession to find a firm footing in primary care and better articulate its role.

The book provides insights into the community mental health nursing role in dementia care and how it is conceptualized and practised at present. Whilst others may find differing role dimensions, we would propose that community mental health nursing practice in dementia care is a case of 'it's not what you do it's the way that you do it'. Consequently, much of the work of CMHNs expressed in this book concerns the *processes* of professional working. For example, importance is placed on:

- establishing and providing continuity of relationships;
- using a health-orientated knowledge base;
- networking;
- relationship building (with a commitment to a sustained relationship);
- providing friendship.

Indeed, very often these processes are regarded as therapeutic in their own right. This does pose problems when we attempt to define therapy and what is meant by 'being therapeutic'. Processes resist being reduced to and contained in packages that can be tested so that an evidence base can be developed. The visibility and legitimacy of interventions become secondary to the means of their implementation. It is these processes that shape the nature of the community mental health nursing approach to people with dementia and their families from the very outset.

Running throughout this book is a further aspect of community mental health nursing practice. It concerns the 'community' with whom and for whom the nurse works. Nursing is also about maximizing the capacity of each community to be in an optimal state for the management of health. Such an approach to understanding nursing is far from new – even Florence Nightingale referred to the nurses' responsibilities in ensuring that the environment is conducive to health and noted that sub-optimal environments burdened the capacity of individuals to remain healthy.

The 'community' that concerns the CMHN in dementia care is various, each dependent on the breadth of focus on the service:

- The community of the individual with dementia promoting their general health state, their self-management strategies and minimizing the disabling impact of the environment.
- The community of the family – acknowledging and building on the inter-dependency of the person with dementia and their family.
- The community of the neighbourhood – recognizing the role of public health, transport and health care access among other issues that mediate social inclusion and the promotion of health.
- The community of those co-located – ameliorating the differentiation of 'them and us' promoted by the non-confused and encouraging respect for diversity and difference.
- The community of service providers – sustaining the organization, respecting the support and learning needs of all staff and advancing multi-disciplinary and inter-agency working.

This would suggest that community mental health nursing practice in dementia care needs to evidence itself across a broad range of activity, but specifically focus on processes and define the community for whom it is orientated. This is a significant lesson we have learnt whilst developing the book, but there is so much more that can and must be learnt about community mental health nursing practice. We hope that this book will provide you with the encouragement to do so.

References

Adams, T. (1998) The discursive construction of dementia care: implications for mental health nursing, *Journal of Advanced Nursing*, 28(3): 614–21.

Adams, T. (2001) The social construction of risk by community psychiatric nurses and family carers for people with dementia, *Health Risk and Society*, 3(3): 307–19.

Adams, T. (2002) Developing partnerships in dementia care, in S. Benson (ed.) *Dementia topics for the millennium and beyond*. London: Hawker, pp. 58–60.

Ainsworth, D. and Jolley, D. (1978) The community psychiatric nurse in a developing psychogeriatric service, *Nursing Times*, 74(21): 873–4.

Audit Commission (2000) *Forget Me Not: Mental Health Services for Older People*. London: Audit Commission.

Barker, C. and Black, S. (1971) An experiment in integrated psycho-geriatric care, *Nursing Times*, 67(45): 1395–9.

Barton, R. (1966) *Institutional Neurosis*. Bristol: John Wright.

Brooker, C. (2001) Personal correspondence.

Carradice, A., Shankland, M. and Beail, N. (2002) A qualitative study of the theoretical models used by UK mental health nurses to guide their assessments with family care-givers of people with dementia, *International Journal of Nursing Studies*, 39(1): 17–26.

Clarke, C.L. (1997) In sickness and in health: remembering the relationship in family care-giving for people with dementia, in M. Marshall (ed.) *The State of the Art in Dementia Care*. London: Centre for Policy on Ageing.

Clarke, C.L. (1999) Family caregiving for people with dementia: some implications for policy and professional practice, *Journal of Advanced Nursing*, 30(4): 975–82.

Davis, R. (1989) *My Journey into Alzheimer's Disease*. Amersham: Scripture Press.

Department of Health (1994a) *Working in Partnership: A Collaborative Approach to Care*. London: The Stationery Office.

Department of Health (1994b) *Better Off in the Community? The Care of People who are Seriously Mentally Ill*. London: The Stationery Office.

Department of Health (1995) *Building Bridges: A Guide to Arrangements for Inter-agency Working for the Care and Protection of Severely Mentally Ill People*. London: The Stationery Office.

Department of Health (1996) *The Health of the Nation: Building Bridges. A Guide to Arrangements for Interagency Working for the Care and Protection of Seriously Mentally Ill People*. Wetherby: The Stationery Office.

Department of Health (1997a) *Developing Partnerships in Mental Health*. Wetherby: The Stationery Office.

Department of Health (1997b) *The New NHS: Modern, Dependable*. London: The Stationery Office.

Department of Health (1999a) *National Service Framework for Mental Health*. London: The Stationery Office.

Department of Health (1999b) *Caring about Carers*. London: The Stationery Office.

Department of Health (2001) *National Service Framework for Older People*. London: The Stationery Office.

Downs, M. (1997) Progress report: the emergence of the person in dementia research, *Ageing and Society*, 17(5): 597–607.

Ferguson, C. and Keady, J. (2001) The mental health needs of older people and their carers, in M. Nolan, S. Davies and G. Grant (eds) *Working with Older People and Their Families*. Buckingham: Open University Press.

Fortinsky, R.H. (2001) Health care triads and dementia care: integrative framework and future directions, *Aging and Mental Health*, 5 (Suppl. 1): S35–S48.

Froggatt, A. (1988) Self-awareness in early dementia, in B. Gearing, M. Johnson and T. Heller (eds) *Mental Health Problems in Old Age: A Reader*. Buckingham: Open University Press.

Goldsmith, M. (1996) *Hearing the Voice of People with Dementia: Opportunities and Obstacles*. London: Jessica Kingsley.

Goffman, E. (1961) *Asylums*. New York: Anchor Books.

Gournay, K. and Birley, J. (1998) Thorn: a new approach to mental health training, *Nursing Times*, 94(49): 54–5.

Greene, J. (1968) The psychiatric nurse in the community nursing service. *International Journal of Nursing Studies*, 5: 175–84.

Greenwood, M. and Walsh, K. (1995) Supporting carers in their own right, *Journal of Dementia Care*, 3(2): 14–16.

Gunstone, S. (1999) Expert practice: the interventions used by a community mental health nurse with carers of dementia sufferers, *Journal of Psychiatric and Mental Health Nursing*, 6: 321–7.

Hamilton, H.E. (1994) *Conversations with an Alzheimer's Patient*. Cambridge: Cambridge University Press.

Hannigan, B., Edwards, D., Coyle, D., Fothergill, A. and Burnard, P. (2000) Burnout in community mental health nurses: findings from the all-Wales study, *Journal of Psychiatric and Mental Health Nursing*, 7(2): 127–34.

Keady, J. and Adams, T. (2001a) Community mental health nursing and dementia care, *Journal of Dementia Care* (Research Focus), 9(1): 35–8.

Keady, J. and Adams, T. (2001b) Community mental health nursing in dementia care: their role and future, *Journal of Dementia Care* (Research Focus), 9(2): 33–7.

Keady, J. and Gilliard, J. (1999) The early experience of Alzheimer's disease: implications for partnership and practice, in T. Adams and C. Clarke (eds) *Dementia Care: Developing Partnerships in Practice*. London: Baillière Tindall.

Killick, J. and Allan, K. (2001) *Communication and the Care of People with Dementia*. Buckingham: Open University Press.

Kitwood, T. (1997) *Dementia Reconsidered: The Person Comes First*. Buckingham: Open University Press.

Kitwood, T. and Bredin, K. (1992) Towards a theory of dementia care: personhood and well-being, *Ageing and Society*, 12: 269–87.

Kitwood, T. and Benson, S. (eds) (1995) *The New Culture of Dementia Care*. London: Hawker.

Leopaldt, H., Corea, S. and Robinson, J.R. (1975) Hospital-based community psychiatric nursing in psycho-geriatric care, *Nursing Mirror*, 18 December, pp. 54–6.

Meacher, M. (1972) *Taken for a Ride: Special Residential Homes for Confused Old People*. London: Longmans.

Miller, C., Freeman, M. and Ross, N. (2001) *Interprofessional Practice in Health and Social Care*. London: Arnold.

National Health Service Executive (1993a) *Nursing in Primary Care – New World, New Opportunities*. London: The Stationery Office.

National Health Service Executive (1993b) *A Vision for the Future: The Nursing, Midwifery and Health Visiting Contribution to Health and Health Care*. London: The Stationery Office.

Nolan, M., Davies, S., Brown, J., Keady, J. and Nolan, J. (2001) *Longitudinal Study of the Effectiveness of Educational Preparation to Meet the Needs of Older People and Carers: The AGEIN (Advancing Gerontological Education in Nursing) Project*. London: English National Board for Nursing, Midwifery and Health Visiting.

Robb, B. (ed.) (1967) *Sans Everything: A Case to Answer*. London: Nelson.

Rolland, J.S. (1988) A conceptual model of chronic and life-threatening illness and its impact on families, in C.S. Chilman, E.W. Nunnally and F.M. Cox (eds) *Chronic Illness and Disabilities*. Beverly Hills, CA: Sage.

Silliman, R.A. (2000) Care-giving issues in the geriatric medical encounter, *Clinics in Geriatric Medicine*, 16: 51–60.

Townsend, P. (1962) *The Last Refuge – A Survey of Residential Institutions and Homes for the Aged in England and Wales*. London: Routledge & Kegan Paul.

White, E. (1999a) The 4th quinquennial national community mental health nursing census of England and Wales, *Australian and New Zealand Journal of Mental Nursing*, 8(3): 86–92.

White, E. (1999b) Community mental health nursing: an interpretation of history as a context for contemporary research, in J. McIntosh (ed.) *Research Issues in Community Nursing*. Basingstoke: Macmillan.

PART ONE

Setting the scene

The landscape of contemporary community
mental health nursing practice in dementia care

Voices from the past

The historical alignment of dementia care to nursing

Peter Nolan

Introduction

Although nurses have been caring for older adults with dementia for many years, little has been written about how they first became involved in this area of care. In the evolution of treatments and care of any client group, at least four stages can be discerned:

1   Recognition that a substantial number of people experience a particular condition.
2   An attempt to describe the condition from a scientific perspective.
3   Involvement of clinicians in developing ways of treating the condition.
4   Involvement of nurses in identifying how best to care for those with the condition, and alleviate distressing symptoms for the person and his or her family.

The time required to move through these stages depends on the degree of enthusiasm in society and in the medical and nursing professions to address the particular challenge. This chapter sketches the history of how dementia came to be associated with mental health services, and how nurses became involved in dementia care for older adults. Any exploration of historical developments requires humility on the part of the reader not to succumb to the danger of imposing current perspectives and values on the past. 'Presentism', argues Berrios (1995), is where only the 'achievements' of the present are found to be 'progressive' and all previous efforts and successes within the field are belittled by comparison. History is a process of evolution and requires our empathy to appreciate how every small contribution made its impact on the treatment and care of physical and mental disease.

Berrios (1990) considers that the concept of 'dementia' and the description of the behaviours associated with it have been evolving over centuries and that this process is ongoing today. Pelling and Smith (1991) remind us that in endeavouring to understand the position of the older person in society and health care, we need to be aware that words such as 'old' and 'dementia' are heavily laden with cultural values. The way in which such words are used tells us what it is like to be 'old' in a particular society and what difficulties services which attempt to respond to the cognitively impaired and the socially isolated may face. This book and this chapter, with their declared focus on dementia care, must pay attention also to the society in which people with dementia are leading their lives and how that society prioritizes their needs, apportions resources and determines what are appropriate services.

The story of how dementia has been defined over the years is a complex one, and today ways of describing and diagnosing the problem are again being challenged (Kitwood 1995). Our contemporary understanding of the condition has been shaped by humanity's ancient need to face up to and understand the process of growing old. Porter (1995) notes that senescence has always challenged people to ask whether ageing is inevitable, whether it necessarily entails impairment, incapacity and an increased risk of illness, and whether the more debilitating aspects of dementia can be prevented or retarded. These questions continue to challenge scientists, service providers and individuals today just as they have done in the past. Contrasting with its deep-seated fears of diminished quality of life in old age, humanity has cherished its stories and, indeed, the real-life evidence of elderly people who have capably run families, businesses, cities and governments. Gerontocracies were commonplace in the ancient world and the Bible states that the patriarchs lived to a ripe old age and died in command of all their faculties. Cicero (106–43 BC) wrote in *De Senectute* (45 BC) that old men do many things better than younger men, and achieve greater things. He also observed that 'senile debility' or 'dotage' is not characteristic of all men, but only of those who are 'weak in mind and will'. Paradoxically, he concluded that whilst old age may bring many benefits both to the individual and society, it is in essence an illness.

Anthropological studies from around the world reveal how differently older people are treated in different societies, and how they may find themselves at the heart of their community or society, playing key roles, or pushed to one side and given nothing to do. In our own history, there has been a considerable change in the level of productive activity in the community which is expected, encouraged or allowed from older people. In the past, families and parishes provided care for older people. Today that responsibility has increasingly fallen to the state. Whilst this provides a safety net for those who would have no one to care for them, the expectation that older people will be cared for in specialist facilities, thus freeing their offspring from the obligation of looking after them, has perhaps weakened family bonds. One distressing aspect of the work of caring for older adults in residential and nursing homes is observing how many of the residents never receive any visitors.

As the lifespan of the people in the most affluent societies in the world has increased dramatically during the course of the twentieth century, there has been an accompanying rise in the numbers of those experiencing dementia. In the absence of reliable data concerning the prevalence and incidence of dementia within the British population, health and social services planners must 'best guess' the type and location of resources people will require. There are several reasons why the needs of people with dementia are so poorly served:

1 Continuing disagreement about how dementia can be recognized, with different clinicians observing and measuring a variety of factors in order to make a diagnosis of dementia.

2 Lack of agreement in the literature about how to weight cognitive and non-cognitive factors in formulating a diagnosis.

3 Lack of understanding of the types of environment and relationships that promote social and cognitive functioning in old age.

4 A failure of nurses to develop their role in *promoting health* in older adults as well as in preventing mental health problems.

Historical overview of dementia

From earliest times until the end of the seventeenth century, human life was seen as falling into three stages: youth, maturity and old age (Minois 1989). Old age was not as clearly delineated as the other two, but was generally seen as the period when people were exempted from hard physical work and the period prior to death. For some people and in some societies, it was the time when their insights into life were at their sharpest and when their wisdom about life and living was highly valued and eagerly sought after by their community. From the sixth to the sixteenth centuries, ideas about how to live in communities and how to relate to others were influenced by the monastic system. Religious institutions exercised considerable power over people's lives. The monasteries provided many with a basic education, handed out health care and, in times of hardship, provided the food that enabled families to survive. Immediately prior to the dissolution of the monasteries by Henry VIII, there were over 800 religious foundations in Britain, serving and controlling their local communities, and setting the tone for how older people were treated. Although there was a variety of monastic traditions, many followed more or less closely the Rule of St Benedict. Benedict (AD 480–547) was born in Italy and his Rule aimed to formulate a way of living that would provide people with a sense of purpose, a livelihood, and increase their happiness. He advocated the 'golden mean', which meant that no activity should be carried to excess. The Rule was taken up by thousands of monasteries in Europe over the centuries, and even today is followed by many men and women who have dedicated themselves to the Christian religious life.

Benedict paid particular attention in his Rule to how the sick, the infirm and older people should be treated. He felt that the vulnerable in society should be shown the respect that one would show to Christ Himself and provided with facilities to suit their needs and maximize their happiness, and with companionship to prevent loneliness and heighten their involvement in the community. Whilst they were to be exempted from certain duties and given special food at certain times of the day and night, they were also expected to exercise regularly 'within their capabilities' and to assist younger members of the community with their problems. The monastic community had a responsibility to visit the old regularly, and being such a visitor carried with it a special status. There was no nobler calling than that of 'infirmarian', the person designated by the abbot to care for the older members of the community.

The decline of the monasteries heralded the demise of a culture of care for older people, which was replaced by a radically different one based on scientific rationalism. Industrialization and urbanization reshaped the place of older adults in society and the way in which they were seen. Those who were unable to work, or not required to work because jobs were reserved for the young, came to be seen as burdens, especially if sick. There was interest in understanding the aetiology of dementia but little interest in how people suffering from it should be cared for or treated. The old became objects of study and sources of information gained at post-mortem. Among the many new terms, mostly now regarded as derogatory, which came into use shortly before 1700 to refer to old age and senility were 'amentia' (without a mind), 'imbecility', 'morosis' (condition of dying) and 'fatuitas' (idiocy).

The earliest entry for the adjective 'demented' can be found in the *Oxford English Dictionary* of 1664. In 1684, Thomas Willis used the word 'dementia' to refer to people deemed to be out of their mind. Elsewhere in his work, he uses it synonymously with stupidity or foolishness (Berrios 1987). Dementia is first referred to as a condition in Blancard's *Popular Physical Dictionary* (1726) in which it is described as 'extinction of the imagination and judgement'. The suggestion here is that dementia destroys the essentially human aspects of the person, and the dictionary goes on to explain that dementia entails 'paralysis of the spirit which is always accompanied by abolition of the reasoning faculty'. Those with dementia could not exercise their judgement and hence were incapable of entering into contracts, signing wills or being members of a jury. The incremental effect of such definitions slowly but surely reshaped social attitudes towards older people who were increasingly seen as totally dependent on others because they were incapable of managing their own affairs or of functioning socially.

The beginnings of the science of old age

The early nineteenth century was a period of intense scientific activity. Dementia was closely observed and attempts were made to distinguish it from the inevitable decay of old age and from other diseases with similar symptoms. Among those who took a specialist interest in the condition was Pinel, whose book *Nosographie* (1818) was one of the first to describe a systematic study of older people with a view to establishing what they had in common. Pinel based most of his findings on multiple post-mortem investigations carried out on the bodies of elderly people, but his aim was to be able to identify the early signs of dementia in the living. He concluded that characteristics of 'disordered activity, forgetfulness and concerted attempts to compensate for loss of functioning' were common in those deemed to have dementia. Esquirol (1838) also conducted observations and found that 'grandiosity, disinhibition, motor symptoms and terminal cognitive failure' were common in those thought to have been suffering from dementia for some time. Calmeil (1835) cautioned against attributing a particular cluster of symptoms to a condition not yet clearly defined, arguing that there were many conditions, such as venereal disease, which boasted similar symptoms. His own post-mortem studies concluded that there was little to indicate any organic dysfunction of the brain in those thought to have dementia. In 1860, Morel stated that dementia constituted a progressive weakening of the faculties and was an irreversible terminal state. Commenting on all of these studies, Berrios and Freeman (1991) point out that, in the absence of a clear definition of what the condition was, researchers were probably looking at different diseases and many were almost certainly describing general paralysis of the insane rather than dementia.

Charcot (1881) linked dementia to disorders of circulation, noting that cerebral haemorrhage was a condition which occurred frequently in old people. He argued that *senile haemorrhage*, when blood clots formed in the brain, resulted in poor oxygenation of brain tissue and consequent poor physical and mental functioning. Speculating on the possible importance of exercise and diet as preventative measures, he was one of the first and the few to suggest that certain conditions of old age could be prevented. Yet his ideas echoed (unconsciously no doubt) the advice given in the Rule of St Benedict. Pick, another pioneer in the field, concluded from his observations that dementia was related to dysfunction of language and praxis caused by atrophy of the temporal lobes (Pick 1901). For Pick, dementia was the inevitable result of ageing, which in turn was caused by irreversible deterioration in various parts of the brain. Like Charcot, Alzheimer (1911) considered that dementia was closely associated with cerebrovascular problems. He described the case of a 51-year-old woman with cognitive impairment, delusions, hallucinations and focal symptoms whose brain at post-mortem showed plagues and arteriosclerotic changes. Kraepelin (1910) was the first to coin the term 'senile dementia' and stated that the condition was due to changes in the cortical cells of the brain. In subsequent studies, he found that some people in their early forties showed similar changes and described their condition as senium praecox. The overall effect of these studies was to persuade scientists and doctors that dementia was irreversible and was due mainly to arteriosclerosis of the blood vessels in the brain. Yet it is not surprising that researchers from the field of the biological sciences should conclude that dementia was caused solely by biological factors. Their repeated assertion that dementia was irreversible provided the perfect excuse to make no attempts to limit, mitigate or indeed cure the condition. Some British psychiatrists, however, felt that there was more that could be done for those with dementia than the biological scientists claimed, as this next section will attest.

Early responses to dementia in Britain

The debate running up to the establishment of the British asylum system in 1845 made no mention of older adults or of how they should be cared for. Presumably, the planners believed that older people would be catered for in other institutions (although the infirmary wards in the workhouses were full to capacity at this time), or that being old would preclude people from being admitted to a psychiatric institution. Once built, however, the asylums were asked to admit many more older people than had been anticipated. Of the 75 patients who died at Coney Hatch

Asylum in 1859, 36 were elderly people who had been confined to bed in excess of six months, were ill-nourished and had some degree of paralysis. By 1884, over 10 per cent of a patient population of 2585 patients at Coney Hatch were over 65 years of age, and the oldest patient admitted in 1887 was 83 (Hunter and Macalpine 1974). Accounts from other asylums suggest that this was typical of what was happening elsewhere. The work of caring for older people was hard and it was difficult to recruit and retain staff for the 'geriatric' wards. It seems likely that whatever care patients received constituted no more than a very basic form of nursing. In addition, there were no senior nurses with sufficient knowledge and skills to oversee the work of the wards. Whereas on other wards in the asylums, staff/patient ratios were 1 to 12 for males and 1 to 11 for females, on the geriatric wards they were only 1 to 20.

By the end of the nineteenth century, the work of neurologists, mostly in Germany and France, suggested that the medical field best suited to treating those with dementia was, indeed, psychiatry. However, it was some time before the debate was taken up by clinical personnel in England. The first manual for asylum nurses published in 1885, the *Red Handbook for Attendants upon the Insane*, made no reference to the care and treatment of older people with dementia. Among the first to point out that dementia was a much bigger issue in Britain than had been acknowledged was Wilcox (1902), whose paper in the *Journal of Mental Science* noted that much more was known about dementia than was currently reflected in practice. Wilcox claimed that British doctors and nurses were far behind their American colleagues in the provision of treatment and care for older people with dementia, and accused them of leaving these patients to spend their last years in neglect and isolation.

Wilcox's reading of the American literature may have given him a somewhat inaccurate idea of the situation regarding care of dementia patients in the United States at this time. Commenting on the plight of older people in hospital, Rosenberg (1987) remarked that whilst doctors might be busy debating and writing about dementia in their professional journals at the beginning of the twentieth century, their deliberations were having little impact on practice. He concluded that in most parts of the United States, in the voluntary and municipal hospitals, and even in the religious hospitals, there was little interest in aged and chronic patients.

Substantive papers on dementia were not to appear in England in the *Journal of Mental Science* for another 20 years, and even then were of a discursive nature. A typical paper was that by Phillips (1920) who debated at length what Kraepelin meant by senile dementia and how it might differ from dementia praecox (schizophrenia). He alluded to 37-year-old twin sisters in his care whom he thought both had dementia and hypothesized that this was a case of *folie à deux*. He suggested that dementia might possibly be transmitted from one person to another and that it might therefore be best to segregate dementia patients. He went on to suggest that dementia was probably closely allied to melancholia and that blood sugar levels and the size of the heart were probably more significantly correlated than had previously been appreciated. Whilst papers such as this indicate interest on the part of some doctors, the relatively few mentions of dementia in the *Journal of Mental Science* during the first quarter of the twentieth century demonstrate that there was insufficient commitment from the whole body of psychiatrists to trigger a coherent approach to diagnosis, treatment and care.

By 1927, London County Council appears to have realized that the growing numbers of older patients were being inadequately cared for. Its pamphlet *Introduction to Mental Nursing* (1927) constituted a recruitment drive. The role of the mental nurse was described as being diverse. The section headed 'Types of patients' contains an interesting insight into current, perhaps popular, opinion on senile dementia:

> There is a number of types of patients which the probationer will learn to recognise when taught during training. Some patients are excitable or manic in reaction, others are dull or depressed. Others are dull and apathetic and may be suffering from schizophrenia, leading to a permanent deterioration and dementia. Many of the older people may show forgetfulness and neglect of their person consequent on mental deterioration or senile dementia, and these require special nursing care, especially when bed-ridden.

Evidence that nurses were receiving some education and training in dementia by the end of the 1920s can be gleaned from questions appearing on examination papers set by the Royal Medico-Psychological Association which had sole responsibility at this time for accrediting mental nurses. Question 3 of the Final Examination Paper in November 1928 read: 'Give an account of the mental symptoms that may be met with in a case of senile insanity. Discuss the nursing requirements of senile patients.' There are no records of how many candidates answered this question, or of how satisfactorily they answered it, but it can safely be concluded that the only students to attempt the question would have been those taught by the relatively small number of doctors with an interest in the area. The term 'senile insanity' is interesting in that it was not one used in the literature of the time, and it can only be inferred that those who set the examination felt free to devise whatever term they chose. Nonetheless, the fact that the question appeared on the Finals paper implies that the nursing profession was expected to be aware of and cater for the needs of elderly patients with dementia.

Similar questions regularly appeared in the written examination for nurses, but in May 1930 one question seemed to imply that thinking (and perhaps practice) in nursing circles had made a significant advance. The question was: 'Describe a case of Dementia Praecox. In what way can a nurse assist in delaying or preventing the onset of dementia in such cases?' First, the question suggests that the terms 'dementia praecox' and 'dementia' were closely aligned in England at this time, although Kraepelin saw them as two distinct nosological categories. And secondly, it would appear that, by the 1930s, it was considered that dementia could be prevented or delayed by the kind of care that nurses might offer. This was quite a departure from the Kraepelin position that dementia was irreversible and deterioration was inevitable. What had happened in the space of ten years to lead the examiners to suggest that dementia was treatable and could be influenced by nursing care? First, the number of older people in mental hospitals had grown considerably: in some hospitals more than half the patients were over 65 years of age. The need to cater for these patients was overwhelming, and many doctors and nurses must have become aware that far more could be done than simply feeding and washing them. Lack of emotional and intellectual stimulation coupled with monotonous routines clearly served to suppress individuality and hasten the social deterioration of patients, and the environment of the average mental hospital was more likely to promote psycho-pathology than alleviate it (Martin 1984). Secondly, some doctors were already seeking to better the conditions of patients and establish therapeutic relationships with them. At De La Pole Hospital in Hull, Bickford (1955) demonstrated how, with very little effort and no expense, great improvements in the lives of older people and relief of many debilitating symptoms could be achieved simply by means of compassion, understanding and attention. Nurses, he argued, should be at the forefront of care for elderly people and more skilled care was preferable to simply having more staff. Thirdly, a small band of general nurse tutors who had been teaching in psychiatric hospitals since the early 1930s were teaching their students about the importance of good physical care in reducing the mental confusion and bodily discomforts of geriatric patients (Nolan 1993).

Outside the institutions, the number of older people was increasing, and politicians were becoming aware of some urgency in the need to tackle the key issues for this section of the electorate. In 1901, the number of people in England over 65 years of age constituted 5 per cent of the population; in 1931, 7.4 per cent and in 1951, 11 per cent. Apart from the passing of the Old Age Pension Act in 1908, which attempted to buffer people from poverty in the later years of their lives, little of any consequence was done for the elderly until the advent of the National Health Service in 1948. Then it was found that most of the 4.6 million people aged 65 and over in the UK had lived or currently lived in deprived housing, were in receipt of primitive health care, and had been exposed to occupational hazards or experienced injury during the two world wars. The vast majority had lost their teeth and those in need of glasses relied on Woolworth's where spectacles could be obtained for sixpence (Webster 1991).

The 1960s – a new era in treating the disorders of older people

Whether it was due to recognition of how widespread the 'problem' of dementia had become, or to the fact that health professionals had become more aware of the needs of older people, the 1960s was the decade when the deficits within existing health and social services for older people were highlighted. Concerted attempts were made by professionals to find new ways of managing the disorders of old age other than those suggested by the 'scientific method'. Kitwood (1997) explains how efforts were made to respect the 'personhood' of people with dementia by aiming to understand and empathize with their experiences and those of the families with whom they lived. The Royal College of Nursing (RCN) established a working party in 1960 to look at the problems associated with older people, and ways of providing care so as to improve their quality of life. The working party included ward and departmental sisters, and Section 2 of its report (Royal College of Nursing 1960) lists the main concerns:

- An increased population of older people in mental hospitals owing to patients living longer and the fact that there was nowhere to transfer 'long-stay, stabilised and infirm patients'.

- Poor level of provision for older people in both the social services and the voluntary sector although the Mental Health Act 1959 had advised that the needs of older people with dementia should in future be met by hostel accommodation, training centres, follow-up schemes, social centres, day and night hospitals, and 'in and out hospitals'. As psychiatric hospitals would no longer be required to admit 'elderly senile patients', alternatives had to be identified.

- The need to improve care for the 'residue' of older patients currently in psychiatric hospitals and who must remain indefinitely.

The working party expressed concern that old people's homes and hospitals could easily become communities of forgotten individuals. Whereas older patients had fared poorly in psychiatric hospitals, the nurses feared that they would be even worse off in 'specialist centres' in the community. The Royal College called on nurses to become more active in improving facilities for older people:

> ... by emphasising more staff training, implementing recent advances in therapeutic practice and dietetic treatment. More research should be undertaken into habit-training of groups of patients. Nurses should be supported in carrying out experiments into better nursing, how patients could be encouraged to live more inspired and fuller lives. There is far too much segregation of geriatric and long-stay patients into 'specialist wards', with the result that the interests of neither groups are met.
>
> (Royal College of Nursing 1960: 12)

Nurses were urged to bring the needs of elderly patients to the attention of hospital managers and regional and national health officers.

Research on old age now began to attract researchers of distinction such as Townsend (1962) and Townsend and Wedderburn (1965), who drew the problems of the elderly to the attention of the public and the political parties. In 1965, the London Conference of the World Psychiatric Association was devoted entirely to 'mental disorders of old age'. Contributors from all over the world addressed ways of raising the standing of 'psychogeriatrics'. As a result, improvements in practice were made and new research swelled the volume of literature in the field (Arie and Jolley 1999).

Alongside professional developments, a series of 'scandals' had a considerable impact. The first of these was the publication in 1967 of Barbara Robb's book, *Sans Everything: A Case to Answer*, which documented highly distressing abuses in public institutions for the aged and included a number of chapters by experts suggesting reforms. In the wake of the book, regional hospital boards were charged with appointing committees made up of a doctor, a nurse and a lay member with experience of health service administration to investigate the allegations. Their reports acknowledged that some hospitals gave cause for concern, but otherwise attacked the book for gross exaggeration and dishonest emotionalism. Robb complained to the Council of Tribunals of bias in the way in which the committees had been set up and lack of commitment on the part of the Department of Health and Social Security to taking seriously the issues raised in her book.

Also in 1967, a nursing assistant at Ely Hospital in Cardiff went to the *News of the World* with serious allegations about the treatment of elderly patients at the hospital and pilfering by members of staff. In response, another committee was set up and its findings corroborated the nursing assistant's account. Details were provided of incidents with names of patients and staff involved and dates and times of day. The committee's report was taken seriously by government (Crossman 1972) and it was noted that the most damning criticisms were directed against the nursing administration:

> Standards were low, supervision was weak, reporting of incidents was inadequate and the training of nursing assistants was non-existent. Though some members of the nursing staff at Ely were concerned about conditions, many had come to feel that it was almost more than their jobs were worth for them to voice their feelings and concerns. Nursing had become a defensive organisation, unable to identify poor nursing practice and reluctant to do anything about it when it did.
>
> (Martin 1984: 8)

The growing involvement of nurses in dementia care

When, in the mid-1970s, the author of the present chapter was appointed charge nurse to an older adult ward in the south of England, there was little evidence of progress consequent to the events outlined above. The ward was euphemistically referred to by both staff and patients as 'God's waiting room'. Nearly 50 per cent of the patients in the hospital were over 65 and there were five wards (comprising 35 beds each) for patients who were confined to bed. Many of the bed-bound patients were in the tertiary stage of syphilis, and dying in great pain. None of the nurses and doctors attached to the author's ward had any specific training in care of older adults, or in the types of conditions, such as severe pressure sores, intractable pain, incontinence and impaired cognitive functioning, with which the patients presented. Although the wards were clean and tidy, and the nurses did their best, the care they provided was restricted to meeting the physical needs of patients. On their ward rounds, senior nurses were more likely to comment on the appearance of the wards than the quality of care provided for the patients.

The need to improve clinical nursing skills in specialist areas was recognized by the new Clinical Board of Nursing Studies set up in the early 1970s. Dementia care was one of the areas targeted. Initially, there were few courses because there were few nurse tutors with the appropriate knowledge, skills and experience to teach on them. Further courses became available with the establishment of the English National Board in the early 1980s. This second wave of courses was designed to enable nurses not working in the large cities to attend. Although the impact of the courses took time to make itself felt, nevertheless the requirement that nurses taking on senior positions in older people's services should have attended an appropriate course marked a significant change in the culture and expectations that had prevailed in the psychiatric hospitals.

Froggatt (1995) believes that it was the closing of the mental hospitals and of the geriatric wards from the 1980s onwards that most significantly contributed towards progressing the care of older people. Alternative ways of caring for the elderly had to be found. A new culture had to be engendered not derived from the traditional view of dementia as a progressive, degenerative illness leading to a terminal vegetative state (Bell and McGregor 1995). Social and health care attitudes that conspired to perpetuate negatives attitudes towards older people had to change (Webster 1991). Older people needed purposeful activity to keep them stimulated, and small specialist units supported by family involvement were found to be far superior to large, anonymous institutions.

There is a growing recognition that many people manage the latter parts of their lives extremely well, although understanding of the key factors which contribute to this is in its infancy (Lieberman and Tobin 1983). Within this new culture of valuing older people, the nursing profession has found that it has much to contribute and that levels of job satisfaction can be high. Nurses working in primary care have an important role to play in the early identification of dementia, initiating physical and neurological investigations, and arranging and delivering sessions on reality orientation, communication, self-maintenance and social involvement. Ward and Dewing (2001), among others, note that when older people are consulted in a sensitive and non-patronizing way, they can become valuable allies in identifying appropriate services and assisting nursing personnel to deliver them. Thornton and Tuck (2000) report that nurses in community settings are well placed to deliver mental health promotion to disadvantaged groups and to engage carers and family members in providing purposeful activities for older people. Nurses are also able to detect depression in older people and initiate treatment and care regimes to prevent deterioration (Tucker *et al.* 2001).

Meetings and conferences proliferate to share new ideas on best practice, and the nursing literature on care of the elderly is growing. A lively and robust literature is essential for bringing new ideas to practitioners, highlighting areas that need developing and encouraging service providers to contribute to the debate. The time may soon be here when there exists a critical mass of nurses with wide-ranging and relevant skills who can make a significant contribution to changing the attitudes and practices of colleagues working with older adults.

Conclusion

> Britain's getting older. The number of people aged over 65 has doubled in the last seventy years. The number of people over 90 will double in the next 25 years.
>
> (*National Service Framework for Older People* 2001: 1)

There are today many more and better-informed nurses involved in the care of older people than was the case two decades ago. Progress has been made, but there are still problems to overcome. Even though people over the age of 75 consume five times the normal per capita average of NHS resources, evaluation of the effectiveness of such services is scarce and users are far too infrequently involved in planning and developing services. Schell (2001) points out that ageism still permeates the health care system and there is a woeful lack of health and social care provision for older people with multiple and complex needs. Cooper and Coleman (2001) report that older patients are still commonly perceived by nurses as being mentally and physically dependent, and, where pressurized work schedules prevail, nurses tend to give greater priority to the meeting of physical needs only.

The literature suggests that where nurses have advanced the care of older people, they have done so by utilizing psychological approaches rather than medical. Nurse consultants and advanced nurse practitioners will need to bear this in mind when using their positions to influence the types of service provided for older people in line with *The National Service Framework for Older People* (2001). The Framework is based on four tenets:

1   High quality care and treatment, regardless of age.

2   Older people treated as individuals, with respect and dignity.

3   Fair resources for conditions which most affect older people.

4   Easing the financial burden of long-term residential care.

The care which older people require in order to optimize and prolong their physical and mental functioning would appear to lie in the psycho-social domain rather than in the biomedical. People whose lives have a sense of purpose, who are involved in the community, and who have regular time with their families, enjoy a better quality of life and are more likely to maintain cerebral competence for longer than those who are isolated from social contact. The skills and understanding of nurses are, therefore, especially appropriate for caring for older people. Nolan *et al.* (2001) urge nurses to champion better care for older people and insist that their basic rights be met. These authors express concern that 'person-centred care', so often quoted in government policies, is not sufficient in the case of older people. Instead, they advocate 'relationship-centred care'. The challenge is to transcend the rhetoric of client-centredness, and to work to enhance the quality of relationships so that they are stimulating, consistent and life-enhancing and not just preoccupied with meeting needs or solving problems.

At the beginning of this chapter, four stages in the evolution of treatment and care were identified. Today, the extent of the challenges presented by old age has been identified (stage 1); the conditions associated with old age and dementia have been described in the scientific literature (stage 2); and clinicians have started to develop ways of treating older people (stage 3). Now it is time for nurses to focus on care, involving older clients in planning and carrying out their own care, and drawing on the knowledge, experience and concern of members of their family. The literature abounds with descriptions of useful approaches to dementia, but nurses need to become more skilled in experimenting with them and more creative in how they approach and assist older people (Schell 2001). Although much has been achieved, there is still much more to do if nurses are to contribute to the improvement of care for all clients with dementia and agitate effectively on their behalf. In the chapters that follow, the reader will encounter what is being achieved in the care of people with dementia and how nurses can play a central part in improving services for this vulnerable section of society.

References

Alzheimer, A. (1911) Uber eigerartige Krankheitsfalle des spateren Alters' Zeitschrift für die gesante, *Neurologie und Psychiatrie*, 4: 356–85.

Arie, T. and Jolley, H. (1999) Psychogeriatrics, in H. Freeman (ed.) *A Century of Psychiatry*. London: Mosby/Wolfe Medical Communications.

Bell, J. and McGregor, I. (1995) *A Challenge to Stage Theories of Dementia*. Bradford: Hawker Publications.

Berrios, G.E. (1987) History of the functional psychoses, *British Medical Bulletin*, 43: 484–98.

Berrios, G.E. (1990) Alzheimer's disease: a conceptual history, *International Journal of Geriatric Psychiatry*, 5: 355–65.

Berrios, G.E. (1995) Dementia – clinical section, in G.E. Berrios and R. Porter (eds) *A History of Clinical Psychiatry: The Origin and History of Psychiatric Disorders*. London: Athlone Press.

Berrios, G.E. and Freeman, H. (eds) (1991) *Alzheimer and the Dementias*. London: Royal Society of Medicine.

Bickford, J.A.R. (1955) The forgotten patient, *The Lancet*, 1: 917–19.

Calmeil, L.F. (1835) Demence, in *Dictionaire de Medicine – Repertoire General des Sciences Medicales*, 2nd edition, Paris: Bechet, 70–85.

Charcot, J.M. (1881) *Clinical Lectures on Senile and Chronic Diseases*. London: New Syndenham Society.

Cooper, S.A. and Coleman, P.E. (2001) Caring for the older person: an exploration of perceptions using personal construct theory, *Age and Ageing*, 30: 399–402.

Crossman, R.H.S. (1972) A politician's view of health service planning, *The Times*, 9 August.

Esquirol, E. (1838) *Des Maladies Mentales*, Paris: Baillière.

Froggatt, A. (1995) *Introduction: Widening Our Vision of Dementia Care*. Bradford: Hawker Publications.

Hunter, R. and Macalpine, I. (1974) *Psychiatry for the Poor*, London: Dawsons of Pall Mall.

Kraepelin, E. (1910) *Psychiatrie: Ein Lehrbuch für Studierende und Arzte*. Leipzig: Johann Ambrosius Barth.

Kitwood, T. (1995) Dementia – social section, in G.E. Berrios and R. Porter (eds) *A History of Clinical Psychiatry: The Origin and History of Psychiatric Disorders*. London: Athlone Press.

Kitwood, T. (1997) *Dementia reconsidered: the person comes first*. Buckingham: Open University Press.

Lieberman, M.A. and Tobin, S.S. (1983) *The Experience of Old Age: Stress, Coping and Survival*. New York: Basic Books.

London County Council (1927) *An Introduction to Mental Nursing*. London: London County Council.

Martin, J.P. (1984) *Hospitals in Trouble*. London: Basil Blackwell.

Minois, G. (1989) *History of Old Age: From Antiquity to the Renaissance*. Cambridge: Polity Press.

Morel, B. A. (1860) *Traité des Maladies Mentales*. Paris: Masson.

National Service Framework for Older People (2001) http://www.doh.gov.uk/nsf/olderpeopleshortsummary.htm (accessed 29 January 2002).

Nolan, M., Aveyard, B. and Keady, J. (2001) Nurses must now be the champions of older people, *British Journal of Nursing*, 10: 418.

Nolan, P. (1993) *A History of Mental Health Nursing*. London: Chapman & Hall.

Pelling, M. and Smith, R.M. (eds) (1991) *Life, Death and the Elderly: Introduction*. London Routledge.

Phillips, N. (1920) Clinical psychiatry: discussion on dementia praecox and Kraepelin's position, *Journal of Medical Sciences*, XLIX: 360.

Pick, A. (1901) *Senile Hirnatrophie als Gundlage von Herderscheinungen*, Wiener Klinische Wochenschrift, 14, 403–4.

Porter, R. (1995) Dementia – social section, in G.E. Berrios and R. Porter (eds) *A History of Clinical Psychiatry: The Origin and History of Psychiatric Disorders*. London: Athlone Press.

Rosenberg, C.E. (1987) *The Care of Strangers*. New York: Basic Books.

Robb, B. (ed.) (1967) *Sans Everything: A Case to Answer*. Edinburgh: Nelson.

Royal College of Nursing (1960) *A Comprehensive Mental Nursing Service*. London: RCN [copies stored in the library of the Royal College of Psychiatry, London].

Schell, E.S. (2001) Nurses' perceptions of elderly patients, *Age and Ageing*, 30: 367–8.

Thornton, K.A. and Tuck, I. (2000) Promoting the mental health of elderly African Americans: a case illustration, *Archives of Psychiatric Nursing*, xiv: 191–8.

Townsend, P. (1962) *The Last Refuge: A Survey of Residential Institutions and Homes for the Aged in England and Wales*. London: Routledge & Kegan Paul.

Townsend, P. and Wedderburn, D. (1965) *The Aged in the Welfare State*. London: G. Bell.

Tucker, S., Darley, J. and Cullum, S. (2001) How to detect and manage depression in older people, *Nursing Times*, 97: 36–7.

Ward, A. and Dewing, J. (2001) A sharper focus. *Nursing Older People*, 13: 11–13.

Webster, C. (1991) The elderly and the early National Health Service, in M. Pelling and R.M. Smith (eds) *Life, Death and the Elderly*. London: Routledge.

Wilcox, A.W. (1902) Clinical neurology and psychiatry, *Journal of Mental Science*, XLVIII: 779.

2

Integrating practice and knowledge in a clinical context

Charlotte L. Clarke, John Keady and Trevor Adams

What constitutes evidence in a community practice setting?

Community mental health nursing practice is shaped by many, sometimes competing, forms of knowledge. These range from knowledge that is generated by the process of research through to knowledge that is held by individual practitioners through their professional career of experiences and through the moral and ethical framework of their practice. The role of the practitioner is to make decisions about what knowledge to privilege in what situations in deciding on an optimum course of action for the person with dementia.

This chapter explores some of these forms of knowledge, and in particular considers the role of knowledge that is held by people with dementia. Having considered this evidence for practice, the chapter continues in exploring evidence for the act of practising, and finally outlines broadly evidence of community mental health nursing practice and its associations with philosophies of practice in dementia care. Threading throughout are Mr and Mrs Jones, who act as a focus for us as we explore these issues. Let us start by knowing a little more about their lives.

Case study

Mrs Jones lives in the north east of England. She has always lived there, and for most of her adult life has lived with Mr Jones, her husband. It is not a large house, but they share it with their adult son and have, over many years, filled it with the artefacts of their lives – local pottery is a great favourite. They are a very private family and whilst close to their wider family, are not so welcoming of outsiders into the house. Mrs Jones keeps a secret. It is not so much that her husband is a secret – he is a large and loud person who would be hard to keep under cover anywhere – it is more his level of dependency that she prefers to be known only to themselves. For him to be 'taken away' from her is her greatest dread and so she hides, as much as she can, from the outside world his immobility, his incontinence, his violence and his confusion. Most of these she has managed in her own way for some 40 years for he has been unwell for most of their lives together. It is the confusion only that has gathered pace in recent years but has exacerbated his disabilities. Curiously though, Mr Jones receives substantial amounts of respite care, and the staff in the unit know that it takes, for example, four members of staff to manoeuvre him in the bathroom and that the volume of his shouting can be overwhelming. His level of dependency is not as unknown as Mrs Jones might care to think.

So how can we make sense of the situation? Perhaps there is an unspoken collusion to hide the magnitude of the care problems. The collusion extends to providing Mrs Jones with the pharmaceutical means of rendering her husband relatively placid when he is at home. Perhaps this is an example of good practice, in which nursing and medical staff recognize Mrs Jones's wish to have her husband at home and, to achieve this goal, rationalize the pharmaceutical management as legitimate intervention.

A case such as this challenges us on a number of levels. Where are the ethics of the case? Whatever happened to the rights of the person with dementia? Where are the clinical guidelines and trials to evidence intervention? When we thought community care was a good idea, did we mean the self-imposed isolation of the Jones's? Do we think that a life shared between sedation at home and non-sedation (and distress) in a hospital ward is what community care is all about? Do we think that protecting a family relationship is of primary importance? Let us not be too hasty to condemn this situation – dementia care, community care and evidence-based practice are full of many insoluble situations and it is this inherent challenge that we would now like to explore.

Evidence for practice

Scientific knowledge

There are two forms of 'scientific' knowledge. The most common form is de-personalized to the person using that knowledge and decontextualized from the area in which it is used (Reed and Procter 1995). It is knowledge that is generated by someone else, somewhere else and communicated to the user of the knowledge through research reports and professional or academic publications. This form of scientific knowledge is afforded considerable importance and, indeed, researchers pay a great deal of attention to ensuring that the research is of a high quality. Decontextualized scientific knowledge, and particularly that of quantitative methodologies, is often held to be more absolute in its message than some authors would agree with. For example, Greenhalgh (1999: 323) discusses how population based findings do not hold true for individuals:

> Evidence based clinical decision making involves the somewhat counterintuitive
> practice of assessing the current problem in the light of the aggregated results of

hundreds or thousands of comparable cases in a distant population sample, expressed in the language of probability and risk.

The 'misplaced concreteness' attributed to decontextualized scientific knowledge results in frustrations when trying to apply research-based evidence to individual patients and to services. Practitioners caring for Mr Jones may be using this form of knowledge in deciding the type and mode of delivery of his pharmaceutical intervention.

The other form of 'scientific' knowledge is in the form that is personalized and contextualized (Reed and Procter 1995). This is not a remote form of knowledge but is developed by practitioners for their own client group in their own clinical areas. It may be published and communicated to other people but its primary purpose is to inform the development of local practice to meet local health need (Procter 2002).

Both forms of research may make use of a wide range of research methods and address a range of research questions, for example analysing the needs of service users, or evaluating the effectiveness of a new intervention or service model. What underpins scientific knowledge, and where its strength lies, is the process of its development. This seeks to maximize the quality of the information through systematic and transparent processes that can be clearly articulated to others so that others can make a judgement about the relevance of the knowledge for their own purposes.

Intuitive/experiential knowledge

Nursing, in particular, has developed an understanding of the role of more person-held knowledge that is normally viewed as developing through the experiential processes of working with many people. Indeed, systems have been developed to nurture and make more explicit the experiential knowledge base. For example, in Chapter 16 of this book, Carradice, Keady and Hahn discuss the role of clinical supervision in learning about clinical practice. Blomfield and Hardy (2000) and Procter (2002) argue that the tacit, experiential sources of knowledge that nurses use to inform their practice need to be promoted as important and valid contributors to effective clinical practice.

Benner (1984) goes so far as to attribute this accumulation of experiential knowledge to higher levels of practice in which 'intuitive' knowledge is used in decision making, that unarticulated sense that many nurses speak of when they refer to people 'going off' or when 'something is brewing'. Greenhalgh (1999) describes this as case expertise (the accumulated stories of patient and clinical anecdotes), although this is a term that clearly does not have a universal definition, with Liaschenko and Fisher (1999), in the United States, referring to case knowledge as the general knowledge of more established knowledges such as physiology, pharmacology and therapeutic protocols.

Moral/ethical knowledge

There are two basic principles of ethics for nursing. The first is the universal duty of good clinical care – the use of expertise to protect the life and health of the patient to an acceptable standard. The second is the universal duty to respect the autonomy of the patient. Clearly, these are the two issues that at times conflict with each other when caring for people with mental health needs. This is what Raines (2000: 30) describes as an ethical dilemma: 'when two or more ethical principles apply in a situation, that support mutually inconsistent courses of action'. Ethical decision making and ethical dilemmas permeate even the most fundamental areas of nursing care. Seedhouse (1998: 36) asserts that: 'morality is of such profound importance in health care that it is impossible to understand the nature of health work without also understanding the nature and purpose of ethical reflection'. Manthorpe (2001) provides a very thorough account of ethical practice.

This is distinct from the moral distress experienced by many practitioners who know what is right to do but feel unable to act on or implement that decision in a particular situation (Raines 2000). Reed and Ground (1997: 94) similarly extend ethical consideration beyond the single clinical decision to locating that decision in the political dimensions of health care relationships:

> Many of the moral issues which nurses face are not particular events about which single decisions must be made, but permanent features of the relationships and structures within which nurses and patients find themselves.

Unfortunately, one way to cope with moral distress is to develop an emotional distance to the recipients of care and, as a result, to not even recognize the ethical foundation of an issue. This distancing is fertile ground for the development of the corruption of care (Wardhaugh and Wilding 1993) in which care provision betrays its very purpose of 'caring'. Any form of knowledge for practice has to be located in moral and ethical frameworks to safeguard practice and care provision. There are no aspects of care that are morally neutral despite the technical rationality of evidence-based practice that seduces one into assuming a false neutrality (Trinder 2000). Thus, however effective the pharmaceutical management of Mr Jones, only consideration of any moral dilemmas, such as a possible compromise to Mr Jones's autonomy, can allow practitioners to understand the implications of using this intervention.

Service context knowledge

Knowledge of the context of care and the care environment is critical to the ability of a nurse to deliver effective care. Nursing practice is highly dependent on the interactions between professionals, between agencies and between the patient and their environment. Liaschenko and Fisher (1999) refer to this as a form of 'social knowledge'. Nurses need to match required care (or need) with an appropriate care provider/provision and so they need to know of the skills and working patterns of other providers. Liaschenko and Fisher (1999) argue that knowledge of the other people involved in care provision allows nurses to 'organise care for multiple individuals across time and space'. This knowledge extends beyond a social form of knowledge though, to a knowledge of the care and service infrastructure that may be deployed, and that historically shapes care provision. It is important to recognize, however, that nurses are not the only people who manage the health care system for the benefit of service users. People who have a sustained relationship with services develop their own ability to manage service intervention to help achieve their own goals (Clarke 1999a; Thorne *et al.* 2000).

Person/patient knowledge

Liaschenko and Fisher (1999) identify a second form of social knowledge that emphasizes the ability of the nurse to know of the part that illness plays in the patient's life. This includes knowing about the social environment in which a patient lives; the impact of dementia on the individual's ability to function; the stigma associated with dementia; the extent to which the individual adopts the 'dominant cultural discourse' about dementia. 'Knowing the patient' is something that nurses claim as a unique feature of their practice in a multi-disciplinary field and regard as their vehicle for delivering holistic care (Allen 2000). It is a claim that is being increasingly contested alongside calls for an exploration of its relationship to high quality patient care (Luker *et al.* 2000).

A crucial dimension of this form of knowledge concerns who it is that holds the knowledge. Professional staff draw on the scientific and experiential knowledge base that they have accumulated over several years of professional education and practising with people with dementia. The holders of person/patient knowledge, however, are people with dementia themselves. It is a knowledge that is specific to their own life and is rich in their personal biography rather than rich in scientific knowledge. Thorne *et al.* (2000) highlight how people with a chronic disease come to understand their own situation 'in an infinitely more sophisticated manner' than health care professionals.

The dominance of scientific evidence, in particular, to legitimate practice has four major consequences:

1   It stifles the creation of knowledge by practitioners.

2   It fails to match the pace of change in practice such that practices often operate beyond a known evidence base.

3   It compromises the accountability of practitioners to service users, imposing professionally defined evidence.

4   It silences the knowledge base of the service user such that care may fail to build on self-management strategies.

These last two points indicate a strong influence that is antagonistic to being responsive to patients and to engaging people with dementia in their own decision making and care prioritization. The knowledge base of practitioners is very different in its origin and orientation from the knowledge base of service users and carers (Clarke and Heyman 1998).

Locus of expertise

A final aspect of knowledge for CMHNs in dementia care that must be considered is the locus, of point of location and control, of that knowledge. Traditionally, medical and nursing staff have assumed the locus of expertise, and indeed this is reinforced by holding exclusive access to scientific and experiential knowledge. However, it is a position that is being challenged, in part through the increasingly open access of the public to knowledge, and in part through the drives to recognize the level of expertise held by patients with long-term health needs and carers. Allen

(2000) describes how 'expert carers' are challenging nurses' control over caring processes, nurses' claims to expertise and their authority to define standards of care. Drawing on patient/person knowledge undermines the nurses' claims to professional identity and challenges the ability of nurses to be the only people who can 'know' the patient. The increasing dilution of registered nurses through skill mix reviews further challenges nurses' claims to know the patient since it is increasingly non-professionally qualified staff who work most closely with patients (Allen 2000).

Evidence for practising

Evidence-based practice

Delivering patient care in a way that is evidence based has become critical to contemporary health care practice and it is an approach that underpins clinical governance. The nature of evidence-based practice is complex, with Sackett *et al.* (1996) highlighting that research-based knowledge must be applied to the clinical environment and individual patients, and that clinical decision making must accommodate patient preference. One central feature of an evidence-based practice approach is that it is a logical decision-making process in which as much of the proposed intervention is informed by good quality research as is possible. However, at all times, an acknowledgement and accommodation of the patient's opinion as well as other factors temper this. Greenhalgh (1999) argues that understanding the patient's experience of illness is the only way in which a practitioner can make use of all aspects of evidence (including, but not exclusively, research studies) to 'reach an integrated clinical judgement'. It is not 'cookbook' decision making but rather it is a process in which decision making is explicit. It aims to make practice defensible. However, it is an approach that has been subject to misunderstanding, and rather than creating defensible practice has at times been seen to create defensive practice. Defensive practice is not good quality practice since it tends to privilege one form of knowledge over others, and inevitably that privileged form is the most visible to the practitioner and the one that requires least interpretation by the individual practitioner: scientific knowledge.

The approach to professional accountability that requires demonstration of 'best practice', 'evidence-based practice' and 'clinical effectiveness', becomes particularly problematic in some areas of care and for some client groups, not least where there are differences of perspective between the practitioner, service user and family as in dementia care (Clarke 2001). Viewing decision making as only a series of cognitive steps has also received criticism from Martin (1999), with Sleep and Clark (1999) referring to the 'tyranny of external evidence'. Indeed, French (2000) highlights the individual and organizational risks associated with implementing evidence-based practice that result from the research findings being generated in a place that is different from the place of implementation.

Knowledge chains

There are, in effect, three 'knowledge chains' in operation: that of practitioners that is derived from sources other than their immediate practice environment (for example, research); that of the practitioners derived from their practice; and that of the service user. Each of these 'knowledge chains' is explored in a little more detail below:

1   The knowledge for practice results in the drivers for developments in practice being derived from outside any specific care environment. This 'distal' knowledge (Clarke and Wilcockson 2002) is relatively prescriptive and is not owned by practitioners themselves;

2   Knowledge *from* practice is that which is derived from within a specific care environment. It is, therefore, dependent on the contextual issues within that environment such as staffing levels, the nature of the service and the process of engaging service users in care provision. This 'proximal' knowledge is derived by practitioners, who consequently have a strong sense of ownership of that knowledge. Most importantly, proximal knowledge is able to be sensitive to service users at both an individual and a local level. However, one of the more major concerns about evidence-based practice is that the dominance of quantitative science may devalue, or even exclude, other sources of knowledge such as proximal knowledge (Trinder 2000);

3   The knowledge of service users is that which is derived from the individual's own experiences of self-management and the acquisition of information from family, friends and lay sources of information.

There are high expectations of evidence-based practice, but Trinder (2000) regards it as no panacea. Distal knowledge may be a tool but it is the proximal knowledge that allows practitioners in health and social care to know whether it is the right tool for the job, whether it is the right knowledge for the needs of their patients. As a result, there is relative stability of distal knowledge but instability in decision making based on rapidly fluctuating proximal knowledge. Clarke and Gardner (2002) describe this as situated decision making. Similarly, Martin (1999) highlights how 'clinical judgements made by mental health nurses are time- and situation-dependent and consequently are unique'.

It is in the area of bringing together proximal and distal knowledge that there is most concern expressed within the literature. Trinder (2000: 214) writes that 'comparatively little attention has been given to the question of how to combine evidence with clinical expertise or consumer perspectives'. Greenhalgh (1999) also calls for the integration of individual patient narratives with population-derived evidence in the context of evidence-based practice, and Rolfe (1998) argues that most desirable is a synthesis of scientific, theoretical, experiential and personal knowledges.

The complex interrelationship of these various forms of knowledge is highlighted by Greenhalgh (1999). Best practice is achieved when the different forms of evidence, such as clinical anecdote and systematic reviews, are viewed as mutually supportive and informative rather than in competition. Professional practice is a complex process that involves juggling situational demands, intuition, experience and knowledge. Proximal knowledge is generated through the critical examination of care and service provision in relation to the needs of the service users (Clarke and Wilcockson 2002). In a wider context, Brechin *et al.* (2000: xi) argue that 'critical practice draws on an awareness of wider ethical dilemmas, strategic issues, policy frameworks and socio-political contexts'.

Crucially, proximal knowledge involves understanding how one's practices and care interventions are reflective of little more than the philosophy that we sign up to. For example, in dementia care, the biomedical model leads to care interventions such as pharmaceutical and behavioural management, whilst a socio-critical model leads to interventions such as family nursing and systemic practice (Clarke 1999a). Distal knowledge is unable to help us make choices between such philosophical underpinnings of our professional practice. Indeed, the more the shift towards the reductionist approach and technical rationality of evidence-based practice, the less practice becomes theoretically explicit (Im and Meleis 1999). Philosophical guidance is more likely to be derived from policy developments, and here it may not concur with the assumptions about practice held by individual practitioners or teams. However, this has created the space for value-driven approaches to have a transformative effect on dementia care (see, for example, Kitwood and Bredin 1992) and there are parallels in learning disability with the UK White Paper *Valuing People* (Department of Health 2001).

Making best use of the knowledge that is located in each of these chains requires knowledge to be exchanged. However, the factors described below make this hard to achieve fully, and in particular affect the ability of knowledge to move from people with dementia and carers in the direction of professional staff.

The inequalities of knowledges

One consequence of emphasizing technical-rational knowledge (Department of Health 1996) is to locate expertise in those who have the evidence – that is, the health and social care practitioners (Hansson 1989). Alaszewski (1998: 152) argues that a technical evidence base may enhance the skill base of practitioners but will 'not necessarily ensure that the decisions were sensitive to the specific circumstances of each case'. Such a position also erodes the opportunity for lay people to have their own knowledge base (and their own expertise) valued. Further, placing family carers in the role of co-client or resource (Twigg and Atkin 1991) renders their own knowledge base irrelevant to the care of the person with dementia, negating their opportunity to be regarded as experts in care.

Constraints in exchanging knowledge

Mechanisms for exchanging knowledge make research-based knowledge the most easily accessed. The recent explosion of concern about getting evidence to the practitioner has led to the development of facilitatory mechanisms such as clinical guidelines. Mechanisms for knowing of lay perspectives has lagged far behind. The perspective of people with dementia and family carers is disadvantaged by their lack of a collective voice and of a critical mass to describe and develop their common experiences. Despite policies which are increasingly emphasizing the importance of user involvement in service planning (see, for example, Department of Health 1994) and a known divergence between lay and professional perspectives on health and health care (Heyman 1995), little attempt is made to ensure that users have a full contribution in decision making (Clarke 1999a). Price (1996) describes the shift in professional practice to understanding the client's own goals as necessitating a change in the care relationship from that of client and teacher, to that of client and facilitator. Yet to fail to access the knowledge of people with mental illness is to 'shut ourselves off from their wisdom' (Barnett 1997).

A one-sided story: perpetuating social inequalities

The dialogue of the white middle classes and middle aged is most audible to professional carers, and so responding to the service user's perspective may perpetuate social inequalities. The loudest voices and those with most power squeeze out the stories of the less powerful. For people with dementia, there are a number of reasons why their contribution to a shared knowledge base, their own knowledge, is squeezed out (Clarke 1999b). Very often it is their mental health status itself which oppresses them (Frank 1995). Central to our ability to appreciate the knowledge base of someone with dementia is whether they are perceived to have any 'personhood' (Kitwood and Bredin 1992; Goldsmith 1999) or whether the dementia has resulted in a death of 'self' (see Sabat and Harré 1992; Sweeting and Gilhooly 1997). At last, this oppression of people with dementia has started to be tackled, with texts such as Goldsmith (1996) and Wilkinson (2002) creating a path to engaging with people with dementia that we would be well advised to follow.

The fragmentation of care and knowledge

Any knowledge base is incomplete: it tells us as much about what we do not know as what we do know. However, 'not knowing' is obviously problematic in practice and results in a patchwork of knowledge about care which has holes in it. The fragmentation of knowledge into 'bits' that can be evaluated perpetuates a task-orientated interpretation of health and social care practice (Kendall 1997). For example, a reductionist approach to interpersonal communication (for example, maintain eye contact, sit at the same level) obscures the context of that communication as being within a practitioner–client relationship, to the detriment of its therapeutic potential. Similarly, it is necessary to consider the context in which the evidence is being applied. Ross and Meerabeau (1997: 5) argue that service delivery is dependent on the context and process of change: 'robust evidence . . . will not produce real health gains if the factors associated with patient compliance and the organisational issues implicit in the process of care are not understood'. There is a lack of knowledge about some quite fundamental issues concerning the care of people with dementia. The lack of knowledge about the relationship between practitioners and family carers and the person with dementia has resulted in care interventions that have been unknowingly abusive of the relationship between the person with dementia and their carer because of assumptions of involvement based on gender and kin relationships (Ungerson 1987; Parker 1993; Carter 1999).

Evidencing community mental health nursing practice in dementia care

Fundamental to understanding community mental health nursing practice and the nature of its evidence base, is the prerequisite need to comprehend just what the CMHN does and seeks to achieve. The earlier discussions of different forms of knowledge that may be used, and their effect on decisions that are made, point to some of the difficulties that there are. It is clearly insufficient to understand community mental health nursing practice on the grounds of a research evidence base of its interventions alone. There must also be recognition of the philosophical and ethical base of the profession, that in turn defines the extent to which the knowledge base belonging to the person with dementia is accessed and valued. Critical to understanding the evidence of community mental health nursing practice is the coherence between the philosophy of practice and the specifics on the interventions and the processes of delivering those interventions. There are multiple interventions with people with dementia, just a selection of which can be detailed here.

Practice philosophy and practice action

Emphasizing individuality and biography

Approaches that focus on the biography of the person with dementia include life review and reminiscence therapy. Hargrave (1994) describes making videos with older people to capture and create meaning of their past, and Murphy and Moyes (1997) describe the wide variety of media such as photographs which can be used to provide a multi-sensory approach. Whilst life review and reminiscence have the ostensible purpose of helping the individual come to terms with their past, they also allow others, be they family members or professional staff, a window into the past world of the older person. Basing care delivery on a respect of the individuality of each person requires a regard for them as people in the present as well as in the past. This requires us to regard their present existence as of value. However, the pathology-orientated health care system and problem-led approach to care delivery implicitly views ability as irrelevant to care unless it is absent. Consequently, people are gradually stripped of their abilities as their health fails, with little recognition of that which is left (Reed and Clarke 1999). Rather than deliver care which is problem driven, one alternative is to adopt a strengths perspective in assessment and care management, as described by Perkins and Tice (1995).

Emphasizing norms

One quite dominant approach to care management values the social norms of society as a 'benchmark' for the value and activity of people with dementia. There has been a long, if now rather discredited, tradition of interventions which seek to keep people 'in contact' with reality (or at least that reality known to others). Reality orientation, for example, strives to reinforce the 'facts' of time, place and person (see Holden and Woods 1982). There is no room for any other reality, for acknowledgement that people may work within a differing framework in which time and place become irrelevant. Behaviour that 'we' find problematic, such as wandering and agitation, have been subject to symptomatic management through techniques such as behaviour modification. Such approaches require the behaviour to be controlled, and Kitwood (1995: 10) wrote that 'managing the behaviour of another means a disregard of that person's own frame of reference, their struggle for life and meaning'. The alternative is to regard the individual as having a right to agency and a purpose in their actions. The meaning of the action is as much our responsibility to discover. In Chapter 14 of this book, Weaks and Boardman describe how they use a theory of normalization to frame their interventions based on a respect for the family unit and its members' own understanding of what is important for that family.

Emphasizing social connectedness

This approach emphasizes people as social beings, connected to society rather than disengaged from it. Knowing of, understanding and working with a wider social group is the philosophy underpinning family-centred modalities of care which do not displace the individual or their family from the attention of care but rather seek to work within the system. For example, family systems therapy, for all its potential for therapeutic effectiveness in this field (Benbow 1997), remains little researched and therefore an unknown intervention (Richardson *et al.* 1994). Some care interventions actively seek to allow the person to engage with others. For example, Gibson (1997: 134) describes how the use of 'knowledge of a person's past to hold them in present relationships is one of several creative means which can be used to maintain warm caring mutual relationships and stave off encroaching frightening retreat into isolation'. Reminiscence and life history work clearly play a part, as do approaches that stimulate and help understand communication with someone with dementia (see, for example, Crisp 1995, 1998). The therapeutic function of interaction between people with dementia is uncertain, although Foster (1997) suggests that there is the potential for enhancing the well-being of older people, and in Chapter 11 of this book Lowery and Murray describe the use of group work for carers and for people with dementia.

Emphasizing activity

Phair and Good (1995) use the term 'personal therapeutic intervention' to describe activity that intends to create a sense of purpose and well-being. However, people do need to be prepared for therapeutic activity, and the ability of the individual, their readiness to participate and the nature of opportunities for interpersonal interventions need to be considered. Personal therapeutic interventions are not just about doing special activities with people; they are mainly about incorporating activity into normal daily routines and maximizing existing opportunities. This may be something as simple as talking about what is on the radio or about the headlines in the daily papers. Activity therapy can incorporate a range of physical and educational activities as well as more distinct therapeutic entities such as reminiscence therapy. One form of activity therapy might be pet therapy, with Furstenberg (1988) describing how pet therapy improved mood, alertness, reality orientation and interaction in people with dementia. Other activity therapies include music therapy, art therapy, creative writing and many more variations that seek to provide sensory stimulation and purposeful, pleasurable activity.

Emphasizing psychosocial aspects of being

Psychosocial management of older people with mental health needs is an enormous and diverse field that has gained popularity in recent years. Broadly, interventions take a supportive approach, an analytical approach or a cognitive approach. Miesen and Jones (1997) identify a range of psychotherapies, psychomotor therapy, behaviour modification, remotivation and resocialization therapy, reminiscence therapy, reality orientation training, activity groups, validation, normalization of living patterns and living environment. Other interventions include family therapy (or systemic practice) and creative therapies (for example, music therapy). These interventions may be focused on the older person alone, their family carer alone or the family unit.

The therapeutic relationship

Community mental health nursing is perhaps about more than a set of actions, or direct interventions, with people with dementia and their families. In all aspects of nursing practice, many authors emphasize the importance of the relationship between the nurse and the patient as therapeutic in itself and certainly as a vehicle for delivering other interventions. In this way the relationship becomes an important aspect of the way in which nurses work (Luker *et al.* 2000) and an aspect of the therapeutic effectiveness of their actions. Luker *et al.* (2000) emphasize that developing this familiarity with a patient is emotionally draining and depends on good communication skills and continuity of the caring relationship. The way in which the nurse accesses and comes to know of the knowledge base that derives from the individual patient and that concerns the patient as a social being, allows them to act in an advocacy role with service users (Liaschenko and Fisher 1999; Thorne *et al.* 2000).

One model that makes best use of the relationship between the practitioner and the person with dementia has been developed in Australia by Garratt and Hamilton-Smith (1995): the ELTOS (Enhanced Lifestyle Through Optimal Stimulus) model. ELTOS provides a useful framework for guiding activity with people, emphasizing communication, teamwork, validation, lowered stress and positive stimulus. The key areas of action are:

1   Focus on the person whom you care for rather than on the tasks you are performing.
2   Get to know the people in your care – who they are, who they have been, their likes and dislikes, their families and their friends.
3   Accept the reality of those people you support as being 'real' to them. Do not make value judgements when you try to interpret their actions and thoughts.
4   Remove or minimize the stimuli which obviously distress those you care for and support.

5   Use your knowledge of the people you are caring for to build for them a meaningful daily routine. Where possible give them some choice about things that have to be done, for example the time for getting up or having a shower. Identify pastimes and activities which have a special meaning for them. Where possible, arrange for such activities and pastimes to occur in the community where the person would normally undertake them.

6   The final action is to use your knowledge and understanding of the people you are caring for in a cooperative manner and share this knowledge with your co-workers. Do not underestimate the amount of knowledge that care workers as a team possess collectively.

Brokering services

Liaschenko and Fisher (1999) emphasize the role of nurses in coordinating care and in linking the patient to resources. In this way, nurses do not necessarily deliver care directly themselves but act more as a broker to ensure that the patient receives the right services at the right time. This is all the more important in dementia care because of the changing needs of the individual over time and the transitional nature of their care requirements and services response (Clarke 2001; Cook *et al.* 2001). As Liaschenko and Fisher (1999: 36) go on to explain:

> Although the recipient of care is situated in a particular time and space, the goal of the health care system is to move the individual from one level of care, usually more intense, to a less intense level. Yet the resources of the health care system can be temporarily discontinuous and are often geographically dispersed.

Conclusion

There are several sources of knowledge that inform community mental health nursing for people with dementia: scientific, intuitive/experiential, moral/ethical, service context, person/patient. It is essential to effective and acceptable practice that all forms of knowledge are considered in making decisions about care, and to achieve this requires an exchange of knowledge between the practitioner, the person with dementia (and carer) and the written 'evidence' base.

The nature of the evidence base required for community mental health nursing is varied and depends on what we understand the practice to concern. It is proposed that this involves three core areas: the philosophy and practice of interventions, the therapeutic nature of health care relationships, and care coordination.

Let us take a moment to think again of Mr and Mrs Jones. The pharmaceutical management of Mr Jones whilst he is at home is something that may well make us shudder a little with professional unease. We know that this is not right – it does not accord with our ethical base that requires us to respect him as an individual rather than as an appendage of Mrs Jones; it takes away from him some of his own autonomy; and it is not in itself an act that is therapeutic. But it does allow him to remain at home. We know that Mrs Jones wishes this and that Mr Jones appears to object to periods of respite care when he is not in his own home. Perhaps we can assuage some of our unease by considering it as a means to an end and that the end (remaining at home) is something that is wanted by Mr Jones. There is no 'right' way of responding to this situation, but we must remind ourselves that people with dementia and their families, like Mr and Mrs Jones, must live with the consequences of our professional decisions. The least we can do is to understand the basis on which we make those decisions.

References

Alaszewski, A. (1998) Health and welfare: managing risk in late modern society, in A. Alaszewski, L. Harrison and J. Manthorpe (eds) *Risk, Health and Welfare*. Buckingham: Open University Press.

Allen, D. (2000) Negotiating the role of expert carers on an adult hospital ward. *Sociology of Health and Illness*, 22(2): 149–71.

Barnett, E. (1997) Collaboration and interdependence: care as a two-way street, in M. Marshall (ed.) *The State of the Art in Dementia Care*. London: Centre for Policy on Ageing.

Benbow, S.M. (1997) Therapies in old age psychiatry: reflections on recent changes, in M. Marshall (ed.) *State of the Art in Dementia Care*. London: Centre for Policy on Ageing.

Benner, P. (1984) *From Novice to Expert: Excellence and Power in Clinical Nursing Practice*. Wokingham: Addison-Wesley.

Blomfield, R. and Hardy, S. (2000) Evidence-based nursing practice, in L. Trinder and S. Reynolds (eds) *Evidence-based Practice: A Critical Appraisal*. Oxford: Blackwell.

Brechin, A., Brown, H. and Eby, M.A. (2000) Introduction, in A. Brechin, H. Brown and M.A. Eby (eds) *Critical Practice in Health and Social Care*. London: Sage.

Carter, C.E. (1999) The family caring experiences of married women in dementia care, in T. Adams and C.L. Clarke (eds) *Dementia Care: Developing Partnerships in Practice*. London: Ballière Tindall.

Clarke, C.L. (1999a) Dementia care partnerships: knowledge and ownership, in T. Adams and C.L. Clarke (eds) *Dementia Care: Developing Partnerships in Practice*. London: Ballière Tindall.

Clarke, C.L. (1999b) Partnership in dementia care: taking it forward, in T. Adams and C.L. Clarke (eds) *Dementia Care: Developing Partnerships in Practice*. London: Ballière Tindall.

Clarke, C.L. (2001) Understanding practice development, in C. Cantley (ed.) *A Handbook of Dementia Care*. Buckingham: Open University Press.

Clarke, C.L. and Gardner A. (2002) Therapeutic and ethical practice: a participatory action research project in old age mental health, *Practice Development in Healthcare*, 1(1): 39–53.

Clarke, C.L. and Heyman, B. (1998) Risk management for people with dementia, in B. Heyman (ed.) *Risk, Health and Health Care*. London: Arnold.

Clarke, C.L. and Wilcockson, J. (2002) Seeing need and developing care: exploring knowledge for and from practice, *International Journal of Nursing Studies*, 39(4): 397–406.

Cook, G., Reed, J., Sullivan, A. and Burridge, C. (2001) *Moving In and Moving On: Transition of Older People Between and Within Care Homes*. Newcastle: Centre for Care of Older People, University of Northumbria at Newcastle.

Crisp, J. (1995) Making sense of the stories that people with Alzheimer's tell: a journey with my mother, *Nursing Inquiry*, 2: 133–40.

Crisp, J. (1998) Towards a partnership in maintaining personhood, in T. Adams and C.L. Clarke (eds) *Dementia Care: Developing Partnerships in Practice*. London: Ballière Tindall.

Department of Health (1994) *Working in Partnership: A Collaborative Approach to Care*. London: The Stationery Office.

Department of Health (1996) *Promoting Clinical Effectiveness: A Framework for Action In and Through the NHS*. London: NHS Executive.

Department of Health (2001) *Valuing People*. London: Department of Health.

Foster, K. (1997) Pragmatic groups: interactions and relationships between people with dementia, in M. Marshall (ed.) *State of the Art in Dementia Care*. London: Centre for Policy on Ageing.

Frank, B.A. (1995) People with dementia can communicate – if we are able to hear, in T. Kitwood and S. Benson (eds) *The New Culture of Dementia Care*. London: Hawker Publications.

French, P. (2000) Evidence-based nursing: a change dynamic in a managed care system, *Journal of Nursing Management*, 8: 141–7.

Furstenberg, F.F. (1988) Short term value of pets, *American Journal of Nursing*, 88(1): 57.

Garratt, S. and Hamilton-Smith, E. (1995) *Rethinking Dementia – An Australian Approach*. Melbourne: Ausmed.

Gibson, F. (1997) Owning the past in dementia care: creative engagement with others in the present, in M. Marshall (ed.) *State of the Art in Dementia Care*. London: Centre for Policy on Ageing.

Goldsmith, M. (1996) *Hearing the Voice of People with Dementia*. London: Jessica Kingsley.

Goldsmith, M. (1999) Ethical dilemmas in dementia care, in T. Adams and C.L. Clarke (eds) *Dementia Care: Developing Partnerships in Practice*. London: Ballière Tindall.

Greenhalgh, T. (1999) Narrative based medicine in an evidence based world, *British Medical Journal*, 318: 323–5.

Hansson, S.O. (1989) Dimensions of risk, *Risk Analysis*, 9(1): 107–12.

Hargrave, T.D. (1994) Using video life reviews with older adults, *Journal of Family Therapy*, 16: 259–67.

Heyman, B. (1995) Introduction, in B. Heyman (ed.) *Researching User Perspectives on Community Health Care*. London: Chapman & Hall.

Holden, U.P. and Woods, R.T. (1982) *Reality Orientation*. London: Churchill Livingstone.

Im, E. and Meleis, A.I. (1999) Situation-specific theories: philosophical roots, properties, and approach, *Advances in Nursing Science*, 22(2): 11–24.

Kendall, S. (1997) What do we mean by evidence? Implications for primary health care nursing, *Journal of Interprofessional Care*, 11: 23.

Kitwood, T. (1995) Cultures of care: tradition and change, in T. Kitwood and S. Benson (eds) *The New Culture of Dementia Care*. London: Hawker Publications.

Kitwood, T. and Bredin, K. (1992) Towards a theory of dementia care: personhood and well-being, *Ageing and Society*, 12: 269–87.

Liaschenko, J. and Fisher, A. (1999) Theorizing the knowledge that nurses use in the conduct of their work, *Scholarly Inquiry for Nursing Practice: An International Journal*, 13(1): 29–41.

Luker, K.A., Austin, L., Caress, A. and Hallett, C.E. (2000) The importance of 'knowing the patient': community nurses' constructions of quality in providing palliative care, *Journal of Advanced Nursing*, 31(4): 775–82.

Manthorpe, J. (2001) Ethical ideas and practice, in C. Cantley (ed.) *A Handbook of Dementia Care*. Buckingham: Open University Press.

Martin, P.J. (1999) Influences on clinical judgement in mental health nursing, *Nursing Times Research*, 4(4): 273–80.

Miesen, B.M.L. and Jones, G.M.M. (1997) *Care-giving in Dementia: Research and Applications*, Vol. 2. London: Routledge.

Murphy, C. and Moyes, M. (1997) Life story work, in M. Marshall (ed.) *State of the Art in Dementia Care*. London: Centre for Policy on Ageing.

Parker, G. (1993) *With This Body*. Buckingham: Open University Press.

Perkins, K. and Tice, C. (1995) A strengths perspective in practice: older people and mental health challenges, *Journal of Gerontological Social Work*, 23: 83–97.

Phair, L. and Good, V. (1995) *Dementia: A Positive Approach*. London: Scutari Press.

Price, B. (1996) Illness careers: the chronic illness experience, *Journal of Advanced Nursing*, 24: 275–9.

Procter, S. (2002) Whose evidence? Agenda setting in multi-professional research: observations from a case study, *Health, Risk and Society*, 4(1): 45–59.

Raines, M.L. (2000) Ethical decision making in nurses: relationships among moral reasoning, coping style and ethics stress, *JONA's Healthcare Law, Ethics, and Regulation*, 2(1): 29–41.

Reed, J. and Clarke, C. (1999) Older people with mental health problems: maintaining a dialogue, in M. Clinton and S. Nelson (eds) *Advanced Practice in Mental Health Nursing*. Oxford: Blackwell Science.

Reed, J. and Ground, I. (1997) *Philosophy for Nursing*. London: Arnold.

Reed, J. and Procter, S. (1995) Practitioner research in context, in J. Reed and S. Procter (eds) *Practitioner Research in Health Care: The Inside Story*. London: Chapman & Hall.

Richardson, C.A., Gilleard, C.J., Lieberman, S. and Peeler, R. (1994) Working with older adults and their families – a review, *Journal of Family Therapy*, 16: 225–40.

Rolfe, G. (1998) Advanced practice and the reflective nurse: developing knowledge out of practice, in G. Rolfe and P. Fulbrook (eds) *Advanced Nursing Practice*. Oxford: Butterworth-Heinemann.

Ross, F. and Meerabeau, L. (1997) Editorial: Research and professional practice, *Journal of Interprofessional Care*, 11(1): 5–7.

Sabat, S.R. and Harré, R. (1992) The construction and deconstruction of self in Alzheimer's disease, *Ageing and Society*, 12: 443–61.

Sackett, D.L., Rosenberg, W.M.C., Gray, J.A.M., Haynes, R.B. and Richardson, W.S. (1996) Evidence based medicine: what it is and what it isn't, *British Medical Journal*, 312: 71–2.

Seedhouse, D. (1998) *Ethics: The Heart of Health Care*, 2nd edn. Chichester: Wiley.

Sleep, J. and Clark, E. (1999) Weighing up the evidence: the contribution of critical literature reviews to the development of practice, *Nursing Times Research*, 4(1): 306–13.

Sweeting, H. and Gilhooly, M. (1997) Dementia and the phenomenon of social death, *Sociology of Health and Illness*, 19: 93–117.

Thorne, S.E., Nyhlin, K.T. and Paterson, B.L. (2000) Attitudes towards patient expertise in chronic illness, *International Journal of Nursing Studies*, 37: 303–11.

Trinder, L. (2000) A critical appraisal of evidence-based practice, in L. Trinder and S. Reynolds (eds) *Evidence-based Practice: A Critical Appraisal*. Oxford: Blackwell Science.

Twigg, J. and Atkin, K. (1991) *Evaluating Support to Informal Carers – Summary Report*. York: Social Policy Research Unit, University of York.

Ungerson, C. (1987) *Policy is Personal – Sex, Gender and Informal Care*. London: Tavistock.

Wardhaugh, J. and Wilding, P. (1993) Towards an explanation of the corruption of care, *Critical Social Policy*, 37: 4–31.

Wilkinson, H. (ed.) (2002) *The Perspectives of People with Dementia*. London: Jessica Kingsley.

3

Multi-disciplinary teamworking

Trevor Adams, Mark Holman and Gordon Mitchell

Introduction

Community mental health nurses (CMHNs) have often been seen, and perhaps have seen themselves, as lone practitioners: mental nurses who have not only cut themselves loose from the restrictions of the mental hospital, but also freed themselves from the dominating power of the psychiatric profession. This view of their work has led to various studies that have focused on the work of CMHNs in isolation from that of other health and social care professionals (see Adams 1999; Gunstone 1999; Carradice *et al.* 2002). Whilst these studies are wholly appropriate and contribute to our existing understanding of community mental health nursing practice, they do not acknowledge the reality that many CMHNs work within multi-disciplinary teams such as community mental health teams (CMHTs). This chapter goes some way to address this shortcoming by examining the work of CMHNs with people who have dementia and their carers within the context of community multi-disciplinary teamwork.

Throughout this chapter, examples of the issues associated with multi-disciplinary teamwork will be given from the everyday experience of two NHS Trust areas. First, the Derwentside Practice Development Unit, County Durham and Darlington Priority Services NHS Trust based in Consett in the north-east of England. Secondly, the intensive community treatment team based in Hull and East Riding Community Health NHS Trust.

The development of multi-disciplinary teamwork within dementia care

Traditionally, and as Peter Nolan explained in Chapter 1, mental health care was based on the binary relationship between the psychiatrist and the mental nurse. Accounts of what happened in mental hospitals reveal the dominating, though infrequent, presence of the medical superintendent alongside the subservient, though continual, presence of the mental nurse. The emergence of other professionals such as clinical psychologists, occupational therapists and social workers after the Second World War, each with their own account of mental health and distinctive contribution to care, gave rise to the need to coordinate the contribution of each profession to the provision of mental health care.

In the 1950s and 1960s other changes were occurring within mental health care, the most important of which was the relocation of existing service provision from mental hospitals to the community. Within this context, multi-disciplinary teamwork became an important feature of mental health care to people with severe and enduring mental health problems, including people with dementia. As *Building Bridges* (Department of Health 1995: 35) notes:

> Specialist services working in hospitals and the community are increasingly working in teams. This is recognised as the most effective way of delivering multi-disciplinary, flexible services which the principles outlined demand.

As a result of the wider trends towards community care and multi-disciplinary teamwork within mental health care, comprehensive multi-disciplinary community 'psychogeriatric' teams emerged.

Two additional reasons for the emergence of community psychogeriatric teams should be noted. First, the impetus for the development of these teams came from a number of young and innovative psychiatrists working in various parts of the UK. Secondly, the move towards multi-disciplinary teamwork within the context of community care was supported by a long line of policy documents from *The Rising Tide* (Health Advisory Service 1982) to the more recent *The Handbook on the Mental Health of Older People* (Department of Health 1997). Whilst the *National Service Framework for Older People* (Department of Health 2001) did not specifically address multi-disciplinary teamwork, it did strongly advocate at a senior managerial level multi-disciplinary and inter-agency working, and supported systems such as joint investment plans (JIPs) and the idea of a single assessment, joint planning, investment and implementation of service provision. In this way, the *National Service Framework for Older People* outlined the infrastructure required to support multi-disciplinary teamwork within dementia care.

Overall, the development of multi-disciplinary teamwork became a means of coordinating the proliferation of health and social care professionals. The fear was that, without proper coordination, community care might fall apart. Another way that these concerns were addressed was through the introduction of the Care Programme Approach (CPA) (Department of Health 1991). The key feature of the CPA was that care or case management should be employed with users of mental health services. This approach was initially developed in services to younger people with severe and enduring mental health problems. However, various recent policy documents such as *A Handbook on the Mental Health of Older People* (Department of Health 1997) and the *National Service Framework for Older People* (Department of Health 2001) clearly advocate that case management should be applied to older people with dementia. For example:

Recent policy guidance addresses the integration of the Care Programme Approach with Care Management for adults of working age in contact with secondary mental health services, and stresses that the same principles are relevant to the care of older people with mental health problems.

(Department of Health 2001: 91)

Whilst many CMHTs have applied case management to people with dementia and their family carers, few writers have described how case management can be applied to people with dementia in the context of multi-disciplinary teamwork.

Characteristics of multi-disciplinary teamwork

Working with other health care professionals is not new to CMHNs; even in mental hospitals 50 years ago, mental nurses worked with psychiatrists. What is new, however, is that the emphasis is not upon maintaining the medical/psychiatric dominance, but rather on developing collaborative, inter-professional teamwork within dementia care. This being the case, various new ideas and concepts need to be introduced into the discussion about community mental health nursing practice that take the subject beyond its traditional concern with people with dementia and family carers, to include multi-disciplinary teamwork.

Writers such as Øvretveit (1993) and Payne (2001) describe different types of health and social care team that might contain CMHNs. Payne highlights the problematic nature of defining the idea of a team. However, a simple definition offered by Øvretveit is that a team is 'a small group of people who relate to each other to contribute to a common goal' (p. 55).

In addition, Øvretveit (1993: 55) defines a community multi-disciplinary team as 'a small group of people, usually from different professions and agencies, who relate to each other to contribute to the common goal of meeting the health and social needs of one client, or those of a client population in the community'. Defining community mental health teams in this way neglects the possibility that there may be other systems beyond the community mental health team. Payne (2001) addresses this issue by developing the idea of the 'open team' in which team members participate with other systems and teams. This is a particularly useful concept within the provision of dementia care as CMHNs usually work closely with other systems, such as the family system and the welfare system.

Miller *et al.* (2001) describe three styles of teamwork. The first is integrated teamwork which is characterized by a high degree of collaborative working in which there is stability and predictability. This type of working is achieved when each professional is assigned to a particular specialism, and is not 'called away' to other teams. A further characteristic of integrated teamwork is that all the professionals are focused on the same client group, and thus there is one focus of practice within the team. In addition, the structure of integrated teams allows joint working that gives rise to the assessment, monitoring and evaluation of client work. Underpinning integrated teamwork is the openness of communication between team members together with a high level of understanding about what each member contributes to the team. Miller *et al.* (2001) identify the benefits of integrated team-working which include continuity, consistency, reduction of ambiguity, appropriate and timely referral, an holistic approach, and actions and decisions based on problem solving.

The second style of teamwork described by Miller *et al.* (2001) is fragmented teamwork. In this style of working, many aspects of client care such as problem solving, decision making and accountability are carried out by single-profession groups. Moreover, communication is short and often consists merely of giving information rather than of sharing professional perspectives. In addition, in fragmented teamwork there is often only a superficial understanding of each other's role. This lack of understanding is usually compounded by team members' protecting their own role and is reinforced by the mono-professional nature of their practice. There is also usually a mixed awareness of the benefits of collaborative working to client care. The nature of teamworking on fragmented teams can lead to either autocratic leadership, without consultation, or 'steered' leadership, without consensus. Each of these leadership styles can lead to the fragmentation of client care through the development of mono-professional groupings. Furthermore, fragmented teams often display a failure to meet 'as a team' and do not make collaborative decisions about either client care or their team.

The third style of teamwork described by Miller *et al.* (2001) is core and periphery working; this combines features of integrated and fragmented teamwork. In this third style, there is a core membership, displayed by collaborative working, and a remainder that are peripheral to that core. Whilst, within the core, integrated practice occurs, the dislocation of the team means that communication between the two parts of the team, the core and the periphery, is constrained and tenuous. This maintains a lack of understanding about each other's roles and how team members may display collaborative working.

Whilst each of these styles displays elements of collaborative teamwork, they do not all provide the same possibility of collaborative working. Miller *et al.* argue that, of these styles, integrative teamwork is most likely to offer effective teamwork. The main concern of this chapter is about the development of collaborative teamwork within community mental health nursing practice with people who have dementia and their carers (Miller *et al.* 2001). Consequently, the rest of the chapter sets community mental health nursing practice within the context of teamwork. Of necessity, there is a tendency to discuss integrated teamwork and community mental health nursing as 'ideal types', as pure forms that exist outside of practice. As an antidote to this tendency, the remaining text provides illustrations taken from everyday practice within the Derwentside Mental Health Service for Older People that will enhance the possibility of the development of practice.

Derwentside Practice Development Unit

Mental health services in County Durham are provided by the County Durham and Darlington Priority Services NHS Trust. Services across the Trust have evolved to meet the needs of the local communities and have developed at differing rates. The Trust covers a large geographical area with mixed urban and rural areas and there are marked differences in the levels of economic development. Furthermore, the Trust was formed from two pre-existing mental health services that had developed differing strategies based around existing services. These factors have made the development of a common Trust-wide model of service difficult and have allowed locally based services to develop to meet the needs of their immediate populations.

The Derwentside locality lies at the northern edge of the Trust. Derwentside is a mainly rural area in north-west Durham with a population of about 85,000 people, most of whom live in Consett and Stanley. Historically, the area was supported by steelmaking in Consett and coal mining throughout the district. With the decline of these industries, the area suffered economically and now features regularly on most of the deprivation indices.

The Derwentside Mental Health Service for Older People is based in Consett on the site of an ex-district general hospital. It comprises a 15-bed admission ward and a day hospital with 25 places. There is also a small continuing care unit comprising 13 beds in Stanley, about nine miles from the core service. The service's community team is drawn from medical staff, community mental health nursing, occupational therapy, physiotherapy and psychology staff, and is based at Shotley Bridge. Referrals are made to the psychiatrists who act as gatekeepers to the service. The psychiatrists screen patients for physical health problems, the consequences of which may have led to the mental health referral; they also assess their mental health needs and present cases at the community team meeting where they are accepted by team members for further assessment or treatment. One of the authors (MH), in collaboration with other members of the team, looked at the patients' experience of the service as part of the accreditation of the service as a practice development unit for the University of Teesside. This involved mapping out the pathway and its features that patients undertake as they pass through the service. As part of this exercise, the team developed a single set of records that follow the patients. Moreover, the team started an evidence-based practice group, made up of existing team members, in order to develop and refine a single package of assessment tools.

The team does not have an attached social worker, but has regular meetings with the local social services team for older people to review the links between services at both a management and a practitioner level. The team has also developed close links with colleagues in acute medicine and the non-statutory services in the locality. Many people with dementia live in care homes and the CMHNs have developed links with the local homes to offer training and advice in the care of residents.

Key areas of multi-disciplinary teamwork

Leadership

Øvretveit (1993) emphasizes that community teams must have good leadership, an issue reiterated later in this book by Mawhinney, McCloskey and Ryan (Chapter 17). Øvretveit argues that teams in which all members are managed by the same person, such as CMHTs, should be managed by someone acting as a team manager. In this role, team managers are responsible for their own work and for delegating work to their team members. Team managers are responsible to their line manager for their own performance and that of their staff. CMHTs can attract charismatic team leaders, particularly when it is a new and innovatory project, and this may give rise to problems when they leave their post and an attempt is made to find a replacement.

Team management may occur in one of three ways. First, teams may be managed by a team leader. In this case, teams members from different professional backgrounds will be managed by someone who, for some team members, is not from the same professional background. Sometimes, when team managers do not have relevant expertise to provide management for a particular professional group, help is obtained from someone who has relevant experience. Nevertheless, in these cases, full managerial responsibility remains with the team manager. Secondly, team members may be managed by a line manager who is outside the CMHT and manages people from the same professional group. In this case, a contract or 'service agreement' between the team leader and the professional leader should exist. Thirdly, the team may operate a system of joint management in which team members are jointly managed by the team manager and a professional leader. Whilst this option provides a diplomatic solution that allows team members to be managed to some extent by members of their own profession, it needs to be carefully implemented to ensure clarity and effectiveness. If it is not successfully accomplished, the team may be open to manipulation that will have a detrimental effect on the quality and extent of the delivery of care.

An important responsibility of team managers is to provide team members with managerial supervision. The aims of managerial supervision are:

- to enable team members to meet standards of service delivery;
- to help team members give a better service;
- to facilitate learning and provide emotional support;
- to reduce the stress incurred by team members.

There are various ways to achieve these aims that usually involve a review of team members' cases either by the team leader or by a peer team member. This form of review is often confused with clinical supervision. Clinical supervision is different from managerial supervision, as it does not have a managerial agenda, but rather addresses emotional issues that arise as the result of team members working closely with clients (this issue is addressed in Chapter 16). From our experience, CMHNs need to have both managerial supervision and clinical supervision. Each of these forms of supervision should remain separate from each other and should be given by different people.

Common problems associated with inadequate leadership include over-control by professional line managers making it difficult to contribute to the team; under-control because they assume that their staff are being managed by the team or professional leaders; managers who are unsure of their accountability, and staff who do not know where to go to get a decision.

Client pathways

Øvretveit (1993) outlines a ten-stage pathway that describes the progression of clients through services (Figure 3.1).

There are various types of pathway, all of which have implications for the work of CMHNs. The first type is the allocation or 'postbox' pathway. In this pathway, referrals are accepted by the team secretary or the team leader and then raised at the team meeting. Alternatively, the referrals may go directly to the team meeting. The referral is then taken on by a team member and is addressed without reference to the team leader.

The second type of pathway is where the referrals are accepted by the team manager, or a secretary, who then decides whether an appropriate referral has been made. Where necessary, they are then discussed at the team meeting and allocated to

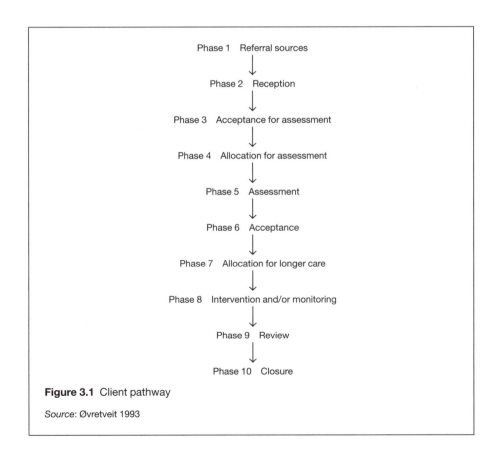

Figure 3.1 Client pathway

Source: Øvretveit 1993

a suitable team member. If it is decided that the team has nothing to offer the case, the team manager or team secretary will either return the referral to the person who made it, or pass it on to another agency. The third pathway allows the case to be reviewed at one or more team meetings after the initial intervention has been made. At these team meetings, the case is fully reviewed and the reallocation of appropriate team members may occur.

A common element to all mental health systems is the use of Care Coordination (Department of Health 2000). On the Derwentside team, when a referral is accepted and acted upon by a team member, that person is designated as the care coordinator, and their case records will constitute both the care plan and subsequent care plan reviews. Several members of a team may take part in a person's assessment or treatment. A care plan will be written at the allocation meeting detailing the actions to be taken by each member of the team and a care coordinator will be appointed. Similarly, the role of other service providers is outlined in the care plan. The care coordinator maintains contact with the patient and other service providers and ensures that regular reviews of the care plan take place. These reviews may occur as part of the team meeting and a new care plan will be completed at the end of the review. Where care is provided by agencies that are not part of the team, the care coordinator will, if necessary, ensure that these agencies are invited to the review meeting along with the patient and/or the informal carers. Risk assessment forms an integral part of this process and care plans must include an assessment of risk and plans that have been made to minimize that risk (see also Chapter 5).

Another important issue is that of 'case finding'. People with dementia and their close relatives often do not know where to get help. Indeed, the Audit Commission (2000) found that many general practitioners (GPs) were unable to give adequate advice and that many felt that they did not have sufficient training concerning dementia care. Moreover, many services were dependent upon people with dementia and their family carers having to find out about their service and how to make a referral. For many people with dementia and their close relatives, finding an appropriate source of care may take some time, possibly months or years. Therefore CMHTs need to have some mechanism by which they find people with dementia who are not themselves able to seek out service provision. One approach that might be developed is assertive outreach.

Assertive outreach

Within services for younger people with mental health problems, systems of case management incorporating the notion of assertive outreach are beginning to develop. One such team is the intensive community treatment team based in Hull and East Riding Community Health NHS Trust. The project started in February 2001 and was scheduled to operate for two years in collaboration with the local Dementia Services Development Centre, Dementia North, based at Northumbria University, Newcastle-upon-Tyne. The project targets people over 65 years of age with new or existing memory difficulties. All therapeutic interventions are focused upon situations where a higher and more intensive level of community treatment is required.

The project aims to prevent admissions to hospital or residential care home environment where possible, by providing intensive community-based assessment and treatment, usually within the individual's own home. Where an admission is necessary, the team facilitates a planned approach to the admission that enables the individual and their carer an appropriate amount of time to consider their options and to achieve the best possible outcome from the admission. An important element in their role is in expediting people's discharge from hospital. People with dementia and family carers receive a comprehensive package of therapeutic intervention that enables them to return home much earlier than is usually possible. Underpinning this work is a focus on maintaining people's independence, choice and dignity. These themes are consistent with the standards outlined in the *National Service Framework for Older People* (Department of Health 2001).

The intensive community treatment team operates on a Monday to Friday, 9.00am to 5.00pm basis. Telephone support is available through a local inpatient unit during out-of-hours periods, with access to an on-call CMHN when required. Two practitioners, one F-grade CMHN and one B-grade health care support worker are employed on the project. The team has full access to existing medical, professional and voluntary support services. The project operates an open referral system, referrals being channelled through existing CMHT bases.

Through a process of assessment and collaborative working with users, carers, voluntary and professional agencies, the team aims to offer realistic, timely and coordinated packages of care to maximize a person's well-being and independence. The team has worked with people and has attained varying degrees of success; much of this success is due to team members being able to work intensively with people for a period of time, rather that the use of specialized interventions. Referrals are received from social services care management teams from across the Trust's locality and also from GP practices.

Assessment

An important aspect of collaborative teamwork is assessment. The teamwork associated with assessment may also be seen within the Derwentside team. The aims of the Derwentside team are twofold. First, to carry out as much of a patient's assessment in their own home as possible, and secondly, to develop an accurate picture of both abilities and risks. Members of a patient's family and other support networks may be included in this assessment. The range and scope of this assessment are discussed at the initial care planning meeting, and details of the planned assessment are included in the initial care plan. The team has developed a set of common assessment tools which allows for comparison of a patient's abilities across time and also across a range of settings. These tools include the following:

- The Mini-Mental State Exam (MMSE) which is widely used for assessing cognitive function (Folstein *et al.* 1975).
- Assessment of Motor and Process Skills (AMPS UK Ltd) used by the team's occupational therapists to assess the quality of an individual's performance of domestic tasks.

- The Behavioural Assessment Scale of Later Life (Brooker 1997). This assessment includes both a checklist version, for completion by health and social care providers, and an interview form which allows a rating both of behaviour and of the impact of that behaviour on carers, who perceive the impact of particular behaviours differently.
- The Brief Assessment Schedule Depression Cards (Adshead *et al.* 1992) which provide a simple mechanism for assessing depressed mood.

Communication

Good communication is an important factor in the promotion of collaborative teamwork. Good communication is helped considerably by all members of the multi-disciplinary team having offices in the same building and it is very beneficial for staff to be accommodated in 'locality teams'. In our experience this helps to break down mono-professionalism and helps prevent members of the same professional group forming a sub-group that may disrupt the development of collaborative team working.

In addition, good communication will be enhanced by the CMHT having a regular team meeting that all the staff are expected to attend. Moreover, it can be worthwhile for administrative staff to attend this meeting, not only because they need to know what is going on but also because in the course of their work they may have contact with users and carers. However, while team meetings should be accommodated within the structure of the CMHT, there is a sense in which good communication between all the team members should be an everyday feature of the CMHT.

In addition to casework, it is important that each team member understands the role of everyone else on the team in order to avoid the misunderstandings and contradictions associated with the ways in which various members of CMHTs understood each other's role (Peck and Norman 1999).

There also needs to be a clear allegiance to a strong and shared philosophy of community mental health care to people with dementia and their carers. Caution needs to be expressed about assuming that because a CMHT has an operational policy, it will command the allegiance of all the team members. Rather, the philosophy should be reinforced by the leadership and should underpin everything done in the name of the CMHT.

Conclusion

As with community care itself, multi-disciplinary teamwork sounds like a great idea but in reality it has proved difficult to implement. Some writers go so far as to suggest that the development of CMHTs is a failed project. Peck and Norman (1999) suggest that there are two alternative explanations for this failure. The first is that the deficiencies of CMHTs, such as overambitious and unfocused aims, and confusion about accountability and responsibility within teams, are attributable to fundamental flaws in the concepts of inter-professional working, and so no amount of improvement in managing CMHTs would reduce their inherent problems. The second is that any failure with CMHTs is simply due to poor implementation.

We believe that multi-disciplinary teamwork has been an important idea within the development of services for people with dementia for some time. Our concern is that many CMHNs have been unwilling, or have found it too difficult, to work in collaborative multi-disciplinary partnerships with other mental health professionals. Up to now very little has been written on community mental health nursing practice within multi-disciplinary settings, and we would hope that this chapter has introduced some new ideas and will encourage CMHNs to work as partners within CMHTs for older people.

Acknowledgements

Acknowledgements are given to Peter Caswell, Hull and East Riding Community Health NHS Trust, Kingston upon Hull.

References

Adams, T. (1999) Developing partnership in the work of community psychiatric nurses with older people with dementia, in T. Adams. and C. Clarke (eds) *Dementia Care: Developing Partnerships in Practice*. London: Baillière Tindall.

Adshead, F., Day Cody, D. and Pit, B. (1992) BASDEC: a novel screening instrument for depression in elderly medical inpatients, *British Medical Journal*, 305: 397.

Audit Commission (2000) *Forget Me Not: Mental Health Services for Old People*. London: The Stationery Office.

AMPS UK Ltd at http://www.amps-uk.com/about.html (accessed 15 November 2001).

Brooker, D. (1997) *Behavioural Assessment Scale of Later Life*. Bicester: Winslow Press.

Carradice, A., Shankland, M.C. and Beail, N. (2002) A qualitative study of the theoretical models used by UK mental health nurses to guide their assessments with family caregivers of people with dementia, *International Journal of Nursing Studies*, 39(10): 1, 17–26.

Department of Health (1991) *Case Management and Assessment: Summary of Practice*. London: DHSS.

Department of Health (1995) *Building Bridges*. London: The Stationery Office.

Department of Health (1997) *A Handbook on the Mental Health of Older People*. London: The Stationery Office.

Department of Health (2000) *Effective Care Co-ordination in Mental Health Services*. London: The Stationery Office.

Department of Health (2001) *National Service Framework for Older People*. London: The Stationery Office.

Folstein, M.F., Folstein, S.E. and McHugh, P.R. (1975) Mini-Mental State: A practical method for grading the state of patients for the clinician, *Journal of Psychiatric Research*, 12: 189–98.

Gunstone, S. (1999) Expert practice: the interventions used by a community mental health nurse with carers of dementia sufferers, *Journal of Psychiatric and Mental Health Nursing*, 6(1): 321–7.

Health Advisory Service (1982) *The Rising Tide*. Sutton: Health Advisory Service.

Miller, C., Freeman, M. and Ross, N. (2001) *Interprofessional Practice in Health and Social Care: Challenging the Shared Learning Agenda*. London: Arnold.

Øvretveit, J. (1993) *Coordinating Community Care: Multidisciplinary Teams and Care Management*. Buckingham: Open University Press.

Payne, M. (2001) *Teamwork in Multiprofessional Care*. Basingstoke: Macmillan.

Peck, E. and Norman, I.J. (1999) Working together in adult community mental health services: Exploring inter-professional role relations, *Journal of Mental Health*, 8(3): 231–42.

4

'We put our heads together'

Negotiating support with the community mental health nurse

Anne Mason, Heather Wilkinson, Elinor Moore and Anne McKinley

Introduction

Recent research involving people with dementia and carers living in Scotland (Mason and Wilkinson 2001a) has provided some insight into what those people feel they need from community mental health nurses (CMHNs). Although this research predominantly focused on the legal needs of people with dementia, respondents discussed these needs within the wider context of how they and others reacted to changing experiences. These reactions included threats to their self-esteem, mood, independence, safety and autonomous status along with a diversity of associated feelings. Within this chapter, the authors suggest that such human responses to this condition are central to determining what the role and scope of community mental health nursing work should be. The work of nursing theorists such as Peplau (1987, 1988), Forchuk (1993) and Reynolds (2001) who are interested in the phenomenological focus of nursing, will be used as a framework to explore this viewpoint.

The personal and legal concepts of autonomy are overriding themes within this chapter. Recent legal reforms within Scotland (Adults with Incapacity Act (Scotland) 2000) have provided a protective framework for people whose autonomy has been threatened in some way, such as those with dementia. CHMNs routinely encounter ethical dilemmas when attempting to uphold the principle of autonomy whilst negotiating appropriate levels of support for both the person with dementia and the carer (McFadyen *et al.* 1998; Gunstone 1999; Adams 2000, 2001). These ethical tensions are supported by findings from the legal study (Mason and Wilkinson 2001a), and this chapter considers such tensions in relation to the CHMN's role in dementia care.

Furthermore, the advantages of working with CMHNs in Scotland to help overcome a wide range of ethical and methodological issues about including adults with dementia in research are outlined using examples from the study. Indeed, a fundamental aim of the study was to identify a method of including people with dementia in the research process. As we found, CMHNs were also seen as 'key gatekeepers' to accessing people with dementia and carers safely and effectively, and unpicking this relationship was vital to the success of the study, and to hearing the voice of people with dementia.

People with dementia and personal autonomy

Personal autonomy is about being the author of one's own behaviour (Levi 1999: 23). In other words, autonomy is about people's rights as individuals to make and sanction their our own decisions and actions. It is a powerful and complex construct creating images of freedom and independence. Collopy (1988: 10) explains six polarities to autonomy and suggests it can be a source of ethical conflict for health professionals that can begin at the level of conceptualization. He claims that how these conflicts are resolved carries inherent risks to the client's autonomy. For people with dementia, the nature of the condition poses an internal threat to autonomy owing to the effects it has on the person's cognitive capacity to make decisions and the potential need for a surrogate (Frolik 1996). However, they may also experience a reduction in their autonomy owing to external factors including decision-making tensions within the family system (Cicarelli 1992, cited by Nolan *et al.* 1996: 134; McFadyen *et al.* 1998). Wetle (1985) argues that this need for surrogate interference by others is sometimes motivated by external paternalistic attitudes. Similarly, Levi (1999) suggests the views held by others about a person's capacity to be autonomous can shape the sort of relationship and extent of public interference required. He claims that a reduction in autonomous status may well equate with a decline in equal respect and advocates that:

> . . . understanding is the cornerstone of respecting autonomous decisions [and] . . . that respecting someone's autonomous decision involves entering into a relationship with that person.
>
> (Levi 1999: 131)

Such a negotiated and interpersonal model is analogous to the therapeutic and problem-solving nurse–patient relationship (Peplau 1987, 1988; Forchuk 1993; Reynolds 2000). The therapeutic role has been well supported within the profession (General Nursing Council for Scotland 1962; Royal College of Nursing 1970; Wilson and Kneisl 1983; Kagan 1985; Pollock 1989). This interpersonal focus requires the skilled application of empathy and its cognitive-behavioural components in order to develop trust (Reynolds 2000).

CMHNs have been described as working within a social model of care that emphasizes such relationship building and individualized care (Pollock 1989). This should facilitate a shared activity with the person needing support, and/or with the primary carer, to plan what interventions are needed that respects the person's preferences, supports self-management and influences health in a positive way. Levi (1999) suggests that learning about an individual's beliefs, practices and values is key to respecting someone's autonomy. Thus, one aspect of community mental health nursing may be to help clarify values and to ensure decisions are authentic. However, Sailors (2001: 191) highlights the difficulty with trying to ascertain decisions that are authentic for people with dementia. She cautions the reader by suggesting that limiting the actions of the earlier self without dementia to benefit the later self with dementia is paternalistic, but limiting the actions to protect the successor self is not paternalistic. This is a somewhat hypothetical argument, but Sailors makes the important point that if a patient makes all the decisions, their treatment choices may fail to serve their well-being. In practice, CMHNs need to know what clients perceive as problems, in order to provide solutions that are considered useful to that person. They also need to recognize when these problems are occurring as a result of the person's difficulty in making functional decisions about their own welfare. When someone's decision-making ability is causing harm to the person, then their legal status can be seen to be in question.

Legal autonomy and Scottish legislation

The legal status of the person with dementia will be challenged by the progress of the condition (Willis 1996; Dickens 1997; Sailors 2001). Willis (1996: 118) describes legal status in terms of a person's functional abilities to make and execute decisions 'necessary for care of oneself and maintenance of one's property'. Once the condition challenges this psychological ability, judgements are made by the legal system about the person's legal status. Thus, the ownership of decisions can be given to others through legal interventions. The criteria used to determine legal capacity is a response 'determined by prevailing values, knowledge, and even economic and political spirit of the time' (Sabatino 1996: 4).

The Adults with Incapacity (Scotland) Act 2000 is an example of such a response to the notion of legal incapacity. Scottish law was outdated and did not meet the needs of specific client groups such as those with dementia (Wilkinson 2001). Creating a more accessible, empowering and protective legal framework for people whose autonomy has been threatened has been a Scottish political priority. The overriding principle of this Act is to acknowledge, respect and uphold the autonomy of individuals whose cognitive capacity to make decisions is vulnerable.

Although this Act upholds this principle, it provides legal interventions that transfer decision making to surrogates. The seductive notion of respecting the autonomy of someone whose capacity to self-govern is in question, is potentially incongruent. However, it is empowering in that it offers opportunities for individuals to make advance arrangements for their welfare and financial affairs, should their capacity deteriorate. It also has legally binding principles and codes of practice (Adults with Incapacity (Scotland) Act 2000) to guide surrogate decision making. Evidence from respondents within this study indicate that the CMHN can be influential in working within this ethical and legal paradigm. This nursing response to current legal principles is an example of how nursing 'changes and fits prevailing social mores' (Peplau 1987: 301). Although nursing's

historical ability to mould itself to changing needs and its ascent to professional-
ization was acknowledged by Peplau, she also recognized the need for the profession to clarify its core identity, and offered a phenomenological focus to the
profession.

A phenomenological nursing focus

The work of the CMHN may offer a unique focus within dementia care but requires
its distinct qualities to be further explored and articulated. Keady and Adams'
(2001) review of the CHMN role communicates the value of their work with carers
and people with dementia. However, they argue that the extent of this value is poorly
understood leaving the profession 'vulnerable and open to misinterpretation' (Keady
and Adams 2001: 35). When examining the specialist and contextual nature of
CHMN's work with people with dementia, it is necessary to consider the role of the
nurse. In 1980, the American Nurses Association (ANA) within its social policy
statement, raised the question 'what is nursing?' (Peplau 1987: 301). Peplau cited the
ANA's definition of nursing as:

> the diagnosis and treatment of human responses to actual and potential
> health problems.

(p. 303)

In response to this, Peplau suggested this definition constituted a major paradigm
shift for nursing work, offering a phenomenological focus to nursing. She makes the
point that there is a need for any profession to identify its unique features that make
it different from other professions and declared that the phenomenon of 'concern'
for nursing would be found in the ANA definition. Some time later, Reynolds (2001)
recovered this key question and unpacked its significance to nurses. Within his
analysis he advances several key points. For example, a starting point for nursing
practice is the need to identify what manifestations are portrayed by the client, that
necessitate support through nursing action. Actions need to be drawn from a theory
base and/or inductive reasoning. The effectiveness of the application of a theoretical
framework needs to be evaluated. Such evaluations will support the efficacy and
authority of nursing practice. Barker and Reynolds (1994) and Reynolds (forthcoming a) maintain the overall aim of such nursing interventions should be to improve
the person's ability to cope with health-related problems within their social context
in a satisfying and empowering way.

The study described in this chapter examines respondents' reactions to
having dementia and what part the CMHN played in providing interventions that
contributed to their health status.

Ethical negotiation: the research design and the role of the CMHN

As a direct result of the legal reforms within Scotland (Adults with Incapacity Act (Scotland) 2000), a qualitative study was funded to ascertain the characteristics of people with dementia who use the Scottish legal system, and to identify what factors influenced the uptake of legal interventions. Semi-structured interviews were undertaken with 62 people mainly by telephone. Out of this sample, 26 were people with dementia and 36 were carers. Numerous ethical issues in accessing and interviewing people with dementia were raised both prior to and during the pilot in relation to:

- their ability to provide an informed consent;
- their use of the telephone;
- their emotional vulnerability;
- confidentiality during access to this group;
- their knowledge of diagnosis;
- the potential distress of being interviewed;
- validity of statements made by respondent;
- the role of carer during consent and the interview.

A more detailed discussion of the research methods and ethical concerns can be found in Mason and Wilkinson (2001a,b). Some of these concerns were raised at the ethical approval stage, which appeared to be motivated by paternalistic attitudes that had the potential to obstruct the opportunity for people with dementia to have their views heard. However, the process of ethical negotiation ensured that the safest and most effective recruitment procedures for accessing a marginalized group were developed.

During the pilot stage of the study, the CMHN was identified as an appropriate and 'safe route' to access people with dementia. The procedures followed by the CMHNs meant an emphasis was placed on protecting the person's identity prior to consent. They were familiar with the person's cognitive and emotional ability to consent to, and participate in, an interview by telephone. The CMHN also had a relationship with the primary carer and/or family and knew what involvement the carer should have in the consent procedure. The researcher was also assured of the continuous relationship that the CMHN would have with the person with dementia and family post interview.

The challenge to interview people with dementia by telephone was carefully monitored and drew on guidance from two key sources: Mishler (1986) and Rosenfield (1997). Mishler (1986) argues that the interview should facilitate a collaborative and participatory role for the respondent with the aim to empower as this promotes a regard for the social and personal context of the respondent. Rosenfield (1997) provided some useful additional insights into how to structure and facilitate the telephone interview using core counselling skills.

Findings: respondents' perceived needs

This section discusses themes that emerged from the data that describe respondents' reactions to their health circumstances. These reactions provide important insights to people's needs and offer direction to the phenomenological focus for the CHMN working with people with dementia. Responses were categorized into the following needs, each of which is discussed within this section:

1   Emotional support and counselling

2   Diagnostic support

3   Threats to autonomy

4   Maintaining the status quo

5   Critical incidents

6   Access to services.

1. Emotional support and counselling

Respondents' reactions to their situation were diverse. The data offered here describe reactions to actual or potential health problems. These reactions include feelings of despair, guilt, and mood changes. Moreover, people with dementia experienced potential or real threats to their self-esteem and identity, as these experiences testify:

> The nurse has helped me to talk about my illness. I can talk to her about how I am managing . . . [silence] . . . I dread it . . . I don't want to be a burden.

> It can be very depressing this Alzheimer's stuff.

> I have even thought of suicide rather than losing my home to pay for my care. The house isn't up for sale because of this. I can't see past this.

> When I was told, I was shattered.

> I don't want to know, I don't want to know. It's a disaster and this is it. I don't want to end up in a place where old women dance around not knowing where they are. I want to die. If this happens I want to die. I will take a pill.

Respondents identified powerful and distressing reactions to their existing or anticipated ill-health. It is these responses that direct the role of the CMHN. The nurse can offer opportunities for people with dementia to talk about these reactions during the therapeutic relationship. This shared empathic understanding can, in itself, offer relief, where the person will feel accepted as someone of worth (Kalkman 1967; Reynolds 2000). It is this understanding of the person that will lead to an accurate assessment of needs by identifying what reactions appear to be harmful and what interventions can be offered to assist with these challenges, a point of focus that is further described in this text. In addition, respecting the person's autonomy is not all about the person making all the decisions independently; it should entail identifying what the person's emotional state is and the effect this is having on their decision-making capacity (Collopy *et al.* 1991, cited in McCormack 2001). This relationship can extend to the carer. The following respondents, who are carers, expressed desires, concerns, difficulties and feelings associated with their caring role:

> I want her to live to the best of her ability and with dignity and with the best possible good care.

> The social services . . . didn't think things were bad enough – and thought he could live well enough on his own and made me feel quite guilty.

> He was quite happy as long as I went along with him. But it was a bit like walking on eggshells.

This commitment to the carer can continue after the person with dementia has moved into a nursing home or has died:

> The nurse understood. She listened to me and the guilt I felt when I was not as understanding as I should have been with my husband [who had recently died] . . . The doctor was going to put me onto the surgery nurse but I asked if I could not have the nurse who had been attending us anyway. So I still see the CMHN.
>
> > (carer)

Some respondents alluded to the emotional and potentially psychotherapeutic support from their CMHNs:

> The CMHN, G, she is a real tonic. We laugh so much . . .
>
> > (person with dementia)

> The CMHN, a friend, we have chats. She has been very good. If I didn't have her I would have gone over the edge a long time ago.
>
> > (carer)

> I open up to her [CMHN]. I talk about our life together.
>
> > (carer)

This potential emotional and counselling role by the CMHN has previously been identified within the literature (Gunstone 1999; Ho 2001). The extended responsibility toward a primary carer/family is acknowledged (Matthew 1990; McCormack 2001). The evolution of the Admiral Nurse project in England (see Soliman's contribution in Chapter 13 of this book, and also Dewing and Traynor's work in Chapter 18) is a response to this extended role offering a specialist service by CMHNs for carers. However, Keady and Adams' (2001) review of the role of the CMHN suggest that meeting the interdependency needs between the person with dementia and carer remains a challenge to the Admiral Nurse profession. To try to understand as completely as possible the needs expressed by both parties requires separate and combined communication between the CMHN, the person with dementia and the carer. Nolan *et al.* (1996) discuss this interdependent state between the caregiver and care recipient who share both congruent and diverse needs. Owing to family members' involvement in the person's care, Adams (2000) supports a family systems approach for the CMHN and suggests that the dyadic nurse–patient relationship is inappropriate. Certainly, it is these tensions that exist between carers and those being cared for that may be a primary focus for the CMHN to unravel. The threat to someone's autonomy when they have dementia, and the paternalistic responses that have been reported to motivate this tension (Wetle 1985; McCormack 2001; Sailors 2001), may well require an intimate understanding of the family dynamics in order to allay anxiety. However, it is argued here that intervention should not be restricted to one treatment modality to the exclusion of another, and that the presenting individual and family reactions should determine the appropriate actions of the CMHN.

2. *Diagnostic support*

For some respondents, recognition of their presenting cognitive difficulties was elusive. The extent of a person's ability and willingness to consider their cognitive difficulties appears to be influenced by the condition, their own outlook and the quality of information and support offered during medical diagnosis; as these extracts suggest:

> I couldn't see there was a problem.

> It has been a gradual progress. I never had a good memory. I have a diary that M [CMHN] gave me – I write everything down.

> No, I don't think I was ever told. Just that it was an impairment – a loss of memory.

> What can you expect at my age? But I am not that stupid [laughs].

This evidence is similar to other recent work exploring the diagnostic experience from the person's perspective (Keady and Nolan 1995; Pratt and Wilkinson 2001). For example, respondents were not given clear or useful information. Yet, Keady and Nolan (1995) reported that people were able to make the best of their situation after receiving a diagnosis. Pratt and Wilkinson (2001) also found individual responses to a diagnosis of dementia included denial, lack of insight, anger, frustration, acceptance, and/or the need to understand more. Furthermore, they reported that respondents from their study generally supported an early diagnosis but with some reservation. Post (1998: 73) advocates 'diagnostic truth telling' claiming that it initiates 'the ethics of autonomy' for someone with Alzheimer's disease. A model for disclosure that is driven by the psychosocial context of the individual (Pratt and Wilkinson 2001) can be a useful framework for supporting a diagnosis. Such a model can be applied through the utility of the nurse–patient relationship, as described by Reynolds (forthcoming a: ch. 19), as follows:

> The nurse, more than the physician must relate positively to the reaction of patients to illness, including the psychological and social changes that illness forces upon the patient.

The varied reactions by people may stem from receiving medical diagnosis, but are not necessarily part of the disease. It is these psychosocial needs, we would suggest, that the CMHN can best respond to using humanistic interpersonal approaches. By developing a therapeutic relationship with the person and the family, information, advice and support can be offered by the CMHN that is useful and meaningful to the client.

The range of reactions among family members/carers was similar to those with the dementia within the present study. Some could not, or were not ready to, accept the diagnosis. Part of the role of the CMHN was to consider the responses of the wider family and offer appropriate nursing interventions. For example, some carers expressed feelings of horror and shock and were unable to accept the diagnosis:

> That was my dad they were talking about . . . But the doctor was throwing too much at us at once . . . I stopped him at that point and told him we have to come to terms with it first, we have to accept that he has dementia. He also gave us some books, but I must admit, the first time I opened it I threw it on the floor.

> I told my sons but they couldn't believe it and were quite indignant thinking that the CMHN was putting ideas into my head. I told the CMHN and she suggested speaking to the son on my phone.

The majority of people with dementia in the study identified the CMHN as a 'key person' to supporting them through their needs in relation to their medical diagnosis:

> I have had a full discussion with R [CMHN] about my memory difficulties . . . there are areas that are working well and some that aren't doing so well now.
>
> (person with dementia)

> I pleaded with the Doctor to find out what was wrong with her. He said it was depression and to make an appointment – but she [the mother] was so dominant and didn't think there was anything wrong with her . . .

> Eventually a new surgery opened and I went along. The CMHN came from the surgery to talk to my husband and me. He came back the next day with Dr L and we were given a diagnosis of frontal lobe dementia of the Alzheimer's type.
>
> (carer)

The efficacy of a specialist dementia team is apparent within the second quotation. The impact of dementia on the wider family/social network is also apparent. Respondents indicated that the timing of information was crucial, as this quote illustrates:

> I didn't get the advice I needed to start with. I couldn't take it in. I like to read and go back to it. The nurse brought me in a book and a smaller book. That was helpful.
>
> (person with dementia)

Broader educational interventions were also part of the CMHN's work:

The course was through the CMHN. It was for six weeks. There are nine carers . . . all ages. We sit and talk. Dementia was explained to us and Dr M came in to talk about dementia.

(carer)

I fell foul of them [CMHNs]. I was supposed to go on a six-week course and meet people like myself and have a cup of tea and a chat. I never went. I didn't fancy it. But the nurse says I am going to the next one. I do think it will be good for me and I should go. I will go on the next one. There is no reason not to.

(person with dementia)

This last quote highlights several important phenomenological issues. First, offering educational courses must be clearly related to the human responses identified during the nurse–client relationship. Secondly, such interventions need to be agreed with the client during the exploitation phase of the relationship (Forchuk 1993: 9). When a person is helped to understand what is happening in respect to a health threat, it can facilitate autonomy. It activates a position of respect and empowerment, by providing the person with the opportunity to consider what present or future changes need to be considered. The following section reports some of the threats that people experienced in relation to autonomy and how these can direct the role of the CMHN.

3. Threats to autonomy

Encouraging a person who has dementia to consider their needs within a legal framework is part of the political and professional agenda within Scotland. The Adults with Incapacity (Scotland) Act 2000 provides a legal infrastructure to be used proactively by people whose autonomy is threatened. An important part of the current CMHN's role within Scotland is to provide legal advice, as these quotes illustrate:

The first professional I had contact with was the CMHN. I was worried about whether I was going to cope further down the line. I wanted to plan ahead.

(person with dementia)

The nurse has been suggesting that I put my money matters in order while I still have control of my affairs and in case of deterioration.

(person with dementia)

The CMHN advised me to seek a Power of Attorney when these things started to happen.

(carer)

However, CMHNs have been criticized for working from their own viewpoint and not collaborating sufficiently with the patient to identify the problem from the client's point of view (Field 1993). It is important that when the CMHN introduces information and advice, it is in response to the client's expressed needs. The CMHN may have a crucial and extended advocacy and/or surrogate role towards their clients as the Act is implemented. Consultation with the person and others is explicit within the Act when legal interventions are required. This would essentially include CMHNs whose primary work should lead to an understanding of their clients' value systems, wishes, expressed responses to health problems and their capacity to self-govern within their daily routines.

However, McFadyen *et al.* (1998) reported CMHNs' tensions between respecting the rights and wishes of people with mental illness and increased legislative powers that could further compromise their relationship. This is an important and growing concern and the impact of the Scottish legal reforms on CMHN's work, and the final picture is still to emerge. However, the principles of the Act and codes of practice (Adults with Incapacity Act (Scotland) 2000) go some way towards ensuring that the interests of the person with dementia are central to any legal intervention. It also provides a legal framework for the CMHN and other professionals to work within and may reduce risk of coercion. However, Adams (2000: 796) argues that social policy alone is insufficient to ensure participation within the decision-making process and argues that it needs 'the subtle and artful use of talk within carer visits'.

Accordingly, CMHNs may influence the autonomy of their clients at both a legal/political and individual level. CMHNs need to observe whether a person's autonomy is being eroded through their relationships with others and/or the environment and take measures to minimize such an outcome. This following quotation illustrates such a tension:

> I look after my own affairs. The nurse did come with me to places – the Post Office. I seemed to have had a wee lapse a wee while ago. It wasn't that I didn't have the money, I just forgot. Now I am managing things myself, once the nurse helped at the Post Office.
>
> (person with dementia)

As discussed earlier, Levi (1999) suggests that a reduction in autonomous status may well equate to a decline in respect by others, including professionals, family and friends. The following example relates a respondent's experiences with family relationships:

> The son-in-law and grandson, they used to torment me and say, 'oh you've forgotten again'. But since the diagnosis they don't do that any more. I miss that. I had a word with my daughter about it. I don't want them to treat me differently.
>
> (person with dementia)

It is argued here that family reactions affecting the person's self-esteem and image are a nursing responsibility. Together, the CMHN and person with dementia can decide what actions to take that are acceptable to the person. Wetle (1985) advises each participant in surrogate decision making to clarify their assumptions, values and ethics. The following respondent aptly illustrates a situation that would have benefited from this advice:

> I called a summit meeting with the CMHN and GP and Social Worker. The Social Worker still maintained Mum should stay at home. My husband and I started to wonder if it was to do with funding . . . The nurse and I put our heads together and Mum went for two weeks' respite . . . Mum said 'I love it here'.
>
> (carer)

The appropriate level of care and the autonomous status of the mother are in dispute here. The collaboration and decision made between the CMHN and family carer may have been appropriate and correct. The CMHN may have identified responses by the mother that warranted this course of action. Chenitz's theory of relocation (Nolan and Grant 1994: 61) might be useful for the nurse to draw on here. Chenitz (1983) offers a framework to help nurses anticipate a person's reactions to respite care and suggests ways in which the experience can be made more positive and beneficial for the person. Clarifying the reasons as to why there was some dissent between the different parties in the previous quote, examining the available options, what the potential health outcomes would be, and how to balance the involvement of the mother in these discussions without undue distress, would go some way towards respecting the mother's personal autonomy.

Adams' (2001) contribution to the work of the CMHN raises some sobering thoughts about the power and control that occurs during discourse between the CMHN and family carer. He identified communication strategies used by CMHNs that exert power through the family carer to the confused relative. Analysis of conversations between hospital nurses and patients reported similar findings (McCormack 2001). McCormack identified nurses working within an ill-defined information framework, which led to professionals controlling decisions rather than examining the values, personal wishes and desires of the patients. To assert such power without due consideration and understanding of the individual needs of each client raises questions about whether the nurse has been equipped with the necessary communication skills to meet the needs of clients. Reynolds (2000: 22) reported considerable evidence to suggest that nurses lack the appropriate interpersonal skills required to establish helping relationships. Reynolds concluded that nurse education was ineffective in preparing nurses to build therapeutic relationships and that such a deficiency in communication skills will perpetuate a failure to assess clients' needs accurately.

Although other disciplines may establish similar types of helping relationship, the phenomenological focus presented by respondents reported here places the CMHN in the position to promote interventions that are protective, but safeguard the person's rights to exercise their personal autonomy as far as possible. The person with dementia must be central to such debates, but how the person is helped to engage in this process, and at what level, requires an understanding of that person's present position. As Kapp (1996: 222) concludes: 'We must ensure that whatever course of action is pursued serves the needs, interests, and, to the greatest extent possible, the preferences of functionally and cognitively dependent elders.' McCormack (2001) suggests that the complexity of the relationships between the health professional, patient and family and organizational constraints prevent a liberal understanding of autonomy and the exercising of individual rights is an untenable option. He advocates a consensus and interconnected decision-making approach where the nurse acts 'as a broker for the consideration of available options' (McCormack 2001: 440).

4. Maintaining the status quo

In our study, maintaining the status quo was a desirable goal for respondents. Some people were able to carry on with their daily living without any, or very little, interference, and the CMHN was seen as a support to this status quo. CMHNs were described as monitors who intervened when necessary:

> E [the CMHN] is wonderful. I think the Doctor asked her to visit when I was diagnosed . . . to monitor the situation.
>
> (person with dementia)

> The CMHN comes in to find out how things are going and sits down and chats with me . . . we have general conversation.
>
> (person with dementia)

> The nurse came in when Dad was dying. Perhaps the CMHN saw Mum (who has dementia) was under the strain and decided to keep visiting her.
>
> (carer)

> He was agitated . . . the CMHN has arranged for medication, which has been a great help.
>
> (carer)

These respondents describe being supported and assessed in an unobtrusive way by CMHNs. This is similar to Gunstone's (1999) single case study that identified assessing, monitoring and socializing as sub-categories of the CMHN's work. Gunstone found that socializing was part of the assessment and relationship process with carers, and that tension, relief and issues of power were being more subtly addressed by CMHNs during social contact with carers. Adams (2001: 102) also identified social interaction as a communication format deployed by CMHNs, which gained access to the 'private and hidden life of the family'. This conversational approach placed carers and the CMHN on a more equal footing.

However, although the friendship and social roles appear to be needed and form a legitimate part of the CMHN's work, this could be misinterpreted at both professional and client level. Being 'too subtle' about the purpose of the relationship, or maintaining a superficial social experience may lead to criticisms, a situation previously observed by Matthew (1990). She reported carers describing health care workers as being fairly ineffectual in dealing with their problems, and some were unaware that it was a CMHN that was visiting. Hence, it is important that CMHNs make their intentions, support, accountability, expertise and genuine concern known to the person with dementia and their family during the progress of the relationship. There is then room to manoeuvre between the different levels of interaction, without confusion.

The monitoring role is considered by respondents from this study and the authors of this chapter as critical to maintaining a person's level of independence within the community. McCormack (2001: 438) suggests that the way dependency is managed can lead to 'feelings of both hope and trust or despair and mistrust'. The basis of the therapeutic relationship is the establishment of trust and acceptance of the person (Kalkman 1967). The effectiveness of 'monitoring' perhaps needs further empirical examination in order that the organization of CMHN work can understand the value of this aspect of its work. It is also a preventative measure against critical incidents occurring.

5. Critical incidents

Crisis intervention was a familiar part of the CMHN role reported by Gunstone (1999). Respondents from the present study reported that access to a community mental health nursing service was inconsistent and some accessed a CMHN only because of a crisis, as these cases illustrate:

> The CMHN was asked to come by the GP because of a crisis situation . . . It turned out to be lupus, we did not realize he was unwell . . . a care package was organized for him through the mental health team.
>
> (carer)

> I looked after him for three years before anyone else was involved . . . but my health deteriorated. A CMHN was sent in after three years by the GP.
>
> (carer)

> It was terrible . . . I asked for an emergency call out from the doctor . . . that's when the doctor got the CMHN to come and visit me.
>
> (carer)

> At Christmas time I had a bath and found I couldn't get out of the bath . . . I must have been in there an hour . . . It was then the CMHN took over.
>
> (person with dementia)

Some critical situations and the adverse effects this can cause for the person and family can be avoided through an unobtrusive monitoring role where relationships are built up with clients. The types of critical situation described were serious and included physical health problems, financial and housing issues, threats of eviction, and essential services (such as the telephone) being discontinued. One recommendation from the study is to encourage the medical profession to open the gateway to information and support, including referral to a CMHN. The implementation of the *Mental Health Framework for Scotland* (1997), which recommends a single point of referral, may help towards this. The implementation strategy for the Adults with Incapacity (Scotland) Act 2000 will also provide further opportunities to raise the awareness of physicians, other health-related and social work disciplines and the public regarding the provisions available to people with potential incapacity. Such awareness raising and increased public knowledge may promote a more proactive public.

6. Access to services

Respondents did offer examples of their needs being met by other providers. Sometimes this was self-investigated. For others, these were accessed through the CMHN during their collaborative work with interrelated services:

> The CMHN gave me some leaflets and put me in touch with the carer's person at Alzheimer's Scotland. I now go to the carers meetings which helps to share things.
>
> (carer)

The CMHN arranged for Mum to go to day care initially which was a great help and gave me a break.

(carer)

I was introduced to a carers group although I didn't want to go – I didn't think I needed it [laughs].

(carer)

The nurses did get him into other day clubs.

(carer)

The relevant issue to draw from this collaboration with other services is whether there was role confusion and/or diffusion between services, and what effects these had on the client's health outcomes. A variety of services will offer advice and information, including the community mental health nursing service; but what specific advice and support needs should the CMHN address differently and more effectively than other professional and community services? In our opinion it should not be to exert professional power and control (see also Adams 2000), but to offer information that is both timely and relevant. Having such an understanding of what a person with dementia and the family can cope with at any one time, and assessing and prioritizing needs, requires skilful application of interpersonal relationship theory (Forchuk 1993).

Further discussion and concluding comments

Respondents (including carers) from this study experienced threats to self-esteem, identity, safety, mood and autonomy. It is identifying and responding to these types of experience that define the CMHN role and phenomenological focus. The CMHN was described by the majority of respondents as a key person to meeting their needs. The CMHN acted as a principal agent that attempted to return or sustain the self-governing skills of both the person with dementia and the wider family that had sometimes been undermined or disrespected by others. The primary work of the CMHN would appear to centre on their ability to gain access to the person's private domain through the development of the therapeutic relationship, and to identify individual reactions that need nursing actions, drawn from a broad range of theories and disciplines. Such actions need to be evaluated as to their efficacy on the well-being and satisfaction of the clients, including the family/primary carer of the person with dementia. This should be applied within an ethical, humanistic and legal framework. However, studies reported within this chapter (for example, McFadyen et al. 1998; Adams 2000; McCormack 2001) have all been critical of the nurse's ability to carry out such a therapeutic role. Reynolds (2000) has also identified low empathy skills in nurses, a core skill for the establishment of the therapeutic relationship (Kagan 1985). Nurse educators should be given every encouragement to provide appropriate learning opportunities that will improve nurses' knowledge of dementia and the starting point for intervention.

These insights into the CMHN role must be considered within the limitations of this non-probability study. However, the data does support similar findings (Matthew 1990; Keady and Nolan 1995; McFadyen *et al.* 1998; Gunstone 1999; Ho 2001; McCormack 2001; Pratt and Wilkinson 2001). Further empirical research is needed to examine the effectiveness of the CMHNs on the health status of people with dementia and their carers. Over a decade ago, Pollock (1989: 193) suggested that CMHNs were expected to 'juggle resources and . . . justify *post hoc* the care that they give'. Yet the need for further evidence about the efficacy of their role is still needed (Keady and Adams 2001). To place a value on community mental health nursing work that promotes the well-being and autonomy of the person and carer would enable planners of nursing services to organize CMHNs that are effective, individual and family orientated. This is even more pressing with the current implementation of the *Mental Health Framework for Scotland* (1997) with its single point of referral, where different disciplines are within a community mental health team. The opportunity for individuals to access support that meets their needs will be largely dependent on the ability of these disciplines to distinguish their own work and collaborate with each other. Hence, within a health system context, Reynolds (2001: 1) directs nursing to identify what human phenomena nurses can 'fix, prevent or ameliorate'. Reynolds argues that it is only then that the separateness and thus interrelation and collaboration between nursing and other disciplines can be addressed in a manner that offers the quality of care and support deserved by its clients. The respondents cited within this chapter go some way to informing us of what their perceived needs are and the value placed on CMHN intervention.

Acknowledgements

Appreciation and thanks to all respondents and carers, all CMHNs, health visitors and managers who supported the study, to Alzheimer Scotland Action on Dementia (especially its Highland staff) and to the Scottish Executive's Research Unit who commissioned the project.

References

Adams, T. (2000) The discursive construction of identity by community psychiatric nurses and family members caring for people with dementia, *Journal of Advanced Nursing*, 32(4): 791–8.

Adams, T. (2001) The conversational and discursive construction of community psychiatric nursing for chronically confused people and their families, *Nursing Inquiry*, 8(2): 98–107.

American Nursing Association (1980) *Nursing: A Social Policy Statement*. Kansas City, MO: American Nursing Association (pamphlet), in H. Peplau (1987) American Nurses Association's social policy statement: Part 1, *Archives of Psychological Nursing*, 1(5): 301–7.

Barker, P. and Reynolds, W. (1994) The proper focus of psychiatric nursing: a critique of Watson's caring ideology, *Journal of Psychosocial Nursing*, 22(5): 17–23.

Chenitz, W.C. (1983) Entry into a nursing home as status passage: a theory to guide nursing practice, *Geriatric Nursing*, March/April: 92–7.

Cicarelli, V.G. (1992) Family caregiving: autonomous and paternalistic decision-making. Newbury Park, CA: Sage.

Collopy, B.J. (1988) Autonomy in long term care: some crucial distinctions, *The Gerontologist*, 28 (Suppl.): 10–17.

Collopy, B.J., Boyle, P. and Jennings, B. (1991) New directions in nursing home ethics, in N. Daniels (ed.) *Duty to Treat or Right to Refuse?* Hastings Centre Report (Special Supplement), 21(2): 1–15.

Dickens, B.M. (1997) Legal aspects of the dementias, *The Lancet*, 349: 948–50.

Field, R. (1993) Patients' and CPN's views of a CPN service, in C. Brooker (ed.) *Community Psychiatric Nursing Research*. London: Chapman & Hall.

Forchuk, C. (1993) *Hildegard E. Peplau: Interpersonal Nursing Theory*. Thousand Oaks, CA: Sage.

Frolik, L.A. (1996) Commentary: Statutory definitions of incapacity – the need for a medical basis, in M. Smyer, K. Schaie and M. Kapp (eds) *Older Adults' Decision-making and the Law*. New York: Springer.

General Nursing Council for Scotland (1962) *Guide to the Syllabus of Subjects for Psychiatric Nurses*. Edinburgh: GNC for Scotland.

Gunstone, S. (1999) Expert practice: the interventions used by a community mental health nurse with carers of dementia sufferers, *Journal of Psychiatric and Mental Health Nursing*, 6: 21–7.

Ho, D. (2001) Role of community mental health nurses for people with dementia, *British Journal of Nursing*, 9(15): 986–91.

Kagan, N. (ed) (1985) *Interpersonal Skills in Nursing. Research and Applications*. London: Croom Helm.

Kalkman, M. (1967) *Psychiatric Nursing*. New York: McGraw-Hill.

Kapp, M. (1996) Alternatives to guardianship: enhanced autonomy for diminished capacity, in M. Smyer, K. Schaie and M. Kapp (eds) *Older Adults' Decision-making and the Law*. New York: Springer.

Keady, J. and Adams, T. (2001) Community mental health nurses in dementia care: their role and future, *Journal of Dementia Care* (Research Focus), March/April: 33–7.

Keady, J. and Nolan, M. (1995) IMMEL: assessing coping responses in the early stages of dementia, *British Journal of Nursing*, 4(6): 309–80.

Levi, B. (1999) *Respecting Patient Autonomy*. Urbana, IL: University of Illinois Press.

Mason, A. and Wilkinson, H. (2001a) *People with Dementia Who Are Users and Non-users of the Legal System in Scotland: A Feasibility Study*, Final Report to the Scottish Executive. Stirling: CSRD.

Mason, A. and Wilkinson, H. (2001b) Don't leave me hanging on the telephone, in Heather Wilkinson (ed.) *The Perspectives of People with Dementia: Research Methods and Motivations*. London: Jessica Kingsley.

Matthew, L. (1990) A role for the CPN in supporting the carer of clients with dementia, in C. Brooker (ed.) *Community Psychiatric Nursing Research*. London: Chapman & Hall.

McCormack, B. (2001) Autonomy and the relationship between nurses and older people, *Ageing and Society*, 21(4): 417–46.

McFadyen, J., Farrington, A. and Piper, J. (1998) Community mental health nursing: the interpretation of roles. *British Journal of Health Care Management*, 4: 1.

Mental Health Framework for Scotland (1997) http://www.show.scot.nhs.uk/publications/mental_health_services/mhs/index.htm (accessed 4 February 2002)

Mishler, E.G. (1986) *Research Interviewing: Context and Narrative*. Cambridge, MA: Harvard University Press.

Nolan, M. and Grant, G. (1994) Mid-range theory building and the nursing theory–practice gap: a respite care case study, in J. Smith (ed.) *Models, Theories and Concepts*. Oxford: Blackwell.

Nolan, M., Grant, G. and Keady, J. (1996) *Understanding Family Care*. Buckingham: Open University Press.

Peplau, H. (1987) American Nurses Association's social policy statement: part 1, *Archives of Psychiatric Nursing*, 1(5): 301–7.

Peplau, H. (1988) Substance and scope of psychiatric nursing. Paper presented at the 3rd National Conference on Psychiatric Nursing, Canada.

Pollock, L. (1989) *Community Psychiatric Nursing: Myth and Reality*. London: Scutari Press.

Post, S.G. (1998) The fear of forgetfulness: a grassroots approach to an ethics of AD. *Journal of Clinical Ethics*, 9(1): 71–80.

Pratt, R. and Wilkinson, H. (2001) *No Diagnosis Has to Be Your Whole Life: The Effect of Being Told the Diagnosis of Dementia from the Perspective of the Person with Dementia*. London: Mental Health Foundation.

Reynolds, W. (2000) *The Measurement and Development of Empathy in Nursing: Developments in Nursing and Health Care 21*. Aldershot: Ashgate Publishing.

Reynolds, W. (2001) The knowledge needed by mental health nurses: implications for the future direction of nursing research/scholarship. Keynote speech delivered at the Pre Nursing Conference, Turku, Finland.

Reynolds, W. (forthcoming a) Developing therapeutic one to one relationships, in P. Barker (ed.) *Psychiatric and Mental Health Nursing: the craft of caring*. London: Arnold.

Reynolds, W. (forthcoming b) Developing empathy within the therapeutic relationship, in P. Barker (ed.) *Psychiatric and Mental Health Nursing: the craft of caring*. London: Arnold.

Rosenfield, R. (1997) *Counselling by Telephone*. London: Sage.

Royal College of Nursing (1970) *Post-certificate Training and Education of Psychiatric Nurses*. London: Royal College of Nursing.

Sabatino, C. (1996) Competency: refining our legal fictions, in M. Smyer, K. Schaie and M. Kapp (eds) *Older Adults' Decision-making and the Law*. New York: Springer.

Sailors, P.R. (2001) Autonomy, benevolence, and alzheimer's disease, *Cambridge Quarterly of Healthcare Ethics*, 10: 184–93.

Wetle, T. (1985) Ethical aspects of decision making for and with the elderly, in M.B. Kapp, H.E. Pies and A.E. Doudera (eds) *Legal and Ethical Aspects of Health Care for the Elderly*. Ann Arbor, MI: Health Administration Press.

Wilkinson, H. (2001) Empowerment and decision making for people with dementia: the use of legal interventions in Scotland, *Aging and Mental Health*, 5(4): 322–8.

Willis, S.L. (1996) Assessing everyday competence in the cognitively challenged elderly, in M. Smyer, K. Schaie and M. Kapp (eds) *Older Adults' Decision-making and the Law*. New York: Springer.

Wilson, H. and Kneisl, C. (1983) *Psychiatric Nursing*, 2nd edn. London: Addison-Wesley.

5

Risk and dementia

Models for community mental health nursing practice

Jill Manthorpe

Introduction

The management of risk is increasingly central to professional practice. Working with people with dementia highlights many current debates about risk and presents a further set of challenges, not only those that seem immediately relevant to practice but also those in respect of law, values and ethics. This chapter sets out a framework for the analysis of risk with a focus on decision making. Whilst the work described is directed to community mental health nurses (CMHNs), it is also germane to the activities of other professionals and the conclusion highlights the increasingly multi-agency and multi-disciplinary nature of risk assessment and risk management.

Risk definitions and concepts

Many texts referring to risk set out the range of definitions that are associated with the term and point to different emphases (for example, Heyman 1998; Parsloe 1999; Alaszewski *et al.* 2000). Within health and welfare services – ranging from areas of work such as probation to child protection and from HIV/AIDS work to smoking and heart disease – professionals are encouraged to identify, manage and reduce risk. In this way, their practice is based upon an equation of risk as harm. In dementia services, such harms are readily illustrated through examples of 'wandering' leading to harm, to dangers in the home and to self-neglect and accidental self-harm.

Such ideas about risk as harm permeate much practice and policy guidance. The risks associated with people with dementia are related more to their perceived vulnerability than to potential harm to others. There are some exceptions to this: 'leaving the gas on', a common fear among practitioners and family carers, presents risks to the broader neighbourhood, but in the main the risks or harms associated with people with dementia relate to the greater likelihood of harm to themselves.

This stands in contrast to perceptions of other groups of service users, particularly adults with mental health problems who are increasingly seen as presenting danger or harm to the public following media reports of their 'dangerousness' and accusations of professional inabilities to contain the risks they present in terms of violence.

These different definitions of risk impact on nursing practice. In a study of nurses' management of risk in the community funded by the English National Board for Nursing, it was found that most nurses interviewed acknowledged risk as an important aspect of their work and accepted that it permeated all aspects of their practice and decision making (Alaszewski *et al.* 2000). Most treated its definition as unproblematic and associated it with negative consequences. However, a substantial minority referred to an element of risk that is so important: the crucial role of chance, probability or likelihood. It is this uncertainty and unpredictability which distinguishes risk from negative outcomes, and, as this chapter argues, CMHNs supporting people with dementia have much to contribute to debates about risk and shifting the balance to accept that harm is not inevitable if certain actions are taken.

In conjunction with this assessment of risk is the professional role in recognizing the positive aspects of risk taking. These can be readily neglected. Risk taking can be an important expression of individuality and is central to notions of adult status (Manthorpe *et al.* 1997). Within dementia care, new conceptualizations of wandering as exercise, for example, offer potential for reframing activities that appear inherently hazardous into actions which may be positive and life enhancing (Alaszewski and Manthorpe 2000).

In the study referred to above (Alaszewski *et al.* 2000), nurses working with older people were often aware of the possibility of negative outcomes – such as falls – but most wanted to balance these against positive aims, such as respect for the older person's autonomy. Many worked in the spirit of the *National Service Framework for Older People* (Department of Health 2001) which has emphasized this idea of risk taking as a sign of independence.

In the next section we explore practice examples, but we conclude this section with a brief discussion of what has been termed the 'risk society'. This helps to explain why handling uncertainty challenges experts and identifies an important link between risk assessment and management and the concepts of trust and confidence. Risk is managed and negotiated in a political and social context (Lupton 1993) as well as with professional or care-giving domains. For many practitioners, risk is part of conversations and processes of decision making: it is less the imparting of information from expert to patient.

Ideas of a risk society (see Giddens 1991; Beck 1992) acknowledge that risk taking is pervasive. A modern, or postmodern society, is increasingly risk aware and places, simultaneously, pressure on experts and professionals to diagnose and contain risks whilst doubting their pre-eminent status in defining and management of these same hazards. In dementia care there are several examples of these competing notions – is risk, say of self-neglect, something that should be defined by objective measurements and assessments? Or, on the other hand, is 'self-neglect' a socially constructed idea which depends on different perspectives? How do we assess whether the risk is greater in supporting a person at home in unhygienic and (to our eyes) unpleasant circumstances compared with the risk of moving from home to a clean but unfamiliar environment? And who is the expert in such a situation?

Shaw and Shaw (2001) have helpfully set out a set of key critical themes around risk which relate to risk perception and its grounding in social psychology, to risk definitions and their philosophical links and to sociological understandings of risk and its cultural influences. Briefly, these centre around:

- lay versus expert knowledge of risk;
- the social dimensions of risk;
- risk and its political context;
- trust in and the credibility of experts;
- the regulation of risk;
- risk within ethical systems such as human rights and accountability.

In the next section we explore the first of these: lay and expert knowledge of risk in dementia.

Living with risk: lay and expert views

Exploration of risk in relation to dementia has long been seen as related to both carers and the person with dementia (Jefferys and Jennings 1982). Carers may be seen as facing threats or risks to their well-being by continuing to care when alternatives would be in their best interests. For example, carers may risk future benefits, such as employment chances or income, by choosing to care. Conceptualization of caring as a burden rather than the work of experts in the context of a relationship (Brown *et al.* 2001) represents this rather simplistic way of seeing caring as solely linked to outcome and perceiving outcomes negatively. Recent work on care giving has challenged such approaches by listening to carers' accounts of the risks of caring and how they manage or cope with possible harms (Clarke 2000). Such work suggests that a carer builds on their individual knowledge of a particular person with dementia to frame particular risks (Clarke 2000). And, as Adams (2001) has observed, carers can influence how risks are constructed. In their conversations with CMHNs, for example, he found some carers were able to avoid attempts by nurses to classify behaviours of their family members as hazardous.

Lay perceptions of risk in dementia care remain dominated by family members' accounts, although the voices of people with dementia are emerging (see Wilkinson 2002). Clarke's (2000) study, for example, illustrated how some carers made judgements about possible dangers in light of a person's past activities and preferences:

> The benefits of allowing the person with dementia to continue their accustomed activities often outweighed the perceived risks, for example Ms Y continued to allow her father to wander out of the house because she perceived the risks of

containment (particularly by pharmaceutical measures) to be more significant for him than the risk of an accident while out.

(p. 87)

Like carers, practitioners sought to see how risk related to a person's past wishes or drew implications from what was known about their way of life. Such a perspective links to the interest in biographical work, not simply as a means of communicating with people with dementia, but as a process of finding out what the person valued previously or the choice of activities they made. Notions of character or the 'type of person' are often voiced in services to explain elements of practice. Whilst these can be sensitive and case specific, they may also be overdeterministic and not relate to change or development.

Clarke (1999) also argued that three factors mean that services often fail to deliver person-centred care and employed risk as a means of illustrating these systems difficulties. Firstly, she observed that many practitioners or services only encounter either the person with dementia, or the family member. In day care, for example, staff may not know the carer and thus have little idea of the relationship and its dynamics. In such contexts, similar to work with people with learning disabilities, it can be argued, it is possible to develop one-sided views of risk and to portray families as risk averse. They may be characterized as overprotective and cautious. Work within learning disabilities has much to offer in exploring carers' perspectives on risk (see, for example, Heyman *et al.* 1998 and Alaszewski *et al.* 2000).

Secondly, Clarke (1999: 299) argued that practitioners 'judge risk-taking in relation to their knowledge of the illness', and consequently view the person with dementia as having incapacity and inability to make judgements. They see people with dementia as unable to act rationally. Risk is associated with calculation and logic, with weighing up likelihood and recognizing consequences as discussed earlier. Dementia, by definition, is seen as a condition affecting all such rational assessment and management processes. This puts professionals in the position of feeling they must compensate for such deficits, particularly if they have the responsibility to 'care for' vulnerable people.

Thirdly, Clarke (1999) pointed to the difficulty of managing risk because practitioners work around 'aggregated' rather than individualized knowledge. This, however, can be seen as an advantage. Practitioners can make more realistic assessments of likelihood by thinking around the chances of events occurring. Risks are often judged more likely if the consequence envisaged is vivid and imaginable (Pigeon *et al.* 1992). In dementia care, this may help to explain the fears around gas explosion, for example, or catastrophe. Risks that have low probability but high consequence may be feared out of proportion. However, as Clarke (1999) observed, family carers possess knowledge of the person with dementia and share a history with them. This makes it difficult if professionals assess risk in a vacuum. Their knowledge in relation to the likelihood of a harmful, even fatal, consequence may not concur with others' emphasis on the consequence or outcome itself.

Such different interpretations of risk may relate to practitioners' difficulties in providing support to family carers. Working within organizations that manage risks by placing great store on professional accountability means that nurses and social workers can feel under pressure if 'things go wrong'. They are also perceived to be at some distance from the practical experiences of caring, as illustrated by Pickard and Glendinning's (2001) study of CMHNs' perceptions of older carers. In this study, CMHNs were the professional group most likely to be supporting family carers, but this support centred around giving advice, referral, education and counselling. Carers themselves would have preferred more assistance in practical support, such as help with personal or health care activities. It is possible that this would give carers greater confidence in CMHNs' 'knowledge' and that CMHNs might be able to instil trust in their ability to link generalized expertise to specific individuals and their circumstances.

Risk policy at agency level: proactive and reactive

It was noted above that many community nurses (and other welfare professions) experience work as a process of risk management which leaves them vulnerable to criticism and censure. For those working within mental health services, public and media attention to homicide has contributed to a climate of concern and the NHS has responded at various levels to the criticisms of professional practice – notably through the creation of a clinical governance framework (NHS Executive 1999). Within organizations, another key response has been the creation of risk policies and these serve to link practice and organizational imperatives. Whilst some documents name 'risk' as the subject of their concern, other documents can be usefully analysed as 'risk policies'. These help to identify the messages that are given to professionals about risk management.

In this section, two documents are used to consider risk at agency level. The first is a government document which has the status of policy: *No Secrets: Guidance on Developing and Implementing Multi-agency Policies and Procedures to Protect Vulnerable Adults from Abuse* (Department of Health 2000) sets out a framework for the protection of vulnerable adults, starting with the prevention of abuse but developing guidance on the systems that need to be in place to respond to abuse if it is suspected. Whilst the document focuses on vulnerable adults, people with dementia are widely accepted as falling within such a category. Indeed, public and professional concerns about the difficulties of protecting people with dementia lie behind some of the moves to develop policy and response in this area.

However, looking at *No Secrets* through a 'risk lens' helps to identify some of the challenges in balancing calls for protection with equally weighty calls for empowerment. People with dementia, if they are portrayed as vulnerable – with mental disability, unable to care for themselves or protect themselves (to draw down some of *No Secrets*' definition of vulnerability, Department of Health 2000: 9) – are in danger of being seen as needing supervision or surveillance. Anxieties become heightened that they are 'at risk' within community and institutional settings. Policy and professional practices may overemphasize the need for protection 'in case' there is an abuser. This is not to deny that safeguards have been woefully inadequate in respect of recruitment and employment and in relation to professional practice and research. Standards of care for people with dementia have frequently been criticized as appalling (MacDonald and Dening 2002).

However, close analysis of some of the limited research attempting to assess the relationship between risk of abuse and the heightened risks posed to abuse of people with dementia (Manthorpe *et al.* 1997) suggests that risk needs to be considered more widely. Risk factors among carers seem to be important rather than dementia *per se.* Homer and Gilleard (1990), for example, propose that it is not the degree of impairment or diagnosis of impairment that is significant, but carers' responses and their circumstances. There is no straightforward relationship between dementia and abuse: perceptions, such as stress, and interactions, such as reciprocal violence or aggression between carer and person with dementia, are important.

Thus the 'vulnerability' of the person with dementia needs to be considered in light of a set of risks. It may not be the dementia that by itself enhances the likelihood of the risk of abuse. Carers can present risks – both those related to their own responses to stress and those that are enhanced by difficult or unsupported circumstances. *No Secrets* offers a set of guidelines to help reduce the likelihood of further harm, but it has less to say on the prevention of abuse, particularly in respect of care environments which are of low quality.

Analysis of risk policies, and *No Secrets* can be included within this category, illustrates that one of the roles of welfare agencies is to manage risk. Not all agencies have explicit risk policies (Alaszewski and Manthorpe 1998), and in many areas of work, policies are not called on in response to difficulties in professional decision making. However, dementia is one 'label' which generally connotes vulnerability or enhances propensity to harm. Policies such as local implementation documents relating to *No Secrets* can learn lessons from risk studies. Professionals involved in implementation can broaden the participation circle – by seeking the involvement of their colleagues as well as managers and through the involvement of those classed as vulnerable people. In respect of people with dementia, we have few examples of good practice in their involvement in thinking around systems of protection and how to reduce the risk of abuse. Work from Pritchard (2000), however, suggests the potential of talking to people with dementia about their experiences of abuse and how practitioners can recognize and respond to their needs, especially in the aftermath.

The second type of document considered offers, with benefit of hindsight, a perspective on risk in respect of a single case example. Inquiries into homicide have provided a rich source of evidence about the realities of mental health practice, with CMHNs often key informants about the history, lives and services provided for people experiencing mental health care or treatment. Such inquiries have attracted wide media coverage, often sensational, and have fuelled anxiety about the risks presented by users of psychiatric services (see Stanley and Manthorpe 2001). Such risks are generally seen as synonymous with danger.

A small number of inquiries in the 1990s relate to people with dementia. One of the most widely circulated, the Beech House Inquiry (Camden and Islington Community Health Services NHS Trust 1996), focuses on abuse and injury of patients living in accommodation on a hospital site. This has much to say about indicators of risk, in respect of the patients but also in respect of people who harm others, as well as identifying the particular risks associated with care in institutions, such as isolation, routine, intimidation and secrecy.

However, other inquiries focus on individual 'cases', and one of these has particular relevance to those working in dementia services. The report of the committee of inquiry into the death of William Taylor (Barlow 1996) reports on the care and treatment offered to his son, Keith Taylor (KT), who killed his father at the family home in 1995. Willian Taylor was reported in the inquiry as suffering from multi-infarct dementia. The unexpected death of his mother meant that Keith Taylor took on the main caring role for his father. The inquiry notes that this was particularly stressful for him and that this contributed to his mental health problems, although he had previously been somewhat isolated.

The inquiry report recommended increased use of risk assessment and greater multi-disciplinary working. These conclusions concur with almost all other inquiries' findings. In this particular case, the inquiry (p. 66) was critical of the 'limited attention to the life of the patient [KT] outside hospital and in particular to his own role as a carer' (Keith Taylor had three admissions to psychiatric care). It also identified 'lack of liaison between the mental health teams looking after Keith and William Taylor' as a contributory factor. Problems were also highlighted in respect of confidentiality and information sharing.

This inquiry provides evidence of the ways in which risks are assessed and managed. It sets out the complex systems operating between health and social services and between hospital and community provision. Dementia is often situated in this 'grey area'. The findings suggest the possible risks of separating dementia from other mental health services. They also raise the potential for community mental health nursing practice to be family-focused as well as providing support for people with dementia. As a 'risk' document, the inquiry report is also helpful in conveying the learning from investigation and reflection on practice. Mental health services will never, and should not create the impression that they can, eliminate tragedies. Knowledge is limited and uncertainty endemic. A risk lens is particularly helpful in guarding against ideas that there is a safe system, institution or person.

Working together

Littlechild and Blakeney (1996) suggest that issues of risk in respect of people with dementia fix upon whether they are capable or have insight. They point to the equal importance of examining processes of risk assessment and the ways in which these are conducted and experienced. How can the experience of assessment empower rather than disempower? Must it reinforce a lack of skill or value? Are inabilities and weaknesses solely being assessed? They argue that the process needs to reflect the needs of the person with dementia and suggest that this may mean information collecting takes more time, that alternative ways of communication should be tried and that the practitioner assessing risk should take care to be a familiar face to the person with dementia. In addition they propose that a multi-disciplinary team approach is valuable.

What might such an approach contribute? It may, of course, take further time and complicate matters. However, there is evidence that a range of perspectives can inform decision making in respect of risk (Alaszewski *et al.* 1998a). This can provide fresh perspectives and bring into the risk equation new knowledge and resources. Some practitioners and not others may know about the increasing applicability of home-based technology to dementia care, for example. Technology looks set to be of enormous assistance in reducing much-feared risks about fire or accident (see Woolham and Frisby 2002) and, whilst it will never be a 'safe' or 'risk-free' solution, assistive technology has great potential as a tool to decrease the likelihood of harm and to minimize negative consequences.

In our study of risk in community practice (Alaszewski *et al.* 1998b) we noted that CMHNs worked within teams and this impacted upon their assessment and management of risk. We observed, as many have done, that teamwork can be interpreted broadly (Payne 2000). In most of the teams we studied, nurses and the other professional team members worked relatively autonomously. Each had a 'case load' and most interactions were on a one-to-one level, with home visits an important element of the role. Many such visits (and see Adams 2001 for some helpful direct reporting of conversations with family carers) centred around monitoring. Where risks were identified, CMHNs made decisions based on immediate and past assessments. In the case of one client, for example, a number of risks were known to the CMHN and team, including the person's habit of leaving the front door open, burning pans and going out for walks on her own. However, a burglary or distraction theft had apparently occurred prior to one visit and the CMHN took immediate action to inform home care staff to follow up with further contact and to suggest a possible 'holiday' in respite care to relieve the person's distress.

Whilst working in a team, the CMHN had considerable autonomy. We observed that a framework for joint decision making did exist, in this case a weekly team meeting and review meetings around individual clients or specific circumstances (care management reviews, for example). These were often multi-disciplinary and nurses played a key role. Their contact with individual clients meant they were often prime informants and they often implemented team recommendations, such as further monitoring or a change in services. In one team, we observed that nurses chaired the review meetings, setting the agendas. However, in another team, meetings were led and business managed by the consultant.

Such variability in teamwork approaches to risk raises again the importance of decision making. Some have argued that there is evidence that different professions stress certain matters more than others in their assessment of risk. The Social Services Inspectorate (1997: 4), for example, noted that health professionals sometimes considered social services staff 'as tending to focus too strongly on the civil liberties of service users'. Such a view may affect willingness to work in teams or to approach decision making jointly. Writing from a social work perspective, Stevenson (1999: 203) has acknowledged that 'talk of choice and autonomy' may 'mask an unwillingness to devote attention and resources' to the protection of older people.

Working together in risk assessment and management can equally become caught up in an elusive search for the 'ideal type' risk assessment instrument. Those working with mental health services for people under retirement age (often termed adult services) have been subject to various initiatives to devise all-embracing risk assessment tools in a search for comprehensiveness and certainty. At their worst, these can be 'tick box' forms and operate defensively. At their best, they may have something of use to dementia services particularly when including opportunities for service users and for carers to offer their own perspectives on what they see as risks and their preferred approaches. Whilst not designed for dementia care, the risk assessment learning materials devised by the University of Manchester (1996: 56) make brief mentions of assessment in respect of people with dementia in the context of self-neglect. They recommend broad discussion of concerns and also suggest the value of persevering to establish a relationship and support of the person with dementia. Such risk assessment and management techniques were highly evident in our study of community nurses' practice, although rarely formalized by risk assessment tools (Alaszewski *et al.* 2000).

Risk and rationality

Stevenson (1999: 203) noted the general tendency that 'the more capable old people are mentally, the less likely it is that others will interfere in the choices which they make'. Dementia adds a new element to the general search for balance between empowerment and protection, between choice and the limits of an ageist, disabling and sexist society which can compromise the abilities of older people to live inter-dependently and with autonomy. There is not the space here to discuss how many of the hazards encountered by older people are not distributed equally. The chances of accidents occurring are known, for example, to be unevenly distributed, with limited access to resources and lack of safe environments playing key roles in increasing the likelihood of childhood accidents (Roberts *et al.* 1993). The impact of social class gradient for accidents in the UK needs to be related to the life course more widely.

Such approaches possibly play down the impact of a dementia. But mental confusion plays an important role in risk assessment. Risk analysis assumes a rationality, and 'incapacity' can be assumed to negate this ability. However, individuals' (whether they are lay or expert) concepts of risk are complex and exist in a context where risk is often perceived negatively and partially. Dementia care provides many such illustrations with 'wandering' perhaps the most pertinent as it is currently being reframed from a negative and hazardous activity to one which provides exercise and possibly enjoyment.

Conclusion

In this chapter risk has been presented as a multi-faceted concept and it is one which is increasingly being used interchangeably with that of need. There are a variety of competing perspectives around both terms. More rigour in respect of what is meant by both concepts might help practitioners to achieve greater clarity in decision making, resource allocation and risk management. Risk assessment and management are processes involving multiple conversations, and CMHNs need to ensure that these conversations include people with dementia and their carers. In some cases, CMHNs may need to use their knowledge of, and relationship with, a service user with dementia to advocate on their behalf in respect of their rights to take risks and to be protected from harm. This activity can be considered as an essential element of person-centred practice since well-being is a helpful outcome of risk decision making.

References

Adams, T. (2001) The social construction of risk by community psychiatric nurses and family carers for people with dementia, *Health, Risk and Society*, 3(3): 307–20.

Alaszewski, A. and Manthorpe, J. (1998) Welfare agencies and risk: the missing link?, *Health and Social Care in the Community*, 6(1): 4–15.

Alaszewski, H. and Manthorpe, J. (2000) Finding the balance: older people, nurses and risk, *Education and Ageing*, 15(2): 195–209.

Alaszewski, A., Harrison, L. and Manthorpe, J. (eds) (1998a) *Risk, Health and Welfare*. Buckingham: Open University Press.

Alaszewski, A., Alaszewski, H., Ayer, S. and Manthorpe, J. (1998b) *Assessing and Managing Risk in Nursing Education and Practice: Supporting Vulnerable People in the Community*. London: English National Board for Nursing, Midwifery and Health Visiting.

Alaszewski, A., Alaszewski, H., Ayer, S. and Manthorpe, J. (2000) *Managing Risk in Community Practice: Nursing, Risk and Decision-making*. London: Ballière Tindall.

Barlow, R. (Chair) (1996) *Caring for the Carer: Report of the Committee of Inquiry to Tees Health Authority*. Middlesbrough: Tees Health Authority.

Beck, U. (1992) *Risk Society*. London: Sage.

Brown, J., Nolan, M. and Davies, S. (2001) Who's the expert? Redefining lay and professional relationships, in M. Nolan, S. Davies and G. Grant (eds) *Working with Older People and their Families: Key Issues in Policy and Practice*. Buckingham: Open University Press.

Camden and Islington Community Health Services NHS Trust (1996) *Beech House Inquiry*. London: Camden and Islington NHS Trust.

Clarke, C.L. (1999) Professional practice with people with dementia and their carers: help or hindrance?, in T. Adams and C.L. Clarke (eds) *Dementia Care: Developing Partnerships in Practice*. London: Ballière Tindall.

Clarke, C.L. (2000) Risk: constructing care and care environments in dementia, *Health, Risk and Society*, 2(1): 83–94.

Department of Health (2000) *No Secrets: Guidance on Developing and Implementing Multi-agency Policies and Procedures to Protect Vulnerable Adults from Abuse*. London: Department of Health.

Department of Health (2001) *National Service Framework for Older People*. London: The Stationery Office.

Giddens, A. (1991) *Modernity and Self Identity*. Cambridge: Polity Press.

Heyman, B. (ed.) (1998) *Risk, Health and Health Care*. London: Arnold.

Heyman, B., Huckle, S. and Handyside, E. (1998) Freedom of the locality for people with learning difficulties, in B. Heyman (ed.) *Risk, Health and Health Care*. London: Arnold.

Jefferys, P. and Jennings, R. (1982) Risk and mental disorder, in C.P. Brearley (ed.) *Risk and Ageing*. London: Routledge & Kegan Paul.

Homer, A. and Gilleard, C. (1990) Abuse of elderly people by their carers, *British Medical Journal*, 301: 1359–62.

Littlechild, R. and Blakeney, J. (1996) Risk and older people, in H. Kemshall and J. Pritchard (eds) *Good Practice in Risk Assessment and Risk Management*. London: Jessica Kingsley.

Lupton, D. (1993) Risk as moral danger: the social and political functions of risk discourse in public health, *International Journal of Mental Health*, 23: 425–34.

MacDonald, A and Dening, T. (2002) Dementia is being avoided in NHS and social care, *British Medical Journal*, 324: 548.

Manthorpe, J., Walsh, M., Alaszewski, A. and Harrison, L. (1997) Issues of risk, practice and welfare in learning disability services, *Disability and Society*, 12: 69–82.

NHS Executive (1999) *Clinical Governance: Quality in the New NHS*. London: Department of Health.

Parsloe, P. (ed.) (1999) *Risk Assessment in Social Care and Social Work*. London: Jessica Kingsley.

Payne, M. (2000) *Teamwork in Multiprofessional Care*. London, Macmillan.

Pickard, S. and Glendinning, C. (2001) Caring for a relative with dementia: the perceptions of carers and CPNs, *Quality in Ageing*, 2(4): 3–11.

Pigeon, N., Hood, C., Jones, D., Turner, B. and Gibson, R. (1992) Risk perception, in The Royal Society (ed.) *Risk Analysis, Perception and Management: Report of a Royal Society Study Group*. London: The Royal Society.

Pritchard, J. (2000) *The Needs of Older Women: Services for Victims of Elder Abuse and Other Abuse*. Bristol: Policy Press.

Roberts, H., Smith, S. and Bryce, C. (1993) Prevention is better . . ., *Sociology of Health and Illness*, 15: 447–63.

Shaw, A. and Shaw, I. (2001) Risk research in a risk society, *Research Policy and Planning*, 19(1): 3–16.

Social Services Inspectorate (1997) *At Home with Dementia: Inspection of Services for Older People with Dementia in the Community*. London: Social Services Inspectorate/Department of Health.

Stanley, N. and Manthorpe, J. (2001) Reading mental health inquiries, *Journal of Social Work*, 1: 77–99.

Stevenson, O. (1999) Old people at risk, in P. Parsloe (ed.) *Risk Assessment in Social Care and Social Work*. London: Jessica Kingsley.

University of Manchester (1996) *Learning Materials on Mental Health: Risk Assessment*. Manchester: University of Manchester/Department of Health.

Wilkinson, H. (ed.) (2002) *The Perspectives of People with Dementia*. London: Jessica Kingsley.

Woolham, J. and Frisby, B. (2002) Building a local infrastructure that supports the use of assistive technology in the care of people with dementia, *Research, Policy and Planning*, 20(1): 11–24.

PART TWO

Dementia care nursing in the community

Assessment and practice approaches

6

Assessment and therapeutic approaches for community mental health nursing dementia care practice

An overview

Linda Miller

Introduction

The number of community mental health nurses (CMHNs) has grown since the mid-1980s and their roles are many and diverse (Barr *et al*. 2001). There has been much discussion on issues such as whether CMHNs should specialize, whether they should generalize, and whether specialist services to people with dementia should be located within community mental health teams (Buck and Smith 1998). There is now a uniform approach to a range of specialist community mental health nursing services, including those relating to children and adolescents, people who misuse substances and forensic services. However, the role of CMHNs working with people with dementia is less well defined and there is a debate about whether dementia should be included as constituting a severe and enduring mental illness (Keady and Adams 2001).

This lack of definition is identified by Keady and Adams (2001) in a review of the literature relating to the role of CMHNs for people with dementia. They argue that the literature comprises 'a number of descriptive accounts about individual or small sample practice, but little in the way of controlled evaluations of such practice or measures of clinical practice' (p. 35). It is not their intention to undervalue any existing 'exciting and innovative' work, but rather to highlight the importance of CMHNs when reviewing past and present practice and, most of all, defining their own distinctive contribution within the context of future mental health care. In addition, Keady and Adams identify the range of skills and competencies that CMHNs use within their practice. Ho (2000) further argues that whilst the role of CMHNs working with people who have dementia has developed and expanded over time, skilled counselling, advising and supporting relatives has remained a constant feature of their work. Other authors make similar observations but set these areas of practice within the context of individual preference or perspective for a specific therapeutic approach (Adams 1996a).

A common theme within the literature is that many of the skills employed by CMHNs are those essential to both the assessment process and any planned intervention or therapeutic approach. The CMHN has an important and significant role to play in the initial and ongoing assessment of people with dementia and their family carers (Audit Commission 2000; Department of Health 2001). The why, where, what and how of assessment depends on where the referral comes from, and the extent to which the dementia has progressed. The effectiveness of the assessment will depend upon the abilities, skills and knowledge of the CMHN.

The aim of this chapter is to explore the role of the CMHN working with people who have dementia and their carers in the context of existing service provision, particularly in terms of assessment and the implementation of therapeutic approaches. Underpinning the chapter is the idea of partnership. This means that CMHNs do not just work with people who have dementia or their carers, but rather work in partnership with people who have dementia and their family carers (Adams 1998, in press). As such, their work is underpinned by a family-orientated approach to dementia care. As was noted in Chapter 1, a family orientation that includes not only the person with dementia but also the rest of the family has been a common feature of community mental health nursing practice from its beginnings (Barker and Black 1971). Indeed, this chapter argues that there are three agencies involved in the provision of dementia care: the person with dementia; one or more family carers; and service agencies themselves, in this case, the CMHN. Moreover, an extended understanding of partnership recognizes that it is not only people with dementia and their carers that have needs: CMHNs too have needs which must be recognized. It is quite legitimate for CMHNs to share the pain of having dementia, and this raises the question of the need for the provision of clinical supervision within community mental health nursing practice, an area that is explained further in Chapter 16.

The CMHN's role in assessment

Whatever therapeutic approach the CMHN chooses to employ, the approach or intervention will only be as good as the assessment process it follows. A thorough and appropriate assessment will provide a firm basis upon which a care plan may be developed or intervention delivered. Assessment can be a complex and difficult process and can create great anxiety for the person being assessed and their family carers. Authors such as McWalter *et al.* (1994), Holden (1995) and Knight (1996) point out that assessment should continue throughout the whole involvement of the CMHN with the 'case'. Indeed, this way of working was identified by Adams (1996a) in a study of CMHNs working with people who have dementia and their carers. Moreover, it is argued that people undertaking assessments should understand the purpose of the assessment. It is further argued that the importance of an holistic approach to assessment that takes full account of a mix of biomedical, psychological and social issues relating to people with dementia and their carers, should be stressed (Holden 1995; Knight 1996). It is for that reason that the success of community mental health nursing assessment is dependent on their knowledge of a range of underpinning disciplines relating to the biological, psychological and social sciences (Holden 1995; Pritchard and Dewing 2000).

Burns *et al.* (1999) provide a review of 150 assessment scales. These scales include those that assess a person's memory function, global functioning in dementia, deterioration in dementia, and behavioural disturbances in dementia. They do warn, however, that the book should be used as a map rather than a guide, and stress that the choice of a particular scale will depend on the question being asked. Similarly, McWalter *et al.* (1994: 214) outline a number of standardized assessment tools that they describe as 'widely employed among those working with dementia . . . [which] generally attempt to quantify the person's difficulties along some dimension'. Among these tools are two that are familiar to many practitioners working with older people with mental health problems: the Mini-Mental State Examination (MMSE) (Folstein *et al.* 1975), and the Clifton Assessment Procedure for the Elderly (CAPE) (Pattie and Gilleard 1979). The MMSE assesses people's intellectual and cognitive functioning, whereas the CAPE assesses behaviour and dependency ratings as well as intellectual functioning. The Mayo Clinic Rochester (2001) suggests that whilst the evaluation of mental status is essential, it is important to remember that scales such as the MMSE are not without their problems. They identify the 'lack of sensitivity to mild cognitive impairment, and its failure to discriminate between normal subjects and those with mild AD [Alzheimer's disease]'. They also add that 'it is important to recognise that dementia can still be present despite a normal score on cognitive assessment'.

The focus of such assessment scales is on the difficulties a person has, and they tend to overlook any strengths or attributes that remain. Focusing on problems or difficulties is, Watkins (2001) suggests, disempowering and detrimental to the individual's sense of 'self esteem and hopefulness'. In terms of the work of Kitwood (1997) on malignant social psychology, the attention to assessing what the person with dementia cannot do may have an adverse affect on their sense of self and personhood. As Cheston and Bender (2000: 204) argue: 'Assessment procedures need to be guided by a philosophy of care that places the emotional and social needs of the sufferer at the forefront of clinical work.' However, the limitations of assessment tools do not undermine their usefulness as a measure of cognitive ability, but rather indicate that they should be used cautiously and not in isolation.

There is, therefore, a need to develop a comprehensive picture of the person with dementia, to gain a sense of who they are, the life events that have shaped them and 'what makes them tick'. The importance of applying a biographical approach to the assessment process is well documented and is an underlying idea within the approach of Kitwood (1997) to dementia care. Knowing something about the uniqueness of a person's life story makes it easier for CMHNs to develop a successful therapeutic relationship that does not simply focus on either the limitations of the person with dementia or their carers. As Bond (2001: 48) notes:

> An understanding of dementia has to be located within a framework which takes account of the life histories of people and their informal caregivers, their material circumstances, the meaning dementia has for the individuals and the struggle they experience to be included as citizens of their societies.

Watkins (2001: 45), however, expresses a word of caution with respect to building a picture of people's private, personal world and argues that '[to] think that through an assessment process, we would come to "know" a person in all their complexity would be disrespectful arrogance'. People who think they know others well cannot mind making subjective value judgements, something that is inappropriate to the assessment process.

CMHNs may at times find themselves in a 'cleft stick' when trying to balance the needs of the person with dementia with those of the carer. This can be difficult because, as Keady and Nolan (1994) point out, not all family relationships are positive. However, in many cases the carer is often the one who best knows and understands the subtle personality traits of the person with dementia. Carers often experience a sense of loss similar to that of the person with dementia themselves, and as a consequence will have important needs to be met. Keady and Nolan (1994) and McWalter *et al.* (1994) highlight the lack of appropriate assessment tools that focus on assessment of needs either for the person with dementia or their carers and have developed assessment of need frameworks that are worthwhile of exploration by CMHNs. Keady and Nolan (1994) developed the carer-led assessment process (CLASP) which they suggest is 'very useful in the preliminary and on-going assessment of individuals with dementia who live on their own in the community' (p. 106). McWalter *et al.* (1994) developed the care needs assessment pack for dementia (CarenapD) that is described as focusing on unmet needs rather than on their eligibility for services. Both CLASP and CarenapD provide an assessment framework for the collection of information of need that is not readily available through the use of many of the assessment tools previously referred to.

It is, however, important to note that neither Keady and Nolan (1994) nor McWalter *et al.* (1994) view these frameworks as a panacea for assessment but rather as a means of complementing and supporting other assessment tools. Stanley and Cantley (2000: 113) comment on the diversity of assessment tools and argue that 'different levels of assessment should be interdependent and inform each other'. However, they note that assessments, despite their obvious interrelationship, are often 'conducted in isolation one from the other'. This often means that people with dementia and their carers are subjected to a battery of assessment processes, carried out by 'strangers' in unfamiliar environments which are anxiety provoking and confusing, requiring the repetitive recounting of personal information. Holden (1995: 27) comments that by being subjected to a battery of tests which are often 'impersonal, usually irrelevant, stressful and an invasion of dignity and privacy', the person being assessed may be made fearful that they may be shamed by their inability to respond accurately to questions or to complete particular tasks appropriately. The CMHN can be pivotal in terms of informing and supporting the person with dementia and their carer(s) through assessment processes. However, assessment that puts diagnosis first and the person second can result in the person with dementia experiencing a reduced sense of self and the relationship between themselves and the CMHN becoming non-therapeutic and simply a means to an end (Cheston and Bender 2000).

CMHNs typically visit people with dementia and their carers in their own homes. As Adams (in press) has noted, this places CMHNs in a powerful position and provides them with the ability to exert surveillance over not only the person with dementia but also their relatives. In addition, the presence of the CMHN in the home allows the CMHN to have more control over what is happening. This provides the CMHN with the ideal opportunity to develop a relationship that is therapeutic rather than purely functional. As I have already noted, a person-centred approach to assessment is essential to establishing a relationship from which a foundation for therapeutic interventions or approaches can be developed. However, it is important to consider that it is not sufficient simply to understand the importance of developing a therapeutic relationship. Having the skills and abilities as described by Keady and Adams (2001) and Pritchard and Dewing (2000) is also essential to moving beyond the initial stage of the relationship. The CMHN who is both knowledgeable and skilled can work in partnership with people with dementia and their informal carers to develop therapeutic approaches based on effective initial and ongoing assessment of their needs.

Therapeutic approaches

Traditionally, the role of the CMHN working with people who have dementia has focused on monitoring the mental state, supporting the carer, and liaising with other organizations to provide services in the community until such time as referral to continuing care was necessary (Adams 1996b). Supporting the carer was understandably seen as the priority, as services were dependent upon the ability (and willingness) of carers to provide care to the person with dementia within the home (Adams 1996b).

Working 'therapeutically' with clients in terms of psychosocial interventions, family therapy or counselling approaches is often seen as the domain of CMHNs working in other specialities, such as child and adolescent psychiatry and with people who have addictive behaviour. Therapeutic approaches such as reality orientation, reminiscence therapy, validation therapy and snoezelen have been implemented for a number of years within routine inpatient and day care settings but have not been incorporated within community mental health nursing practice. However, the work of Tom Kitwood has greatly influenced the way in which professionals think about the care of people with dementia within both community and hospital settings. His focus on person-centred care and the need to change the old, institutionalized nature of care has stimulated many CMHNs to reflect upon their own practice and has encouraged a more creative response to, and evaluation of, therapeutic approaches (see Adams 1996b; Cheston 1998; Cheston and Bender 2000).

Kitwood (1997) argued that any intervention or therapeutic approach should focus on the individuality of the person with dementia, not the diagnosis of dementia, and give recognition to the influences that their past history may have on their response to the lived experience of dementia. There is a need therefore to have as complete a picture as possible of the person in respect of their:

- past and present functioning;
- hopes and dreams;

- desires, ambitions and frustrations;
- relationships;
- education and work;
- losses;
- coping strategies.

Launching into a therapeutic approach or intervention before obtaining as complete a picture as possible can jeopardize the therapeutic process. Indeed, the gathering of such information can be part of the therapeutic process allowing for the development of a relationship of mutual trust. Using information gained therapeutically can help the person with dementia to maintain a sense of self-worth and a sense of belonging and help them to review their lives in a positive way, and perhaps even resolving past conflict (Wong 1995; Gibson 1996). Gibson's (1996) approach to reminiscence work with people who have dementia stresses the importance of exploring the past and focusing on 'what the person still remembers, not on what she has forgotten' (p. 42).

There are a number of therapeutic approaches that may be used by the CMHN that involve using a person's life story and focus predominantly on its positive aspects, although not necessarily overlooking more negative avenues, particularly if there is unresolved conflict or grieving. Life review, reminiscence therapy and life story work are therapeutic interventions that involve reflection upon, and review of, a person's life history. CMHNs can work with these approaches involving both the person with dementia and their carer. The CMHN must, however, proceed with caution and be aware that past conflicts between the person and their carer may resurface and may require resolution.

Before using any approach involving a person's life story, CMHNs need to ask themselves the following:

- Do I fully understand the concepts behind each therapeutic approach?
- Do I have the appropriate skills required to work with a specific therapeutic approach?
- What is the value of using a specific approach with the person with dementia and/or their carer?
- What do I hope to achieve?

There are common themes and similarities that run through all these approaches using life history that can be confusing to those who are exploring their use in practice for the first time (see Burnside and Haight 1992; Wong 1995). For example, practitioners are often unaware of the different therapeutic levels involved in reminiscence work. They may be familiar with the simple or recreational approach to reminiscence work but not necessarily with approaches that involve an element of evaluation or a review of life events.

For an overview of six types of reminiscence, including examples that help to direct their use in practice, see Wong (1995). In a similar vein, Burnside and Haight (1992) explore the similarities and differences between reminiscence and life review, noting the use of autobiography, life history and oral history with explanations of both approaches.

Cheston's (1998) review of the literature relating to the potential of psychotherapeutic work with people with dementia is also relevant in terms of informing and directing the therapeutic work of CMHNs. He makes the point that, until recently, there has been little evidence of the use of psychotherapy or counselling techniques with people with dementia. In the article, Cheston explores the use of a number of psychotherapeutic techniques that may be appropriate for people with dementia and suggests they will require some therapeutic adaptation before being implemented.

Cheston (1998: 214) stresses the need to be flexible about the environment in which psychotherapy or counselling takes place, and to think in terms of 'being psychotherapeutic' with the individual with dementia, rather than in terms of 'doing psychotherapy'. The very nature of working within the field of mental health care, whatever the speciality, has always required CMHNs to be flexible and adaptable in their approach. However, the skill of adapting therapeutic techniques has not until recently been embraced by CMHNs working with people with dementia. In keeping with a philosophy of person-centred care, Cheston (1998) identifies approaches that can provide a framework for CMHNs to work empathetically with people with dementia. He cites the work of Goudie and Stokes (1989) on resolution therapy and Feil (1993) on validation therapy. Both approaches utilize Rogerian principles of counselling and are underpinned by a belief that behind the confused verbal and behavioural expressions of persons with dementia are hidden meanings, feelings and emotions that need to be acknowledged. Both approaches work on the premise that the feeling content of the language and behaviours of the person with dementia are seen to be more important than the accuracy of any statement they may make. The interpretation by the CMHN, for example, about the content and feeling aspects of the communications between a person with dementia, verbal or non-verbal, can be verified by the process of validation (Kalman and Waughfield 1993; Benjamin 1995; Miller 1995). The techniques involved in these approaches can help the CMNH to reach out to the person behind the label of dementia, to tap into their world, their reality, rather than to force them into ours.

It is important here to return to the notion of partnership and the family orientation of the CMHN's work. CMHNs will rarely work solely with the person with dementia. Most of the time there will be a close family member who is the primary carer, often supported by other social networks such as family members, friends and neighbours. Families need the opportunity to express their own feelings and emotions, to be helped to have some understanding of what the future may hold for the person with dementia and themselves. The CMHN is in a privileged position for offering family carers the opportunity to learn the techniques involved in therapeutic approaches that might enhance the caring relationship.

Indeed, there is a need for CMHNs to work with carers in order to develop strategies for caring and coping in as positive a way as possible, whilst at the same time being given credit for the skill and knowledge that they bring to the caring relationship. In any caring situation there is undoubtedly the possibility of crisis occurring which may lead to the carers' personal resources failing them, leading to a breakdown in the home situation (Adams 1990; Wilford 1996). These authors suggest family-orientated approaches are appropriate interventions in such circumstances. Wilford (1996), for example, explores the implementation of

Falloon's psychosocial family management programme as a framework for family support in the care of a person with dementia. He describes how using Falloon's six-step problem-solving process enabled each family member to define what they saw as the major problem or problems and to identify possible solutions (Falloon 1985). Wilford (1996: 22) found that working with this approach helped to make 'significant change in the dynamics of the family' within a short period of time.

Adams (1990) also advocates the employment of psychosocial interventions by CMHNs at times of carer crisis, outlining the use of a psychotherapeutic approach that allows for:

- clarification of issues: helping the carer become aware of why the crisis has occurred;

- validation of normality: helping the carer understand that the experience of anxiety, tension and loss of control is a normal reaction to stressful circumstances;

- confrontation: helping the carer accept the reality of the situation – Adams stresses that confrontation should only be used in the context of a supportive relationship;

- ventilation of feelings: enabling the carer to speak freely about the stresses and strains of the caring situation;

- exploration of alternatives: helping the carer to think through ways of resolving the crisis.

Adams (1990: 11) suggests that following a psychosocial approach to carer crisis 'will be one of the ways in which community nurses will meet anticipated need with appropriate skills'.

A further model for working with carers' worthy of consideration by CMHNs is Zarit's stress reduction model (Zarit *et al.* 1987). This model involves two stages:

- information giving;
- promoting problem solving with the family.

The first stage is aimed at minimizing carer stress by providing information about the nature of dementia, specific problems that may be encountered and the availability of relevant services. The second stage focuses on the identification of the problem, its causes and consequences and an exploration of possible solutions (Miller and Soliman 1998). The model is explored in Chapter 13 when Soliman looks in detail at the assessment and intervention base of Admiral Nurses.

There are similarities or common themes reflected within each of the afore-mentioned approaches which indicate that there are clearly identified aspects of carer stress that should be addressed whatever the framework used. Moreover, it is important to add that the sense of loss and grief is an issue for both the carer and the person with dementia, and to note the importance of CMHNs using an appropriate grief therapy approach. The CMHN needs to identify possible frameworks for working with loss and grief issues, and for further discussion the reader should see the work of Worden (1993) as developed by Wilford. Worden's (1993) tasks of mourning can provide a useful tool for CMHNs when working with loss and grief situations.

Conclusion

Assessment and therapeutic approaches are interdependent. Neither should be rushed, and consideration of the where, when and how of implementation is paramount to the well-being of the person with dementia and their carers. Both the assessment and the therapeutic intervention should be the main focus. Moreover, attention should be focused on the abilities of people with dementia and their carers rather than on the disabilities of the person. The nature of the work of CMHNs best places them in a position to coordinate assessment approaches and to develop therapeutic working relationships. However, the literature does indicate variations in the training experiences of CMHNs and differences in the ways in which CMHNs view their role (Brooker and White 1997; Keady and Adams 2001). There is, therefore, a need for CMHNs to reflect on their own knowledge and skill base and to identify any training needs before considering whether or not to work with therapeutic approaches involving elements of life review when working with people who have dementia.

References

Adams, T. (1990) Crisis and the confused elderly, *Nursing*, 4(6): 9–11.

Adams, T. (1996a) A descriptive study of the work of community psychiatric nurses with elderly demented people, *Journal of Advanced Nursing*, 23(6): 1177–84.

Adams, T. (1996b) Kitwood's approach to dementia and dementia care: a critical but appreciative view, *Journal of Advanced Nursing*, 23(5): 948–53.

Adams, T. (1998) The discursive construction of dementia care: implications for mental health nursing, *Journal of Advanced Nursing*, 28(3): 614–22.

Adams, T. (in press) The person with dementia, in P. Barker (ed.) *Psychiatric and Mental Health Nursing, The Craft of Care*. London: Hodder Arnold.

Audit Commission (2000) *Forget Me Not: Mental Health Service for Older People*. London: The Stationery Office.

Barker, C. and Black, S. (1971) An experiment in integrated psychogeriatric care, *Nursing Times*, 67(45): 1395–9.

Barr, W., Cotterill, L. and Hoskins, A. (2001) Improving community mental health nurse targeting of people with severe and enduring mental illness: experiences from one English health district, *Journal of Advanced Nursing*, 34(1): 117–27.

Benjamin, B.J. (1995) Validation therapy: an intervention for disorientated patients with Alzheimer's disease, *Topics in Language Disorders*. New York: Aspen Publishers.

Bond, J. (2001) Sociological perspectives, in C. Cantley (ed.) *A Handbook of Dementia Care*. Buckingham: Open University Press.

Brooker, C. and White, E. (1997) *The Fourth Quinquennial National Community Mental Health Nursing Census of England and Wales. Final Report December 1997*. University of Manchester and Keele University.

Buck, D. and Smith, K. (1998) The distribution of psychiatric nurses in England: are they where they should be?, *Journal of Advanced Nursing*, 28(3): 508–16.

Burns, A., Lawlor, B. and Craig, S. (1999) *Assessment Scales in Old Age Psychiatry*. London: Martin Dunitz.

Burnside, I. and Haight, B.K. (1992) Reminiscence and life review: analysing each concept, *Journal of Advanced Nursing*, 17(7): 855–62.

Cheston, R. (1998) Psychotherapeutic work with people with dementia: a review of the literature, *British Journal of Medical Psychology*, 71: 211–31.

Cheston, R. and Bender, M. (2000) *Understanding Dementia: The Man with the Worried Eyes*. London: Jessica Kingsley.

Department of Health (2001) *National Service Framework for Older People*. London: The Stationery Office.

Falloon, I. (1985) *The Family Management of Mental Illness*. Baltimore, MD: The Johns Hopkins University Press.

Feil, N. (1993) *The Validation Breakthrough: Simple Techniques for Communicating with People with 'Alzheimer's-type Dementia'*. London: Health Professions Press.

Folstein, M.F., Folstein, S.E. and McHugh, P.R. (1975) 'Mini-mental state': a practical method for grading the cognitive state of patients for the clinician, *Journal of Psychiatric Research*, 12: 189–98.

Gibson, F. (1996) The use of the past, in A. Chapman and M. Marshall (eds) *Dementia: New Skills for Social Workers*. London: Jessica Kingsley.

Goudie, F. and Stokes, G. (1989) Dealing with confusion, *Nursing Times*, 85(39): 35–9.

Ho, D. (2000) Role of community mental health nurses for people with dementia, *British Journal of Nursing*, 9(15): 986–91.

Holden, U. (1995) *Ageing, Neuropsychological and the 'New' Dementias*. London: Chapman & Hall.

Kalman, N. and Waughfield, C.G. (1993) *Mental Health Concepts*. Florence, KT: Delmar Publishers.

Keady, J. and Adams, T. (2001) Community mental health nurses in dementia care: their role and future, *Journal of Dementia Care*, 9(2): 33–7.

Keady, J. and Nolan, M. (1994) The carer-led assessment process (CLASP): a framework for the assessment of need in dementia caregivers, *Journal of Clinical Nursing*, 3(2): 103–8.

Kitwood, T. (1997) *Dementia Reconsidered: The Person Comes First*. Buckingham: Open University Press.

Knight, B.G. (1996) *Psychotherapy with Older Adults*. London: Sage.

Mayo Clinic Rochester (2001) Dementia: epidemiology, at http:// www.mayo.edu/geriatricsrst/dementia.I.html (accessed 25 November 2001).

Miller, L. (1995) Validation therapy: the human face of elderly care?, *Complementary Therapies in Nursing and Midwifery*, 1(4): 103–5.

Miller, L. and Soliman, A. (1998) Assessment of family carers, *Elderly Care*, 10(1): 22–6.

McWalter, G., Toner, H., Corser, A. *et al.* (1994) Needs and needs assessment: their components and definitions with reference to dementia, *Health and Social Care*, 2: 213–19.

Pattie, A.H. and Gilleard, C.J. (1999) *Manual of the Clifton Assessment Procedures for the Elderly*. Sevenoaks: Hodder & Stoughton.

Pritchard, E. and Dewing, J. (2000) Memory and cognitive assessment, *Elderly Care*, 12(13): 25–7.

Stanley, D. and Cantley, C. (2000) Assessment, care planning and care management, in C. Cantley (ed.) *A Handbook of Dementia Care*. Buckingham: Open University Press.

Watkins, P. (2001) *Mental Health Nursing: The Art of Compassionate Care*. Oxford: Butterworth-Heinemann.

Wilford, S. (1996) Alzheimer's disease: a family-centred approach, *Mental Health Nursing*, 6(5): 20–2.

Wong, T.P. (1995) The process of adaptive reminiscences, in B.K. Haight and J.D. Webster (eds) *The Art and Science of Reminiscencing*. London: Taylor & Francis.

Worden, J.W. (1993) *Grief Counselling and Grief Therapy*, 2nd edn. London: Routledge.

Zarit, S., Orr, J. and Zarit, J.M. (1987) *The Hidden Victims of Alzheimer's Disease*. New York: New York University Press.

7

Cognitive-behavioural interventions in dementia

Practical and practice issues for community mental health nurses

Peter Ashton

Introduction

The overall aim of this chapter is to enhance the practitioners' understanding about how cognitive behaviour therapy (CBT) can be utilized in the support, treatment and management of people who have dementia. Furthermore, the chapter will also illustrate how individual and group application of CBT can be used to support family carers thus supporting further illustrations on the efficacy of CBT within this book, namely Chapter 11 by Lowery and Murray, and Chapter 12 by Pusey.

To achieve this objective, a review of the evidence base for CBT and its application to dementia care is presented. Furthermore, to enable community mental health nurses (CMHNs) to integrate such an approach into routine practice, the chapter also provides an explanation about how CBT principles can be applied. However, it is important to state at the outset that this chapter is *not* intended to be a training manual in CBT, or to produce 'competent therapists'. To achieve this level of practice, CMHNs would need to go beyond this text and undertake more extensive and in-depth training.

Dementia: an outline of need

The Alzheimer's Disease Society (1996), now the Alzheimer's Society, suggests that of the estimated 636,000 people with dementia in the UK, nearly 500,000 are thought to have Alzheimer's disease. Whilst there are some differences in the initial presentation of the different types of dementia, they all erode the person's mental functioning, behaviour and capacity for self-care. Both psychological and behavioural symptoms, such as anxiety, depression, mania, hallucinations, delusions, agitation, aggression and inappropriate everyday behaviours are frequently characteristics of dementia (Purandare *et al.* 2000). For example, in a study of 50 patients with 'mild dementia', Wands *et al.* (1990), using the Hospital Anxiety and Depression Scale, found that as many as 38 per cent of the patients in their sample showed signs of anxiety. Following on from this, Ballard *et al.*'s (1994) study of patients with dementia attending a day hospital reported similar levels of anxiety, with 31 per cent meeting the diagnostic criteria for generalized anxiety disorder. Furthermore, in a more recent study by Ballard *et al.* (1996) of 109 patients attending a memory clinic who met the diagnostic criteria for dementia, 22 per cent had subjective anxiety, 11 per cent experienced autonomic anxiety, 38 per cent experienced tension, 13 per cent experienced situational anxiety and 1.8 per cent had panic attacks. Moreover, there is also a high prevalence of depression in people who experience dementia, with some studies suggesting that between 20 and 30 per cent of people with Alzheimer's disease have a coexisting depression (Reifler *et al.* 1986; Wragg and Jeste 1989; Teri and Wagner 1991; Wagner *et al.* 1997).

Consequently, dementia can be summarized as a multi-faceted disorder that brings about enduring cognitive, emotional and behavioural changes. One of the consequences of these changes is that people with dementia need support, care and treatment from other people to maintain well-being. Frequently, this support is provided in the community by spouses and family members (Wenger 1984; Gilhooly 1986). However, providing this support can be very demanding and stressful. In a study conducted by the Alzheimer's Disease Society (1993), 97 per cent of the carers responding to a 'burden orientated' questionnaire (*n* = 1303) reported having some form of emotional and physical difficulty, such as stress, depression, tiredness and physical pain. In a more recent study, Livingston *et al.* (1996) found that 47 per cent of women carers of a person with dementia were judged to be clinically depressed against only 3 per cent for female carers of a physically disabled older person. These findings help to confirm the view that caring for a person with dementia not only presents physical demands, but can also bring about significant psychological and emotional reactions. It is therefore important for the CMHN to be able to respond to these demands in a comprehensive and therapeutic manner. In addition to practical support, family carers may also need appropriate, and effective, psychological interventions to help them cope and adjust to their role. One such psychological intervention is CBT.

Cognitive behaviour therapy in dementia care

Since the initial development of CBT for depression by Beck *et al.* (1979), CBT has shown itself as an effective form of psychological therapy for a wide range of disorders, including panic disorder (Clark *et al.* 1994), generalized anxiety disorder (Butler *et al.* 1991), obsessive compulsive disorder (Salkovskis 1999), hypochondriasis (Warwick *et al.* 1996), schizophrenia (Haddock *et al.* 1998; Tarrier *et al.* 1999), and cancer (Greer *et al.* 1992). Moreover, a growing number of publications have discussed the effectiveness and processes involved in using CBT with older adults with depression and/or anxiety (see Steuer and Hammen 1983; Yost *et al.*

1986; King and Barrowclough 1991; Wilkinson 1997; Clark 1999; Barrowclough *et al.* 2001; Walker and Clarke 2001).

There is also an emerging body of literature on the use of CBT with people who have dementia, or their carers, using either individual or group therapy. With reference to people with dementia, Teri and Gallagher-Thompson (1991) provided a discussion of their use of CBT with people with an early diagnosis of dementia. In their paper, these authors discuss how patients with mild dementia could be helped to challenge negative cognitions and generate more adaptive ways of viewing their situation and events. Wisner and Green (1986) have also presented a case study to illustrate the adaptive use of cognitive and behavioural techniques in the treatment of anger in a nursing home resident who has dementia. Using a group approach, Kipling *et al.* (1999) discussed how they successfully used CBT with three patients with mild/moderate dementia to help manage unhelpful memory-related beliefs. With regard to carers of people with dementia, James *et al.* (2001) provide a very good discussion and illustration of how the principles of CBT can be used to prevent emotions, such as depression, anxiety, anger and guilt from eroding the capacity of the carer to perform their role. Marriott *et al.*'s (2000) study of 42 patient/carer dyads also demonstrated the effectiveness of CBT in reducing carer distress and depression, a finding also supported by Charlesworth *et al.* (2000), Thompson *et al.* (2000) and Charlesworth (2001).

Although most of these studies relate to the use of CBT by clinical psychologists, the inclusion of CBT in the initial training of mental health nurses (Hughes 1991), coupled with improved access to post-qualification courses and literature, could add to the practice environment of CMHNs in the field of dementia care. It is an opportunity ripe for development.

Principles to practice: cognitive behaviour theory/model

The most significant and influential contributor to the development of cognitive behavioural therapy was Aaron T. Beck. In the early 1960s, Beck developed an approach to psychotherapy that was underpinned by ideas drawn from the field of cognitive psychology. In his influential text, Beck (1976) stated that dysfunctional mood states and behaviour could be better understood from a cognitive, information-processing perspective. An important assumption in cognitive therapy is that information processing plays a primary role in the subjective experience through its mediation and organization of thought, feeling, behaviour and physical sensation. Thus, our experiences of, and responses to, the environment, involve an interaction within the cognitive, affective, behavioural and physiological systems. Throughout life, the person has learning experiences that shape the nature of beliefs held in memory. These core beliefs, and the subsequent assumptions that arise from them, form part of the person's personality and serve to guide the interpretation of life events, resulting in the generation of thoughts, emotions, physiological reactions and behavioural responses. However, any of these parts could act as the 'starting point' for the information-processing activity. Similarly, therapy can also start with any of these elements. However, whilst there is an interconnection between these different elements, the cognitions (memories, knowledge, thoughts, beliefs and assumptions) play a dominant role in the use of this model and in the therapeutic process. Within the cognitive model there are three levels of cognition that are interrelated and play an influential role in information processing and meaning making. First, at the deepest level, are the *core beliefs* or *schemas*. These tend to be global, absolute and relatively stable, and reflect our beliefs about ourselves, others and events in the world, examples include: 'I don't feel valued', 'Others pity me' and 'The world is cruel'. These beliefs enable us to make sense of, and evaluate, experiences, and make predictions about the self and others.

Secondly, arising out of these beliefs at the intermediate level are our *assumptions*. These are related to our core beliefs and can be both functional or dysfunctional. Furthermore, they are often expressed as 'if . . . then' statements; for example, 'If I try hard to look after my husband, then he will appreciate me' or 'If I continue to look after my husband then other people won't think I don't care for him'. The model proposes that these beliefs and assumptions are the product of life experiences.

The third level refers to *automatic thoughts*. These are the spontaneous, unplanned thoughts that emerge within the context of experiences, such as: 'He doesn't love me' or 'They don't think I love him'.

Figure 7.1 provides an illustration of the different elements of the cognitive model with respect to a female spouse carer of her husband with dementia.

Through the interacting process shown in Figure 7.1, the person attempts to give meaning to experiences through the use of existing beliefs, knowledge and memories. These meanings then guide the person to make sense of ongoing events, make appropriate judgements and choose appropriate actions and behaviours. However, this cognitive processing can involve some inaccuracies and inconsistencies brought about by the influence of existing beliefs and assumptions. To assist in this process, Beck *et al.* (1979) identified a number of ways in which our thinking can become distorted or subject to errors:

- *Selective abstraction*: the person selects one aspect of a situation and interprets the whole on the basis of this one detail. For example, the carer says that because she shouted at her husband for his behaviour, it means she is not a caring person.
- *Arbitrary inference*: the person reaches a conclusion without enough evidence to support that conclusion or in the face of contrary evidence. 'People only say I am doing a good job of caring for my husband to keep me happy.'
- *Overgeneralization*: the person draws a general conclusion on the basis of one or more isolated incidents. 'I am a bad wife because I let him go into care.'
- *Personalization*: the person relates to themself external events when there is no basis or only a partial basis for making such a connection. Thus the person may blame themself for an uncontrollable event. For example, the patient has a fall at home and the carer says: 'That was my fault, it would not have happened if I had looked after him properly.'
- *Magnification and minimization*: the person exaggerates or minimizes the significance of an event. 'Allowing my husband to wander off was an absolute disaster', or 'People only visit because they feel sorry for me.'

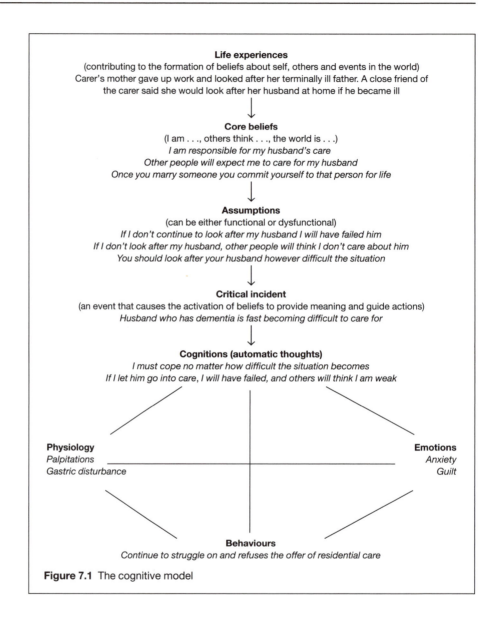

Figure 7.1 The cognitive model

- *Dichotomous thinking*: the tendency to express extremist, black or white, all-or-nothing thoughts, for example: 'I'm evil for sometimes wishing he would die.'

Cognitive behavioural therapy process

CBT is an active, structured, psycho-educational form of therapy which is person centred, collaborative and goal orientated. The therapy process attempts to help the client to develop more insight and awareness into the functional and dysfunctional interrelationship between their thoughts, emotions, behaviour, and through the use of both cognitive and behavioural activities, acquire new skills that will enable them to achieve their goals. Through a collaborative approach, the nurse would guide the client to clarify their difficulties and formulate their goals. Once this is achieved, the process continues with the nurse helping the client to explore their thoughts, interpretations and distorted meanings attached to their experiences, and to adjust them where they are found to be unrealistic, unreasonable or unhelpful. This involves the CMHN (in this instance) helping the client to review the validity and functionality of their thoughts, beliefs and resulting actions, through the use of reality testing, reattribution and behavioural activities. Throughout this process, the client is helped to observe, practise and learn the techniques that will enable them to deal with their life situation in a more effective manner.

Preparation for therapy

Before commencing any therapy, the CMHN would need to decide whether to use individual or group therapy. Clearly, the client's preferences would need to be taken into account, as would the appropriateness of the approach for the client under consideration.

There are advantages and disadvantages to using both approaches. In the case of people with dementia, practical considerations will need to be taken into account. If there are a few people with dementia attending a day centre, for instance, then it may be possible to use a group approach. However, many people with dementia will be living at home, so an individual approach may be more appropriate.

With regard to CBT for family carers of people with dementia, this can be offered on an individual or group basis. However, with appropriate support arrangements, many carers may appreciate the opportunity to meet with other carers away from their home environment. Steurer and Hammen (1983) suggest that this may lessen the experience of social isolation and encourage openness of discussion. Furthermore, the group approach can offer a number of other benefits. Attending a group with other carers experiencing similar difficulties can help validate concerns, and help carers to recognize that they are not alone. By participating in group CBT, carers will have a greater opportunity to gain new insights into their situation, and be able to observe and gain evidence of how others have successfully utilized techniques to help cope with challenging activity, for instance.

In a review of the literature on preparing people for group therapy, Mayerson (1984) concluded that adequate preparation not only promotes appropriate client involvement in therapy and improved attendance, but also significantly affects the outcome of therapy. Careful preparation of clients will help to facilitate the identification and resolution of any anxieties, and deal with any inaccurate preconceptions that clients may have. It will also enable participants to understand what to expect.

If a group approach is to be used, the CMHN would need to decide upon numbers, frequency and duration of sessions, and whether it will be an open or closed group. Given the sensitive nature of what is often disclosed in therapy, a climate of trust and confidentiality is essential. Group size and time allocation would also be important to enable the full participation of all group members. Thus, a group of four to six would seem ideal. A group larger than this may initially feel more threatening to participants, and make it more difficult for all members to contribute.

If it is decided to adopt a group approach for carers, Thompson *et al.* (2000) state that the therapy group sessions adopt the following traditional structure for CBT:

- The building of a collaborative therapeutic relationship.
- Commencing each session with an agreement on how the time should be used (agenda setting).
- A review of previous between-session cognitive and behavioural activities.
- In-session cognitive activities.
- Identification of between-session cognitive and behavioural activities.
- Summary and evaluation of the session.

Irrespective of whether individual or group therapy is to be used, the client's cognitive abilities, such as reading, speaking and comprehension, will need to be assessed. This would apply in particular if the client has dementia. If the client is a carer, the CMHN would need to clarify how the person with dementia is supported whilst the carer is attending the therapy sessions.

When using CBT with older people, Koder *et al.* (1996) have suggested that a small number of special considerations and adaptations may need to be addressed. They suggest that some clients may need to be helped to challenge a commonly held belief that the person is 'too old to change'. They also suggest that sessions have a slower pace, make greater use of handouts and include frequent summaries. When using CBT with people who have dementia, the involvement of spouse, relatives or close friends can enhance the maintenance of achievements. Also, the therapeutic process may not necessarily adhere rigidly to the traditional format of CBT outlined above by Thompson *et al.* (2000).

Whichever approach is chosen, the development and maintenance of a good therapeutic relationship is necessary to encourage a collaborative process in which disclosure and guided discovery can take place.

Developing a therapeutic relationship

Throughout the growth and development of cognitive behavioural psychotherapy, the importance of the therapeutic relationship has been acknowledged. Beck *et al.* (1979) stated that as with other psychotherapies, CBT involves the use of a number of specific techniques within the context of an interpersonal relationship. They suggested that the appropriate display of warmth, accurate empathy and genuineness are likely to substantially increase the effectiveness of the therapeutic process. However, whilst they believe these characteristics are necessary, on their own they would be insufficient to produce optimum therapeutic effect. In support of Beck's position, a number of more recent studies and publications have highlighted and validated the importance of the therapeutic relationship in CBT (Safran and Segal 1996; Raue *et al.* 1997; Sloan 1999; and for a recent review of the potential impact of the therapeutic relationship, see Waddington 2002).

It is therefore essential to start building trust and rapport with the client from the onset of the first session. All aspects of interpersonal skills need to be utilized in a sensitive, attentive and supportive manner. A good way of building rapport is to offer a warm greeting, including a shake of the hand, and to maintain eye contact.

It is important for the CMHN not to interrupt too frequently, particularly in the early stages when the client may feel the need to tell their story. It is also necessary for the CMHN to listen carefully to what is being said. The use of reflective statements, summaries and empathic responses will confirm active listening and also encourage a sense of partnership.

Guided discovery and Socratic dialogue

Guided discovery represents one of the core and central elements of CBT. Weishaar (1993) suggests that this can be seen as the investigative process through which the use of Socratic dialogue, thought diaries and behavioural activities, the client is helped to determine the meaning of their own thoughts, actions and emotions and their interrelationships. Through these processes the client is helped to examine the validity and functionality of their thoughts and behaviour, and test out new and different ways of relating to problematic situations.

Socratic dialogue refers to a style of interpersonal interaction in which the nurse would use a range of questions to help facilitate guided discovery, enhanced self-awareness, cognitive change and problem solving. Beck and Young (1985) state that Socratic dialogue is used to:

- clarify and define problems;

- assist in the identification of thoughts, assumptions, beliefs and possibly images;

- examine the meaning of thoughts and events;

- assess the consequences of specific thoughts and behaviours.

In a discussion of the Socratic method, Overholser (1993) proposed the following examples of types of question that could be used in Socratic dialogue:

- Memory questions used to establish facts and details:

    When did you first notice this difficulty?

    What has changed as a result of your current situation?

- Translation questions in which the client considers information in a different but parallel form:

    How would other people you know think about this?

- Interpretation questions that help the client discover relationships among facts and thoughts:

  I wonder if we can learn anything from the way you think of other people in this situation that might help us here?

- Application questions in which the client thinks about the application of thoughts to a specific problem situation:

  What have you tried in order to cope with this problem?

  So how do you think you could achieve that?

- Analysis questions that help to develop awareness of thought processes used to reach conclusions:

  What do you think is causing this problem?

  What makes you think that interpretation is correct?

- Synthesis questions that encourage the client to solve problems through creative and divergent thinking:

  Could there be any other way to deal with this problem?

- Evaluation questions that ask the client to make value judgements:

  So what does it mean to be a failure?

  When you are think of that situation, what does it mean to be incompetent?

However, Padesky (1993) suggests that Socratic dialogue involves more than just a series of questions. She argues that active listening and frequent summarizing are also needed. If Socratic questioning is to achieve guided discovery, it is important for the nurse to pay attention to all aspects of the client's idiosyncratic responses so that she/he can be truly in tune with the way the client construes the situation or experience. Furthermore, the use of frequent summaries will also help to check whether both parties understand things in similar or different ways and ensure a sense of collaboration, essential for the achievement of guided discovery.

Collaboration can also be demonstrated through the use of agenda setting, particularly if the group approach is to be used.

Agenda setting

Whilst agenda setting may not be used explicitly in individual work with a person with dementia, it would be helpful in group therapy with carers. Agreeing an agenda with the group at the beginning of each meeting is a useful way of prioritizing time to ensure the session focuses on the important issues. It also facilitates collaboration and provides structure to each meeting to ensure the time together is used in a mutually effective manner. By collaboratively agreeing an agenda, quiet and (verbally) restrained clients are encouraged to be more active, whereas verbose clients are more constrained.

Agenda setting would normally be part of both individual and group CBT, and should be used at the beginning of every session. Thus, the process should be part of individual therapy with carers. Typically, the agenda for each session would include a brief review of the previous session, previously agreed out-of-session activities, the main topic for this session, and any activities to be carried out before the next session. This should be explained to the clients within the first session so that they know what to expect and how to prepare for future sessions.

An example of introducing agenda setting could be phrased as follows:

> To help use get the most of our sessions together, I think it would be helpful if we start each session by agreeing what we should talk about. This will provide structure to our sessions and help us keep focused. To help keep track of our issues and monitor progress, I would suggest we try to keep to the following format for each of our sessions. For example, we need to review our previous session and any out-of-session activities carried out. Then we could spend some time on your priority issues and then agree activities to be carried out before the next session. We could then end each session with a brief review. How does this seem to you?

Commencement of cognitive behaviour therapy

If the CBT is to be used on a more formal basis with carers, their expectations would need to be examined and clarified, to ensure that therapy does not proceed with unrealistic expectations. It would also be helpful to start the process of explaining the cognitive model and therapy process. Many older people may not have any previous knowledge or experience of this therapeutic approach.

Within the first session, time should be spent on clarifying the nature of the problems the clients are having, and trying to conceptualize them within the cognitive model. Thus, questions should be used to try to identify relationships between problematic moods, behaviours, thoughts and possible physical sensations. By doing this, the CMHN can start to introduce the cognitive model to the client. Within this process, the nurse should try to get as full a picture as possible of the nature of the difficulties. There will also be a need to establish when the difficulties first started, how often they occur, the effect they are having on the person, and how the person has tried to cope with them. It is important to be as specific as possible so that particular goals can be more easily identified.

Using cognitive and behaviour techniques

In order to help the client develop more insight and awareness into the functional and dysfunctional nature of their thoughts, emotions and behaviour, a number of cognitive and behavioural strategies can be used. One of the first cognitive strategies would be to encourage the client to share the idiosyncratic meanings of their difficulties. This would involve the use of Socratic questioning to draw out thoughts and beliefs relating to their difficulties; these thoughts may be linked with problematic emotions and behaviours. As the client expresses their thoughts, these

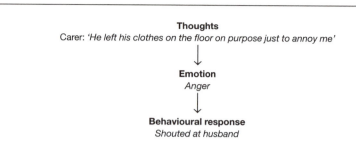

Figure 7.2 Example of the interrelationship between elements of the cognitive model

would be recorded to try to illustrate to the client the interrelationship between the elements of the cognitive model, as Figure 7.2 illustrates.

With reference to Figure 7.2, the client (as carer) could then be asked to re-examine what has emerged in the following manner:

CMHN: So, you became angry and shouted at your husband because you thought he left his clothes on the bedroom floor on purpose.

Carer: Yes, he just wanted to get back at me because I had nagged him.

CMHN: Given what you have learnt about dementia, could there be any other reason for him leaving his clothes on the floor?

Carer: Well, I suppose he could have done that because of his forgetfulness.

CMHN: If that were true, what other thought might you have about that situation?

Carer: I suppose I might think he has forgotten where to put his clothes.

CMHN: Let's assume you believe that thought. What emotional reaction might you now have?

Carer: I might not feel so angry, but more frustrated.

CMHN: OK. And how might you have behaved with that thought in mind?

Carer: I probably wouldn't have shouted at him.

CMHN: If we look at my notes of the two options, what do you notice?

Carer: I suppose the way I think about that situation seems to affect the way I have responded.

CMHN: Good, I am glad you could see that, because that's what this therapy is about. In other words, the way you think about things can have an important influence on how you react. Also, sometimes your initial thought may not be an accurate one, as in this case.

This process would then be used further to help the client review and evaluate other ideas and beliefs. For each questionable or unhelpful belief, the client would be asked to think of the evidence for and against it, and identify alternative beliefs. The client would then be asked to consider evidence that would support the alternative belief. If the client still has doubts about the alternative belief, they could be asked to consider undertaking out-of-session activities that might provide more evidence to support the alternative belief. This is what is referred to as the behavioural aspect of the therapy.

A behavioural activity for a carer receiving CBT could be to try to alter their caregiving behaviour and to notice the response. It could be to talk to other carers to test some specific thought, or to read some material to examine the validity of an initial interpretation of the patient's behaviour.

However, using CBT with people who have dementia can present particular challenges, as many people may have difficulty adjusting to the reality of a diagnosis of dementia. Upon discharge, such knowledge may well generate many negative thoughts, although these thoughts may be *realistic* negative thoughts. In this situation, rather than challenge the negative thoughts, it may be better either to use distraction techniques, such as activity scheduling, or to review the helpfulness of engaging in those thoughts. Whilst the thoughts may be accurate interpretations of the future, continuous expression and rumination may not be helpful to the person themself. In this situation, the person could be encouraged to look at the advantages and disadvantages of their ruminations.

Through this activity, they could be helped to recognize that their ruminations inhibit their ability to enjoy areas of their life still available to them. However, many people with dementia may well 'give up' all activities because of difficulty or failure in one specific area. This may result in an overgeneralization, such as: 'Unless I can do everything I used to do, there is no point in doing anything' or 'I can't cope with that activity, therefore I won't be able to cope with all those others'. By allowing these thoughts to go unchallenged, the person with dementia is likely to deny themself experiences that could contribute to maintaining some sense of control and self-efficacy.

In order to encourage the maintenance of achievements and prevent relapse, some preparation for termination and/or relapse prevention needs to be provided.

Termination and relapse prevention

In working with people with dementia, the CMHN may well remain involved for a considerable time. In this situation, termination would not be so much of an issue. However, the issue of relapse prevention would still be appropriate to consider.

Once the person has achieved benefits from the CBT process, it is important to try to maintain these benefits for as long as possible. Therefore, regular reviews of the patient's use of the techniques may help to slow down the loss of skills. On the other hand, if CBT is to be used in its traditional format for a more defined period of time, such as with carers, preparation for termination and relapse prevention work would need to be addressed.

Beck *et al.* (1979) have suggested that much of the benefit of CBT can be lost through inappropriate and inadequate preparation for termination. They argue that when termination is handled well, clients are more likely to consolidate gains, generalize learnt strategies for possible future problems, and have lower relapse rates. With regard to older people, Yost *et al.* (1986) state that because there may be a greater risk of dependency, it is important to pay attention to this aspect of CBT.

Preparation for termination should begin early in therapy by continued reference to its time-limited and educational nature. Relapse prevention is facilitated by the client being encouraged to see therapy as a training period in which they are coached to learn techniques and strategies that they can use on their own. To help the patient become aware of what they are gaining, regular reviews should be carried out. Within these reviews, the CMHN would encourage the client to reflect on their understanding of the techniques and their role in bringing about change.

The production of contingency plans for dealing with possible future difficulties can also help prevent relapse. Another useful strategy for supporting the client after therapy is to involve significant others. Their understanding of the process will enable them to remind and encourage the client to use the techniques they have learnt. In the final session the following examples of questions put by the CMHN may help prepare the client for life without therapy:

CMHN: To help us evaluate the progress we have made, it might be useful to consider a few issues:

- What have you learnt so far?

- What kind of future problems might you experience, and how could you deal with them?

- Suppose you notice depression creeping back, what do you know about dealing with depression that you didn't know before?

Conclusion

In writing this chapter, it became apparent that despite the wider enthusiasm for CBT, and the extensive research that has been devoted to this form of therapy, there is still a paucity of published material on its application in the field of dementia care. Given the drive towards more holistic and person-centred care (Department of Health 2001), CBT can and should have a place within the services provided for people with dementia and their families. Whilst there may be some limitations to its use as the dementia progresses, it can make an important contribution to meeting the psychological needs of people with mild to moderate dementia, and be of particular benefit to carers.

References

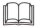

Alzheimer's Disease Society (1993) *Deprivation and Dementia*. London: Alzheimer's Disease Society.
Alzheimer's Disease Society (1996) *Opening the Mind*. London: Alzheimer's Disease Society.

Ballard, C.G., Mohan, R.N.C., Patel, A. and Graham, C. (1994) Anxiety disorder in dementia, *Irish Journal of Psychiatry*, 11: 108–9.

Ballard, C., Boyle, A., Bowler, C. and Lindesay, J. (1996) Anxiety disorders in dementia sufferers, *International Journal of Geriatric Psychiatry*, 11: 987–90.

Barrowclough, C., King, P., Colville, J. *et al.* (2001) A randomised trial of the effectiveness of cognitive-behavioural therapy and supportive counselling for anxiety symptoms in older people, *Journal of Consulting and Clinical Psychology*, 69(5): 756–62.

Beck, A.T. (1976) *Cognitive Therapy and Emotional Disorders*. New York: New American Library.

Beck, A.T. and Young, J.E. (1985) Depression, in D.H. Barlow (ed.) *Clinical Handbook of Psychological Disorders*. New York: Guilford Press.

Beck, A.T., Rush, A.J., Shaw, B.F. and Emery, G. (1979) *Cognitive Therapy of Depression*. New York: Guilford Press.

Butler, G., Fennell, M., Robson, P. and Gelder, M. (1991) Comparison of behaviour therapy and cognitive behaviour therapy in the treatment of generalised anxiety disorder, *Journal of Consulting and Clinical Psychology*, 59: 167–75.

Charlesworth, G. (2001) Cognitive therapy for family carers, *Signpost*, 5(3): 33–5.

Charlesworth, G., Riordan, J. and Shepstone, L. (2000) Cognitive behaviour therapy for depressed carers of people with Alzheimer's disease and related disorders, *The Cochrane Library*, Issue 4.

Clark, D.M. (1999) Anxiety disorders: why they persist and how to treat them, *Behaviour Research and Therapy*, 37: S5–S27.

Clark, D.M., Salkovskis, P.M., Hackmann, A. *et al.* (1994) A comparison of cognitive therapy, applied relaxation and Imipramine in the treatment of panic disorder, *British Journal of Psychiatry*, 164: 759–69.

Department of Health (2001) *National Service Framework for Older People*. London: The Stationery Office.

Gilhooly, M.L.M. (1986) Senile dementia: factors associated with carer-giver's preferences for institutional care, *British Journal of Medical Psychology*, 57: 34–44.

Greer, S., Moorey, S., Baruch, J.D.R. *et al.* (1992) Adjuvant psychological therapy for patients with cancer: a prospective randomised trial, *British Medical Journal*, 304: 675–80.

Haddock, G., Tarrier, N., Spaulding, W. *et al.* (1998) Individual cognitive behaviour therapy in the treatment of hallucinations and delusions: a review, *Clinical Psychology Review*, 18: 821–38.

Hughes, C. (1991) Community psychiatric nursing and the elderly: a case for using cognitive therapy, *Journal of Advanced Nursing*, 16: 565–72.

James, I.A., Powell, I. and Reichelt, K. (2001) Cognitive therapy for carers: distinguishing fact from fiction, *Journal of Dementia Care*, November/December: 24–6.

Kipling, T., Bailey, M. and Charlesworth, G. (1999) The feasibility of a cognitive behavioural therapy group for men with mild/moderate cognitive impairment, *Behavioural and Cognitive Psychotherapy*, 27: 189–93.

King, P. and Barrowclough, C. (1991) A clinical pilot study of cognitive-behavioural therapy for anxiety disorders in the elderly, *Behavioural Psychotherapy*, 19: 337–45.

Koder, D.A., Brodaty, H. and Anstey, K.J. (1996) Cognitive therapy for depression in the elderly, *International Journal of Geriatric Psychiatry*, 11: 97–107.

Livingston, G., Manela, M. and Katona, C. (1996) Depression and other psychiatric morbidity in carers of elderly people living at home, *British Medical Journal*, 312: 153–6.

Marriott, A., Donaldson, C., Tarrier, N. and Burns, A. (2000) Effectiveness of cognitive-behavioural family intervention in reducing the burden of care in carers of patients with Alzheimer's disease, *British Journal of Psychiatry*, 176: 557–62.

Mayerson, N.H. (1984) Preparing clients for group therapy: a critical review and theoretical formulation, *Clinical Psychology Review*, 4: 191–213.

Overholser, J.C. (1993) Elements of the Socratic method: systematic questioning, *Psychotherapy*, 30(1): 67–74.

Padesky, C.M. (1993) Socratic questioning: changing minds or guided discovery? Keynote address at the European Congress of Behavioural and Cognitive Therapies, London.

Purandare, N., Allen, N.H.P. and Burns, A. (2000) Behavioural and psychological symptoms of dementia, *Reviews in Clinical Gerontology*, 10: 245–60.

Raue, P., Goldfried, M. and Barkham, M. (1997) The therapeutic alliance in psychodynamic-interpersonal and cognitive-behavioural therapy, *Journal of Consulting and Clinical Psychology*, 65: 582–7.

Reifler, B.V., Larson, E., Teri, L. and Poulsen, M. (1986) Dementia of the Alzheimer's type and depression, *Journal of American Geriatric Society*, 34: 855–9.

Safran, J. and Segal, Z. (1996) *Interpersonal Process in Cognitive Therapy*. London: Jason Arouson.

Salkovskis, P.M. (1999) Understanding and treating OCD, *Behaviour Research and Therapy*, 37(Suppl. 1): S29–S52.

Sloan, G. (1999) The therapeutic relationship in cognitive behaviour therapy, *British Journal of Community Nursing*, 4(2): 58–64.

Steuer, J.L. and Hammen, C.L. (1983) Cognitive behavioural group therapy for depressed elderly: issues and applications, *Cognitive Therapy and Research*, 7: 285–96.

Tarrier, N., Yusupoff, L., Kinney, C. *et al.* (1999) Randomised controlled trial of intensive cognitive behaviour therapy for patients with schizophrenia, *British Medical Journal*, 317: 303–7.

Teri, L. and Gallagher-Thompson, D. (1991) Cognitive-behavioural interventions for treatment of depression in Alzheimer's patients, *The Gerontologist*, 31(3): 413–16.

Teri, L. and Wagner, A. (1991) Assessment of depression in patients with Alzheimer's disease: concordance between informants, *Psychology and Aging*, 6: 280–5.

Thompson, L.W., Powers, D.V., Coon, D.W. *et al.* (2000) Older adults, in J.R. White and A.S. Freeman (eds) *Cognitive-behavioural Group Therapy for Specific Problems and Populations*. Washington, DC: American Psychological Association.

Waddington, L. (2002) The therapy relationship in cognitive therapy: a review, *Behavioural and Cognitive Psychotherapy*, 30: 179–91.

Wagner, A.W., Logson, R.G., Pearson, J.L. and Teri, L. (1997) Caregiver expressed emotion and depression in Alzheimer's disease, *Aging and Mental Health*, 1(2): 132–9.

Walker, D.A. and Clarke, M. (2001) Cognitive behavioural psychotherapy: a comparison between younger and older adults in two inner city mental health teams, *Aging and Mental Health*, 5(2): 197–9.

Wands, K., Merskey, H. and Hachinski, V. (1990) A questionnaire investigation of anxiety and depression in early dementia, *Journal of American Geriatric Society*, 36: 535–8.

Warwick, H.M.C., Clark, D.M., Cobb, A.M. and Salkovskis, P.M. (1996) A controlled trial of cognitive behavioural treatment of hypochondriasis, *British Journal of Psychiatry*, 169: 189–95.

Weishaar, M.E. (1993) *Aaron T. Beck*. London: Sage.

Wenger, G.C. (1984) *The Supportive Network: Coping with Old Age*. London: Allen and Unwin.

Wilkinson, P. (1997) Cognitive therapy with elderly people, *Age and Aging*, 26: 53–8.

Wisner, E. and Green, M. (1986) Treatment of a demented patient's anger with cognitive-behavioural strategies, *Psychological Reports*, 59: 447–50.

Wragg, R.E. and Jeste, D.V. (1989) Overview of depression and psychosis in Alzheimer's disease, *American Journal of Psychiatry*, 146: 577–89.

Yost, B.E., Beutler, L.E., Corbishley, M.A. and Allender J.R. (1986) *Group Cognitive Therapy: A Treatment Approach for Depressed Older Adults*. Oxford: Pergamon Press.

8

Turning rhetoric into reality

Person-centred approaches for community mental health nursing

Tracy Packer

Introduction

Until the mid-1980s, our understanding of the condition commonly known as dementia has been drawn from a complex examination of the neuropathological, biochemical and genetic components of the disease. For this reason, much of the way we have conceptualized dementia has been informed through images of atrophied brains on a computed tomography (CT) scan, or descriptions of amyloid plaques and neurofibrillary tangles invading and destroying brain tissue. Perhaps we might have witnessed the low scores of those unlucky enough to have the disease on a range of cognitive tests designed to highlight deficits.

The Alzheimer's Disease Society (now the Alzheimer's Society) was predominantly an organization that provided support and care for the carers of people with dementia, tacitly acknowledging that theirs was a thankless task and there was little that could be done for those who had the disease. Within institutions and society at large, people with dementia were spoken about as a category rather than as individuals, and became known as 'sufferers', 'victims' or 'the elderly mentally infirm'. It was widely accepted that although some psychiatric support was possible, dementia was the disease that 'left the body behind', a shell, a shadow of one's former self. The best that could be done, whether in an institution or at home, was to maintain 'basic care' needs and provide support for the carer.

Although a sophisticated understanding of the neuropathological picture of dementia was emerging, up until this time little work had been undertaken to examine the interpersonal or socio-psychological world of people with dementia. It was almost as if they were not expected to have such a world. The paucity of occupational diversity and mental stimulation of any kind within institutional care settings seemed to suggest that this was indeed the predominant view.

This chapter outlines the work of the late Professor Tom Kitwood, and his attempts to address this very question. How can any of us relate to people with dementia, and is it possible for them to relate to us? If so, how can our day-to-day contact be improved, and what can we learn from each other? These questions are important because they go straight to the heart of care. It becomes clear that there is no 'them and us', but simply 'us' (Kitwood 1997a). For community mental health nurses (CMHNs), Kitwood's work presents real challenges, making it clear that addressing the needs of the person with dementia can no longer be superseded by the needs of their carer. Balancing the needs of both, considering one's own impact and facing up to the raw emotions such work may bring, heralds the gateway to an entirely different way of working, one that has become known as 'the new culture of care' (Kitwood and Benson 1995).

Old culture to new

Kitwood became particularly interested in the field of dementia care in the mid-1980s when as an academic psychologist he was invited to become a project supervisor to a clinical psychologist and psychiatrist undertaking work in this area. He subsequently became a member of his local branch of the Alzheimer's Society, and then became involved in work with a small community care scheme in Bradford, Yorkshire. During this time he met numerous people with dementia and their extended families, and developed a further interest in carer support along with the use of detailed life histories to help explain the actions of those with dementia and inform carers about possible ways of addressing them. Kitwood himself states that he began to ask whether 'some of the symptoms that are commonly found [in persons with dementia] might be due more to a failure of understanding and care than to a structural failure of the brain' (Kitwood 1997a: 3; see also Kitwood 1997b).

Together with his colleague Kathleen Bredin, Kitwood suggested that an alternative approach placing an emphasis on the provision of real human contact and communication, rather than neurological deficits alone, would provide a more human approach, one that he was to call 'person-centred care' (Kitwood and Bredin 1992a, b; Kitwood 1993). Drawing on Rogerian psychotherapy among other approaches (Rogers 1961), he began to outline the basic principles of a new approach to the care of people with dementia: one that would recognize first that people with dementia have a right to a status as 'persons', and secondly, would assert that upholding personhood in someone with dementia is not only possible, but also worthwhile.

People with dementia can and do have a right to be 'persons', and as such are morally entitled to a status within society that recognizes their intrinsic worth as members of the human race. This 'worth', Kitwood argues, should not be rigidly defined by criteria offered by conventional western moral philosophy. In particular, he highlights the perspective offered by Quinton (1973) who suggests five criteria for determining whether or not one is a 'person'. These are:

1   Consciousness of self.
2   Rationality, in particular the ability of abstract reasoning.
3   Agency – the ability to determine numerous choices and act upon the ones made.

4   Morality – the ability to live within a set of principles and be accountable for one's actions accordingly.

5   Capacity to form and hold relationships, and in doing so, understand and recognize the needs of others.

Following the publication of Quinton's work, the development of an increasingly individualized lifestyle that rewards intellectual skill and independence has become clearly evident within western value systems. In addition, the advent of sophisticated computer technology that appears (superficially at least) to 'think' for itself has meant that defining what constitutes a 'person' has since been reduced to a focus on just two things: autonomy and rationality. It is at this juncture that the right of people with dementia to be defined as persons is placed seriously under threat. Post (1995) challenges this as a dangerous line of thought and suggests that people with dementia should be viewed as persons because, despite their decreased intellectual function, they are able to respond to feelings, emotions and relationships with others. In other words, Post argues that, as members of the human race, we should all have a sense of 'moral solidarity' with others who 'experience emotions', whatever our differences or degree of mental capacity.

Kitwood drew heavily on the work of the philosopher Martin Buber (1937) to further support this argument. Buber's work is important because he asserts that the central value for being accorded the status of person is that of relationship. As he states: 'All real living is meeting' (Buber 1937: 11). The 'meeting' being referred to here is one of unconditional positive regard, living very much in the present with openness and awareness to feeling and even the unknown. This kind of meeting carries with it risks, for by opening oneself to such an experience, it may result in painful but important self-discovery. Buber calls such a meeting an 'I–Thou' form of relating, as opposed to an 'I–It' meeting which is more detached and superficial. Kitwood argues strongly that people with dementia are often able to engage in an 'I–Thou' meeting, even when severely disabled by their dementia. However, he challenges us with this sobering thought:

> A man or woman could be given the most accurate diagnosis, subjected to the most thorough assessment, presented with a highly detailed care plan and given a place in the most pleasant surroundings – without any meeting of the I–Thou kind ever having taken place.
>
> (Kitwood 1997a: 12)

More recently this view has been upheld by Sabat (2002) who describes how interaction and engagement can be enhanced between the person with dementia and those around them, even when 'in the throes' of a dementing illness. He argues that when a person has dementia they can easily become 'limited' by the poor and often negative expectations of those around them, particularly with regard to their losses in the social and relationship arena. Such views are easily consistent with social construction theory, illustrated by the 'tendency on the part of healthy others to limit the AD [Alzheimer's disease] sufferer to the social persona of "burdensome, dysfunctional patient" . . . thus the person with AD is "defined" by others mainly in terms of attributes which are anathema to him or her' (Sabat 2002). However, the way in which the dominant expectations of those involved in any kind of social relationship with a person with dementia are expressed, could work with, as well as against, the best interests of the person concerned. This is illustrated by Kitwood's definition of personhood, which provides a much more hopeful socially constructed framework within which people with dementia have the potential to flourish. Personhood defined within this context is:

> A standing or status that is bestowed upon one human being, by others, in the context of relationship and social being. It implies recognition, respect and trust.
>
> (Kitwood 1997a: 8)

Nowadays, the perspective offered by Kitwood, but founded on little empirical evidence at the time, has become increasingly supported by the many accounts being provided and published by people who are themselves coming to terms with their own diagnosis and experience of dementia. Diana Friel McGowin, who vividly wrote of her experiences of early onset dementia, provided one of the earliest of these accounts:

> My every molecule seems to scream out that I do, indeed, exist, and that existence must be valued by someone! Without someone to walk this labyrinth by my side, without the touch of a fellow traveller who understands my need of self-worth, how can I endure the rest of this uncharted journey?
>
> (McGowin 1993: 124)

Sterin (2002) graphically writes of her own experience of 'becoming invisible', witnessing a repeated and ever familiar 'gesture of dismissal' from many in the social milieu around her, and often well-meant but misguided 'acts of smothering', particularly from professionals who believed they were acting in kindness towards her. The findings of Keady and Nolan's extensive work with people in the early stages of dementia also support these experiences (Keady and Nolan 1995a,b,c; Keady 1996, 1997).

Some cause for optimism does, however, lie with Peter Ashley's description of his involvement in his own treatment plan following a diagnosis of Lewy body dementia (Ashley and Schofield 2002). The positive impact of the new drug treatment he was suitable to receive, along with his active participation in determining his own life plan and future aspirations, has led to his becoming sufficiently confident enough to become a trustee and council member of the Alzheimer's Society in the UK. That such an opportunity now exists for someone with dementia, in an organization that until recent years focused most of its intervention and support on the needs of family carers, is itself testament to the progression of more person-centred approaches in the field of dementia care. Peter has an electronic and computer engineering background, and uses his computer to stay in e-mail contact through 'jokes, ideas and sympathy' with people around the world who have dementia. He is also drawing on his expertise to work with other professionals in considering ways in which computer technology could help some people with dementia to maintain their ability to communicate.

Admittedly, these examples have been drawn from those in the early stages of their dementia, but work is already under way to develop ways of consulting those who have more severe cognitive disability (Cheston and Bender 1999; Allan 2001;

Killick and Allan 2002). In Peter's case (and others lucky enough to be supported to experience such opportunities), only time will tell what kind of long-term impact upon confidence, trust and social skills this kind of involvement may have. Kitwood controversially went so far as to suggest that the promotion of personhood was not just a psychological task, but was potentially a neurological task as well (Kitwood 1989). In short, if personhood really was maintained from the outset of an early diagnosis, instead of overwhelming brain tissue disruption and loss, the brain (being a plastic organ) might, in certain circumstances, be able to adapt an alternative synaptic circuitry, leading ultimately to some degree of what Kitwood called 'rementia'. This particular assertion has remained controversial, but his contribution to the recognition of the need to encourage and develop a positive social psychology around and including the person with dementia has, despite his untimely death in 1998, left a pivotal and lasting legacy to the field.

Malignant social psychology

Given that his previous psychological work had drawn from the areas of counselling, psychotherapy and moral development, it is perhaps not surprising that Kitwood began to scrutinize what might constitute the subjective experience of dementia. He was particularly challenging in a paper that outlined what he called 'the dialectics of dementia care' (Kitwood 1990). He used the phrase 'malignant social psychology' (MSP) to define, what he argued, was an intrinsic part of the experience of dementia in the UK in previous decades. He described how, once a person began to experience memory loss, a whole sequence of events would take place that, in turn, served to undermine, demoralize and ultimately lead to exclusion. This exclusion was experienced in the person's immediate social milieu, and also in the day-to-day decision making about their needs and desires. Kitwood (1990) argued that such events were closely bound up in a dominant discourse of therapeutic nihilism among health care professionals. These types of response were not in themselves maliciously intended, nor for that matter were they limited to health and social care professionals. Kitwood acknowledged this by writing: 'We should remember that MSP only very rarely springs from malice – from a deliberate attempt to cause hurt. It is part of a culture that we have inherited' (Bradford Dementia Group 1997). He asserted that this culture influenced not only those with professional roles, but also society at large. Family members, neighbours and members of the general public were all likely to be inadvertently contributing to a culture of MSP at some time or other (see Figure 8.1).

Most of Kitwood's published work has focused on recognizing and eradicating MSP when it occurs in formal care settings, such as hospitals, day centres and care homes. As already outlined, his earlier work suggested that the depersonalizing impact of MSP was already well established long before a person with dementia was admitted into a formal care setting. Statistically, we know that a large proportion of people with dementia will never enter any form of institutional care, but that the majority of published work outlining person-centred care has been aimed at care workers in secondary care settings. This leaves a huge gap in knowledge among

Treachery
Disempowerment
Infantilization
Intimidation
Labelling
Stigmatization
Outpacing
Invalidation
Banishment
Objectification
Ignoring
Imposition
Withholding
Accusation
Disruption
Mockery
Disparagement

Figure 8.1 Malignant social psychology

Source: Bradford Dementia Group 1997

those working in primary care, particularly as there has been insufficient development work exploring the relevance and impact of person-centred approaches in such settings and, perhaps importantly, defining what such approaches might consist of.

Iliffe and Drennan (2001: 103–6) have argued that there is still a need to 'eradicate culturally embedded episodes of MSP within Primary Care settings'. This concern is supported by the results of a study carried out among Scottish general practitioners (GPs) which indicated that there is still considerable disparity between what GPs tell the person diagnosed with dementia and what they tell their family carers (Downs *et al.* 2002). From this study it was revealed that people with dementia tended to be given information about the symptoms of the disease, along with an explanation that these are simply 'part of the ageing process'. On the other hand, family members were more often given information about the symptoms, causes, prognosis and support that might be available.

Whilst there may be a number of non-malign reasons for this disparity, not least the wish to protect the person with dementia from loss of hope, it has also been argued (Cheston and Bender 1999: 211) that people with dementia need all of the following:

1   Time to explore the meaning and impact of their diagnosis.

2   The support of a friend or relative during early discussions if the person concerned wishes them to be present.

3   The provision of the right information, at an appropriate time in an accessible format for both persons with dementia and family members.

4   Recognition that people with dementia need to have the expression of emotional distress validated, as well as maintaining the possibility of hope for their future.

CMHNs receive a significant number of referrals from primary care teams and are ideally placed, therefore, to take a leading role in recognizing and working to eradicate episodes of MSP from very early on in the trajectory of dementia. Arguably, this activity should provide a cornerstone to any work that claims to be person-centred, and should form a key component of any therapeutic relationship forged between the person with dementia and those around them.

Positive person work

Clearly, placing the actions and responses of the person with dementia in a bio-psychosocial context, and not attributing them solely to a disease process, must address several significant new aspects of care planning, not least by moving away from accepting unconditionally the professional or family carer's perspective on what has been happening. This is not to say that the account offered by professional and family carers should be politely heard and then discounted. On the contrary, close and careful listening may reveal some root patterns in a person's responses and, if this is the case, then a skilled CMHN will facilitate a more constructive carer–patient dyad in order to establish an agreed way forward.

The core elements of positive person work are not mutually exclusive, and neither should it be expected that they are all present all of the time. However, recognizing the value of a framework for positive person work can provide all concerned with a means of evaluating progress over time, and reviewing the ways in which the changing needs of the person with dementia and their carer can be acknowledged and evaluated in specific ways (see Table 8.1). Should the person with dementia need to enter more formal care settings on a temporary or permanent basis, this same framework could provide a valuable adjunct to their plan of care and help provide a clear value base from which everyone is working.

This particular framework also seems to be consistent with the work of Nolan *et al.* (2002) who call for a 're-appraisal of the ways in which a successful

Table 8.1 Framework for positive person work

Core element	Experience of the person with dementia	Contribution of the CMHN
Recognition	Experiences a sense of 'belonging' and is accepted as an individual with own unique needs for personal space and companionship	Anyone entering the home of a person with dementia should actively acknowledge their presence through appropriate eye contact and sensitive verbal communication. CMHNs recognize that they are important role models for family carers, visitors and other professionals. With this in mind, they should be proactive in formulating and passing on advice about simple communication strategies that may assist in maximizing a person's sense of belonging
Negotiation	Feeling of being in control over what one does or does not do, without fear of being misjudged	CMHNs recognize that all people with dementia, no matter what their level of cognitive disability, need to retain control over some aspect of their daily life. This need may explain why some carers experience difficulties over aspects of care such as hygiene, nutrition and medication compliance. CMHNs can work with the person with dementia and the family carer to plan ways in which they can retain control over some aspect of their lives, in a mutually beneficial manner
Collaboration	Experience of feeling as though one belongs in a partnership of others	CMHNs work with the family carer and the person with dementia to identify ways in which they can both use complementary talents to complete a task or challenge together. This may be a short shopping trip, or something more ambitious such as planning a day out. Later on, it may be a small but significant act of daily living, but the importance of collaboration lies in the view of the person with dementia having something worthwhile to offer as a valued equal to others involved. Care should be taken not to place the person with dementia or their carers in a position where they feel they have somehow failed

Table 8.1 – *continued*

Core element	Experience of the person with dementia	Contribution of the CMHN
Play	Expression of imagination and 'inner child' is recognized and supported	CMHNs recognize that 'playfulness' is not only a strong indicator of well-being in persons with dementia, but also a powerful means of demonstrating their sense of belonging and confidence. For this reason, playful expression should be encouraged rather than stifled, even though some family carers may misinterpret this response as an example of 'disinhibition' that is inappropriate and a sign of the person's increasing dementia. A skilled CMHN, however, will work with great sensitivity to reassure relatives, and in some cases give 'permission' for them to draw on their own 'playfulness' in response
Timalation	Opportunity to explore self-awareness and discovery through a range of sensory experiences	CMHNs explore ways with the person with dementia and the family carer in which day-to-day experiences can provide a range of opportunities for sensory diversity, particularly in the preparation and consumption of food; the exploration of textures, colours and smells of fresh laundry; music; pets; gardening; and tactile contact. Whilst this may not be an obvious need in the first instance, it may help provide a creative route for communication and engagement when words prove to be a more troublesome medium for the person with dementia
Relaxation	No sense of bodily tension, alongside an intrinsic feeling of safety and security	CMHNs use their observational and communication skills to assess this each time they visit the person concerned. Rather than being reactive recipients of reports of increased tension and agitation, they will proactively seek out subtle changes of mood, body posture and engagement. They will recognize that if a person with dementia loses their sense of safety and security then few elements of positive person work will be consistently possible to achieve

Validation	Experience of being psychologically accepted *and* understood by others	CMHNs recognize that all vocalizations and actions of a person with dementia are attempts at communication, and will try to interpret these in this light, rather than viewing them as 'behaviours' that simply need to be 'managed' – usually with pharmacological interventions. It is however, important that the feelings and needs of the family carers are recognized and acknowledged and a compromise achieved, which may not happen quickly or easily
Holding	Feeling of being safe, secure and supported	CMHNs recognize the need of both the person with dementia and their carer to receive support and stress management strategies in order to maximize a sense of safety and security for all concerned. Whilst sensitive observation and probing will be an ongoing part of their work with both individuals, they will also, if necessary, recommend specialist help
Giving	Experience of value and worth in an environment in which you are a contributor along with others	CMHNs work with the person with dementia and their carer to identify ways in which key contributions by the person with dementia are recognized and acknowledged. As the level of cognitive disability increases, sensitive re-evaluation may indicate a need for a delicate rebalancing of such events in order to avoid unnecessary feelings of failure and inadequacy
Facilitation	Opportunities for personal growth and new experiences are made available	CMHNs work with the person with dementia and their carer to devise a risk assessment plan that provides acceptable levels of safety for the individual concerned and the community in which they live, without excluding opportunities for experiencing new sensations and activities
Creation	Opportunity and ability to creatively express self through actions and emotions	CMHNs work with the person with dementia and their carer to explore a range of potential opportunities for creative expression, as well as building on those already present as indicated by sensitive observation, communication and biographical work

Table 8.1 – *continued*

Core element	Experience of the person with dementia	Contribution of the CMHN
Celebration	Opportunity to experience joy and celebration alongside others	CMHNs provide advice about supportive strategies and communication skills that will maximize the abilities of the person with dementia, as well as reduce feelings of anxiety and inadequacy of other family members and friends. By planning for such occasions, the person with dementia is not routinely excluded from larger social and family gatherings, particularly as their dementia progresses

Source: adapted from Kitwood 1997a: 119

intervention [in dementia care] is defined', along with the promotion of a partnership approach with family carers. Five emerging trends have been identified. These indicate the following (amended from Nolan *et al.* 2002: 86–87):

1 People with dementia and their carers should increasingly determine the agenda as far as appropriate interventions and the successfulness of outcomes are concerned, rather than professionals or researchers alone.

2 Working 'with', rather than doing 'to' or 'for' the person with dementia should inform care strategy.

3 Much more attention should be paid to the 'context' of care giving, i.e. in order to promote true support and successful interventions, it is essential that the nature of the care-giving dyad and that of the family are taken into consideration.

4 In order to achieve successful and relevant outcomes, any intervention should be 'reasonable' and 'modifiable', based on negotiation and agreement with the person with dementia and their carer.

5 When determining the impact of interventions and the success of outcomes, all those who are involved in the care planning process should use a commonly understood framework for discussion and debate.

Biography

Kitwood (1997a: 75) argued that the use of life story should be an integral part of care planning in working with people who have dementia. Its use, he argued, would provide care workers with a more multi-dimensional perspective of individuals that would assist them in seeing beyond the disease to a person who has had meaningful life experiences, roles and talents. Indeed, knowing about and valuing such information could contribute towards an improvement in the way in which those around would perceive an individual with dementia. He was particularly interested in the impact of such understanding within formal care settings, where he claimed that many people with dementia were defined, or indeed limited, by expectations related to their diagnosis of dementia. Using a life story approach would not only serve to provide a multi-dimensional view of that individual, but it might also inspire care workers to recognize that there is an innate value in the ongoing experience of the person with dementia. Sensitive life story work would in itself provide a more therapeutic milieu for building a meaningful relationship between the person with dementia and those involved in their care, and it might also explain some of the routines, and responses, otherwise deemed to be a manifestation of the 'dementing process'. Such work may also assist in reinstating a person's intrinsic value as a member of the 'personhood club', rather than an unfortunate recipient of a disease that has rendered them helpless and hopeless.

In England, a team at a continuing care unit in Warrington has argued for the use of lifestyle profiles to be developed for every client who uses their service. Among the numerous issues that such a profile may address, widely recognized questions establishing a person's current and previous sleep pattern, daily routine, eating habits and leisure pursuits are covered. Moreover, the lifestyle profile does not dodge more sensitive questions such as: 'Are you a person who prefers solitude or do you prefer the company of others?' and 'Do your sexual desires still worry you?' Clearly, discussions that contribute to a detailed lifestyle profile cannot be addressed in one meeting, nor should such discussions be treated without great sensitivity as they may 'unearth' any number of issues that the person concerned may not wish to discuss at that moment in time – a point Miller also stressed in Chapter 6 of this book. Neither might they wish to disclose some information to other family members, or anyone else involved in their care. Building up a relationship of trust, along with skills of facilitation, negotiation and re-evaluation, would be essential for any CMHN contemplating such important and sensitive work. It is also important to remember that, by definition, any lifestyle profile should be a constantly changing document and should never be seen as completed. In a brief article outlining their work, the team leader has collaborated with a person with dementia to write that they have 'recognised the fact that people with dementia are individuals with individual needs and do have a choice'. Peter (who has Lewy body dementia) recognizes that he has a choice and is choosing to do something about it. Together they are working to raise awareness among professionals, other people with dementia and family carers so that the person with dementia should be able to choose whether or not to plan for their own individualized care in future (Ashley and Schofield 2002).

Despite a growing body of literature arguing for the use of life story work to be considered an essential part of any care planning exercise for people with dementia across a range of formal care settings, it is clear that by the time the person with dementia requires such services their ability to contribute may already be hampered by several obstacles. For example: the person with dementia may have a failing memory, increased communication difficulties and, in some cases, live alone with the condition so that few surviving relatives can support and corroborate key life events. In some instances, genuine attempts at life story work has resulted in an autobiographical portrayal limited by the expectations and assumptions of a well-intentioned family carer. In others, information provided in this way is seen as helpful, especially when it is the only remaining option. However, an uncomfortable question remains: if asked, how many people could be sure that their spouse or children would give an accurate account of their social needs, likes, dislikes and significant childhood and early adult experiences?

For these reasons, then, it is becoming increasingly likely that the earlier such profiling is undertaken, the greater the contribution a person can make towards the development of their own care-planning needs. Furthermore, such work visibly places the person with dementia at the centre of the care process, proactively engaged in negotiation of all their central needs with those around them (including family carers), as opposed to being passive recipients of a neatly presented collection of photographs and memories that, although attractive, offer little to assist in the recognition of their day-to-day values and needs. Sterin (2002), who has dementia, argues that the process of 'capturing' important information should begin as soon as a person recognizes that they have a memory problem. She advises 'the judicious selection of the most important things that should be written down and remembered on paper, kept always in the same place and consulted frequently' (p. 9).

Clearly, then, CMHNs working with people in their own homes have an important role to play in initiating, facilitating and supporting the gathering of such information. They must also ensure that, wherever possible, the person with dementia maintains control of the selection process and the extent to which that information is used in their individual plan of care – particularly if they enter more formal care settings. There is enormous potential for this approach to be undertaken far in advance of such events, providing an opportunity for the person with dementia to face up to the implications of their changing needs and to the possible choices they may have to face. If taken on board by the CMHN, this will not be easy work, and in many cases may result in the person with dementia's denial of events, their anger, fear and frustration, which in turn has serious implications for the nature of the support provided for the main carer. However, person-centred care does not try to protect people with dementia from such emotions, rather it supports and enables them to acknowledge and face up to them.

Future housing

It is important to appreciate that, along with the increasing recognition that people with dementia can contribute much to plans for their own future, there has also been a period of significant change in thinking around their future housing needs. To be successful, a truly person-centred philosophy of care must apply to the setting within which one lives as well as the skills of family and formal carers. CMHNs will be called upon to use their knowledge in an increasingly varied range of settings, and this may bring with it even greater challenges to their practice base. Increasing consultation with user groups indicates that respite services and housing options will be designed to maximize the unique attributes of people with dementia, rather than expect them to conform to a care approach that limits creativity and freedom of expression (Cox and Minter 1999).

For instance, models of home day care (similar to the principles of the child care model in the UK) will see increasing numbers of people with dementia enjoying respite in a domestic setting near to where they live, instead of attending largely impersonal statutory day centres designed for up to 30 people at each session (Mitchell 1998). Drawing from the learning disability sector, there will be a growth in 'independent supported living' for small groups of three or four people with dementia, providing a person-focused alternative to residential care (Svanberg *et al.* 1999). Homesharing is also a potential development in dementia care that originated as a service for older people without cognitive disabilities, but who felt vulnerable living alone in a large home they did not wish to sell. In this approach, people with dementia who live alone sub-let a room in their home to a 'lodger'. This carefully vetted 'stranger' agrees, via the homesharing agency, to spend a specified number of evenings per week in the house, and carry out a small number of agreed tasks, and in doing so, enables a vulnerable person with dementia to stay in their own home for much longer (Bhandari 1999). Many challenges lie ahead for the CMHN, not least of which is evaluating the efficacy of the person-centred approach in the fast-changing world of community practice.

Conclusion

Community mental health nurses are ideally placed to be at the forefront of shaping and delivering person-centred approaches to working with people with dementia. In a time when assessment and diagnosis are taking place earlier than ever before, such work can, and should, begin early in the trajectory of dementia, and in whatever environment people with dementia may be living. With this in mind, there will need to be even greater flexibility and creativity when facilitating positive person work in collaboration with a range of cohabitees who may not be family carers.

Notwithstanding such developments, CMHNs have a crucial educational and supportive role for all those living in the therapeutic milieu. As Kitwood (1997a) has explained, person-centred care cannot be delivered *by* one person *to* another in isolation, rather it is a philosophy that all those concerned need to understand and own in order to break beyond the traditional boundaries currently limiting the creativity of life experience for many people with dementia. Person-centred approaches to care should not demand that the complex needs of the person with dementia should override those of the family carer, or any other cohabitee. CMHNs certainly have much to learn from some family carers, neighbours and friends. Nevertheless, it must be acknowledged that preparing an equal footing for people with dementia alongside the needs of others around them, well before they enter formal care settings, brings with it its own challenges. If these are faced, then expectations and outcomes for people with dementia and their families in the UK may dramatically improve.

References

Allan, K. (2001) *Communication and Consultation: Exploring Ways for Staff to Involve People with Dementia in Developing Services*. Bristol: The Policy Press/Joseph Rowntree Foundation.

Ashley, P. and Schofield, J. (2002) How to plan your own future dementia care, *Journal of Dementia Care*, Mar/Apr: 20–2.

Bhandari, R. (1999) Close care and companionship, *Journal of Dementia Care*, Jan/Feb: 16–17.

Bradford Dementia Group (1997) *Evaluating Dementia Care the DCM Method*, 7th edn. Bradford: University of Bradford.

Buber, M. (1937) *I and Thou*, trans. R. Gregor Smith. Edinburgh: Clark.

Cheston, R. and Bender, M. (1999) *Understanding Dementia: The Man with the Worried Eyes*. London: Jessica Kingsley.

Cox, S. and Minter, J. (1999) Exploring creative responses in housing and support. *Journal of Dementia Care*. Mar/Apr: 15–17.

Downs, M., Clibbens, R., Rae, C., Cook, A. and Woods, R. (2002) What do general practitioners tell people with dementia and their families about the condition? A survey of experiences in Scotland, *Dementia: The International Journal of Social Research and Practice*, 1(1): 47–58.

Illiffe, S. and Drennan, V. (2001) *Bradford Dementia Group Good Practice Guides: Primary Care and Dementia*. London: Jessica Kingsley.

Keady, J. (1996) The experience of dementia: a review of the literature and implications for nursing practice, *Journal of Clinical Nursing*, 5: 275–88.

Keady, J. (1997) Maintaining involvement: a meta-concept to describe the dynamics of dementia, in M. Marshall (ed.) *State of the Art in Dementia Care*. London: Centre for Policy on Ageing.

Keady, J. and Nolan, M. (1995a) A stitch in time – facilitating proactive interventions with dementia caregivers: the role of community practitioners, *Journal of Psychiatric and Mental Health Nursing*, 2: 23–40.

Keady, J. and Nolan, M.R. (1995b) IMMEL: assessing coping responses in the early stages of dementia, *British Journal of Nursing*, 4: 309–14.

Keady, J. and Nolan, M.R. (1995c) IMMEL2: working to augment coping responses in early dementia, *British Journal of Nursing*, 4: 377–80.

Killick, J. and Allan, K. (2002) *Communication and the Care of People with Dementia*. Buckingham: Open University Press.

Kitwood, T. (1989) Brain, mind and dementia: with particular reference to Alzheimer's disease, *Ageing and Society*, 9: 1–15.

Kitwood, T. (1990) The dialectics of dementia with particular reference to Alzheimer's disease, *Ageing and Society*, 10: 177–96.

Kitwood, T. (1993) Person and process in dementia, *International Journal of Geriatric Psychiatry*, 8: 40–56.

Kitwood, T. (1997a) *Dementia Reconsidered: The Person Comes First*. Buckingham: Open University Press.

Kitwood, T. (1997b) The experience of dementia, *Ageing and Mental Health*, 1(1): 13–22.

Kitwood, T. and Benson, S. (eds) (1995) *The New Culture of Dementia Care*. London: Hawker Publications.

Kitwood, T. and Bredin, K. (1992a) *Person to Person: A Guide to the care of those with failing mental powers*, 2nd edn. Loughton: Gale Centre Publications.

Kitwood, T. and Bredin, K. (1992b). Toward a theory of dementia care: personhood and well being, *Ageing and Society*, 12: 269–87.

McGowin, D.F. (1993) *Living in the Labyrinth*. Cambridge: Mainsail Press.

Mitchell, R. (1998) Home from home by the fireside, *Journal of Dementia Care*, Mar/Apr: 16–17.

Nolan, M., Ingram, P. and Watson, R. (2002) Working with family carers of people with dementia: 'negotiated' coping as an essential outcome, *Dementia: The International Journal of Social Research and Practice*, 1(1): 75–93.

Post, S. (1995) *The Moral Challenge of Alzheimer's Disease*. Baltimore, MD: Johns Hopkins University Press.

Quinton, A. (1973) *The Nature of Things*. London: Routledge.

Rogers, C.R. (1961) *On Becoming a Person*. Boston, MA: Houghton Mifflin.

Sabat, S. (2002) Surviving manifestations of selfhood in Alzheimer's disease. *Dementia: The International Journal of Social Research and Practice*, 1(1): 25–36.

Sterin, G. (2002) Essay on a word: a lived experience of Alzheimer's disease, *Dementia: The International Journal of Social Research and Practice*, 1(1): 7–10.

Svanberg, R., Livingston, M., Fairbairn, A. and Stevenson, C. (1999) Popular solution that can offer 'best value', *Journal of Dementia Care*, Jan/Feb: 24–28.

9

From screening to intervention

The community mental health nurse in a
memory clinic setting

Sean Page

Introduction

There is a paucity of literature about the role of nursing in memory clinics. This
paper aims to partially fill this void by describing the specialist role of a community
mental health nurse (CMHN) in the Manchester Memory Clinic based at Wythen-
shawe Hospital in the UK. This memory clinic was the first to be awarded a Charter
Mark for excellence in public service and is cited by the *National Service Framework
for Older People* (Department of Health 2001), as a positive model of clinical
practice.

The nursing role has developed over a seven-year period and has been discussed
at a number of conferences, and through academic and practice-based articles (see,
for example, Adams and Page 2000; Page 2001). This chapter builds upon this foundation and aims to explore the role of a memory clinic nurse within both the pre- and
post-diagnostic phases of dementia. The broader context of mental health nursing
in dementia care is also discussed with reference to the role of the memory clinic.

Memory clinics

Memory clinics developed in the United States as a means of identifying early cases
of dementia. These memory clinics were in essence outpatient services and provided diagnostic, treatment and advisory services to people with milder forms of
dementia (Lindesay and Morris 1999). These early clinics offered people with mild
memory difficulties a realistic and less stigmatizing assessment than was available in
established dementia services (Fraser 1992).

Memory clinics were initially underpinned by a service-driven model and
addressed the reluctance of many physicians to give a diagnosis of dementia to
someone was either young or whose dementia was in its early stages (Luscombe *et al.*
1998). Quite soon, however, many services incorporated a research-driven model of

service provision. This approach allowed people in the early stages of dementia the opportunity to participate in clinical trials relating to the newly emerging drug treatments for people with Alzheimer's disease (Pitt 2001).

Whilst the only survey of memory clinics in the UK found 22 clinics in operation throughout the country (Wright and Lindesay 1995), the numbers have, since this time, undoubtedly increased. Furthermore, the combination of the service-driven and research-driven models of service provision has become a feature of memory clinics and is becoming increasingly recognized as an integral component of services to people with cognitive impairment (Department of Health 2001).

Nursing in memory clinics

Most published accounts of memory clinics make little or no reference to the role, value and function of nurses (Page 1998). From the early days, memory clinics have been seen as falling within the remit of medicine and were usually within the control of a psychiatrist, geriatrician or clinical psychologist (Hassiotis and Walker 2001). Most references to nursing within memory clinics have characterized them as merely having a supportive or administrative role (Beattie *et al.* 1999) with nurses carrying out clinical tasks, such as blood taking, at the request of the doctor.

However, in recent years it has become increasingly recognized that nurses can make a positive contribution to the quality of the assessments. For example, satisfaction surveys of people attending memory clinics suggest that those clinics which score highly for offering a well-planned, coordinated and anxiety-free experience are those that establish nurses in the role of agents of continuity (Hassiotis and Walker 2001).

Whilst this is to be welcomed, it is important to show that nursing has more to offer to a memory clinic than simply coordinating the activities of other professional disciplines. In particular, the distinctive feature of mental health nursing lies in its holistic practice which ideally places nursing philosophically and practically in a position to encourage medically orientated clinics to develop a 'softer social side'. The move towards a social model of service provision, whilst still embracing the importance of diagnosis, will contribute to the development of innovative pre- and post-diagnostic activities within which the nurse has a pivotal role. It is to a consideration of this area that the chapter now turns.

The Manchester Memory Clinic as a model of service provision

In the 1990s, the Manchester Memory Clinic was based at Withington Hospital, West Didsbury. From the onset, nursing was expected to make a significant contribution to its clinical activity and was seen as a means of developing an innovative and distinctive professional role. In the following years, the clinic has gradually developed into a nurse-led service that operates a unique model of nursing triage (Clark *et al.* 1997).

Whilst it is now used in many specialities, triage is a new development within memory clinics. Its introduction within the Manchester Memory Clinic arose to provide a planned response to a number of pressing issues including: the rapidly increasing referral rate; the lack of new resources; and the desire to maintain high clinical standards. The use of the triage model helps to bring the memory clinic nurse into early contact with people who have dementia and encourages a relationship that provides an appropriate setting for comprehensive assessment. It also engenders the prioritization of scarce resources.

The role of the nurse in triage is to determine what other investigations or assessments may be required to: decide if treatment needs to be initiated immediately; assess the degree of risk; prioritize the action required based upon the person's circumstances; and communicate all this information to the patient, their family, their GP and other members of the memory clinic team.

First contact

The person referred to a memory clinic cannot be separated from the experience that they are going through. Although the memory clinic nurse may be seeing the person for the first time, it should be recognized that many new experiences will have been encountered by the person and they will have realized that they have 'a problem' that needs to be addressed. Usually, by the time of a first contact with the memory clinic, the person will have moved through a stage of striving to hide their concerns from other people, and will have begun to search for meanings for their behaviour and to implement compensatory coping strategies (Robinson *et al.* 1997).

Keady and Gilliard (1999) have attempted to conceptualize this encounter with dementia as the person tries to make sense of their shifting experience of reality. As these authors argue, it is only much later on when people with (undiagnosed) dementia find their situation intolerable that they begin to 'open up' to others and seek to work with them to find answers. At this point, a desire to seek an external (professional) confirmation of events comes to the fore and professionals become involved in what has previously been a personal and private experience.

The traumatic experience of many people with dementia prior to their diagnosis highlights the importance of developing a good and potentially therapeutic relationship between the memory clinic nurse and person with dementia. As rehearsed by Packer in Chapter 8, the development of this type of relationship requires the nurse to instigate a person-centred approach that recognizes that the person with dementia is not merely a passive partner in the process of assessment but an active participant. Indeed, it is now understood that the relationship between the nurse and the person with dementia is a two-way process of exchange in which the nurse learns from the person with dementia and vice versa.

In the author's clinical practice, when the person with dementia first meets the memory clinic nurse they are invited to share their personal experience of memory loss. In this context, there needs to be a mutual sharing of information in order to lessen anxiety. In the first instance, the nurse should identify the expectations that the person with dementia has of the memory clinic. Some people with dementia are unsure about its purpose and most are looking for an explanation about their difficulties and ways to overcome them.

Assessment

The provision of specialist help is based on a thorough understanding of the person through a detailed assessment. This assessment is underpinned by a social model of service provision that begins with an appraisal of the person's history, and move on to consider their:

- understanding and own description of what is happening to them;
- personal biography or life history;
- insights into their social psychology that reflects their own relationships, beliefs and attitudes towards, and about, other people.

The memory clinic assessment draws on Kitwood's concept of personhood. Kitwood (1997) developed the notion of personhood as a new approach that helped people to see the person with dementia as a whole being and not simply as a set of deficits, damages and problems that they had acquired through contact with the everyday world. Understanding the person with dementia helps to provide a suitably empathetic setting for assessment.

Undertaking a detailed assessment at any stage of a person's experience of dementia is not easy. It is a skilled activity that attempts to tease out the threads of evidence that may suggest that a person has a very early dementia. This dilemma is exacerbated when the nurse is presented with patients of all ages, with individual complaints and complicated medical histories.

Health screening suggests that many physical processes can lead to an apparent disturbance in memory or other cognitive functions. It is not uncommon for memory loss to be an expression of an underlying health problem due, for example, to hypothyroidism or depleted levels of vitamin B_{12}. Although the expectation is that medical examination should occur in primary care by the person's general practitioner (GP) prior to referral, it remains an important function of the nurse to take a full and detailed history. This allows recent health changes, medication and family history to be accounted for and considered alongside the later cognitive assessment. In addition, it may also reveal new symptoms, particularly those of a neurological nature, and may indicate the need for a more urgent and detailed medical assessment.

The cognitive functioning of the person with dementia is tested in the assessment to structure their personal accounts through a range of screening tests. This procedure is illustrated in Figure 9.1.

The instruments listed in Figure 9.1 are those used in the Manchester Memory Clinic and are not necessarily the same as those used in other clinics. Each instrument examines a specific cognitive domain such as verbal fluency, concentration and recent memory. These screening tests are administered alongside an open-ended discussion with the person with dementia about their life history and recent events

---

- Mini-Mental State Examination (Folstein *et al.* 1975)
- Kendrick Object Learning Test (Kendrick 1985)
- Test of Verbal Fluency (Spreen and Benton 1969)
- Graded Naming Test (McKenna and Warrington 1983)
- Clock Drawing Test (Agrell and Dehlin 1989)

Figure 9.1 Cognitive screening tests

---

and activities. This enables the nurse to display an interest in the person with dementia, obtaining details about their personal biography, social and occupational life events whilst also assessing their ability to recall and articulate them. Often, remote memories are well preserved and the discussion offers the person with dementia the opportunity to fully participate in an activity that is less anxiety provoking than some, more formal, assessments.

An assessment of mood is also included in the assessment process and recognizes that depression can be expressed through subjective memory complaints. In such instances, a detailed history is often required to elicit the person's feelings of low mood and diminished sense of self-worth. Moreover, it provides an opportunity to counter the fact that people who complain about losing their memory may be experiencing a depressive, rather than a dementing, illness.

Referrals based upon subjective memory complaints are welcomed by the memory clinic particularly as a means of identifying people in the early stages of dementia. The identification of depressive illness is a crucial role for any mental health worker as depression has a negative effect on people's health and quality of life that may, in more severe cases, lead to suicide (Asvall 2001). Assessment reflects the open-ended discussion with the patient. Screening tools for depression, such as the Geriatric Depression Scale (Yesavage *et al.* 1983), are useful for eliciting evidence of the patient's current symptoms but are more important for providing a frame of reference for discussion. The subsequent conversation with the patient addresses how the symptoms identified by the patient affect their everyday life. Often, this conversation will identify relevant symptoms of depression and anxiety that have not been found through the use of screening tools.

Diagnosis

At the end of the assessment, the nurse provides a summary of the information that has been gathered and also gives a brief explanation of the cause and nature of the patient's memory impairment. Many clinics have found that people with memory impairment and their relatives have often been frustrated by clinicians who have not shared this information. Furthermore, various memory clinics have reported the benefits of giving a brief summary to the patient and their family at this point in time. The memory clinic nurse should, therefore:

1   make sense of frequently complex and conflicting information;

2   identify the priorities for the person with dementia;

- No impairment
- Depression
- Dementia syndrome
- A combination of depression and dementia
- Cognitive impairment with no obvious presenting cause

Figure 9.2 Initial memory clinic diagnoses

3   make a provisional diagnosis;

4   offer a rationale for the diagnosis.

Taking on this role represents a major shift in nursing practice and allows the nurse to assume significant clinical responsibility.

By sharing with patient's information about the diagnosis, the nurse responds to their need to know about what is happening to them. By meeting this pressing need, the nurse is also required to practise in a unique way. This practice comprises: working from an initial standpoint of knowing little about an individual who has no previous diagnosis; seeking to establish a relationship with that person; and working in an empathetic way within the context of a comprehensive assessment. This approach will give a framework for any existing diagnosis to be made.

Traditionally, in memory clinics, there are a limited number of potential diagnoses that can be made at the initial assessment (see Figure 9.2). This list helps the nurse to identify a pattern of information, a type of history or a particular person's presentation that are suggestive of a provisional diagnosis.

Although the nursing assessment is comprehensive and forms the main clinical evaluation, it is only the first step in the assessment process within the memory clinic. The aim of that assessment is not only to identify a provisional diagnosis but more importantly, to decide upon the appropriate next step. The following case study attempts to illustrate the continuing nature of this assessment process.

Case study

Arthur, an 84-year-old retired bank manager, had a two-year history of memory difficulties. He had become increasing dependent on his daughter for such things as making decisions and managing his affairs. More recently, he had been forgetting appointments and family birthdays and starting to become repetitive in his speech.

Whilst the changes had been evident throughout a two-year period, his daughter felt that there had been 'something different' about this behaviour for about four years. During the memory clinic interview with the nurse, Arthur admitted that he had had a growing realization that not all was well. He used to be able to keep to himself various changes in his functioning, but recently he had become increasingly frustrated with himself. The decision to share his worries with his daughter led directly to the referral to the memory clinic.

The medical history revealed only a known prostate problem. In contrast, cognitive assessment was more revealing. Even though the Mini-Mental State

Examination (MMSE) score was 29/30, the remaining neuropsychological test results all fell well within the 'organically impaired range'. Talking to Arthur revealed that he had no recall of current affairs or news other than some details of headlines. A careful assessment of mood was undertaken. This included consideration of any previous history of treated or untreated depression, any subjective feelings of low mood, any biological features, particularly changes in appetite or sleep pattern, any loss of pleasure or enjoyment, and some exploration of how Arthur regarded the future. The assessment identified only some subjective feelings of frustration with his forgetfulness rather than any overt symptoms of a depressive illness. A score of 02/15 on the Geriatric Depression Scale reinforced the nurse's belief that depression was not significantly present.

The memory clinic nurse suggested to Arthur and his daughter that there was sufficient evidence that he had been developing a significant memory problem for some time. The nurse explained that further investigations were required to confirm the diagnosis and its cause, which the nurse would now organize. Arthur asked if he had Alzheimer's disease and it was explained to him that this was one possibility that would now be investigated. Arthur was reassured that although having a dementia would be a life-changing event his concerns were now being taken seriously. He was also reassured that he had now embarked upon a programme of assessment, treatment and support and that he would be kept involved in all parts of the diagnostic process.

The triage action was initiated by the probable diagnosis of a dementia syndrome. At this time, there is no need for action by the GP, although if Arthur had been depressed the memory clinic nurse would have liaised with the GP to discuss appropriate treatment strategies. The nurse would have then maintained contact with Arthur to monitor his mood and response to such treatment.

Memory clinics often have access to detailed neuropsychological assessments which are invaluable in helping to make a correct diagnosis in often complex or complicated cases. In this clinic the nurse had already administered some neuropsychological tests as part of the initial assessment. They had all fallen well into the range for an organic impairment. The nurse discussed these results with the clinic's psychologist and it was felt that, in the case of Arthur, further neuropsychological tests were unnecessary. Although the evidence for a dementia syndrome was considerable, there was a need for medical investigations to clarify the type of dementia. These investigations would keep up the momentum and make Arthur feel that something is being done. The triage action would therefore encompass the following:

1   Request medical and radiological investigations. Usually this would include a dementia blood screen, computer tomography (CT) brain scan, electroencephalogram (EEG) and electrocardiogram (ECG).

2   Inform Arthur's GP of the provisional diagnosis and plan of action.

3   Discuss Arthur with the memory clinic team after the investigations.

4   Advise Arthur and his daughter if further assessment is required.

5   Arrange consultation to discuss results and share the diagnosis.

After a series of blood tests and brain scans, the diagnosis of early Alzheimer's disease was discussed with Arthur during a consultation with the consultant psychiatrist in charge of the memory clinic. Following this, Arthur was seen regularly by the memory clinic nurse for post-diagnostic counselling and for monitoring the prescription of an anti-dementia drug.

Post-diagnostic interventions

Making an accurate diagnosis is central to the work of a memory clinic and is one of the main expectations that patients have of the clinic. However, identifying a problem is only one function of a memory clinic – the other is to do something about it.

It has been suggested that it is a poor memory clinic which offers only a diagnostic service (Fraser 1992), and certainly most clinics would aim to offer treatment or intervention relevant to the diagnosis that has been made. Often this is fairly straightforward, such as in the case of depressive illness where an antidepressant can be introduced alongside a psychological intervention, such as cognitive behaviour therapy. However, it is less straightforward with a diagnosis of dementia, where effective treatment has historically been somewhat elusive. Before the introduction of cholinesterase inhibitors (ChEI) in the late 1990s, there was no medical treatment specifically for people with Alzheimer's disease. However, contact with a memory clinic would have opened the door to research trials of potential effective agents. The memory clinic therefore offered people with Alzheimer's disease access to either treatment or participation in research trials investigating potential treatments.

It is in the post-diagnostic phase that nurses have most potential to make a significant impact upon people with early dementia. This is often the period when little is offered to people with dementia and their family, despite the policy emphasis on early intervention seen in recent years (Audit Commission 2000). Typically, health and social services have focused their attention upon 'crisis management' or taking responsibility for people in the later stages of the condition.

In promoting a social paradigm upon which to underpin practice in memory clinics, it is apparent that the early post-diagnostic phase is a crucial period during which nurses can open a window of opportunity by working therapeutically with people with dementia and their families to help them face the new challenges they are encountering. In the memory clinic, there is now a specific role that nurses possess that allows them to support people with Alzheimer's disease and their families and is associated with providing access to ChEI that may bring about a period of stability. It is to this role that the chapter now turns.

Using treatments with people who have dementia

Whilst the search for an effective pharmacological treatment for dementing illnesses remains elusive, significant advances have been made in recent years. In particular, the identification of specific deficits within the cholinergic system found in Alzheimer's disease led initially to the cholinergic hypothesis (Bartus *et al.* 1982) and subsequently to specific treatments. These treatments inhibit the action of acetyl cholinesterase, the enzyme that breaks down acetylcholine and consequently brings about cognitive deterioration (Wilkinson 2000).

The introduction of these cholinesterase inhibitors (ChEI) therapies, Donepezil®, Rivastigmine® and Galantamine®, has had a positive impact upon the management of people with Alzheimer's disease (Burns *et al.* 1999) and the control they can exert over the condition. There is now a clear shift towards establishing services through which the ChEIs can be offered to a wider population of people with Alzheimer's disease. The mechanism for bringing this about is the development of a new model of memory clinic, the dementia treatment clinic, as a service that is firmly rooted in clinical practice.

There is an overlap between a treatment clinic and a memory clinic, and often both will coexist as a single clinical entity. A useful distinction is that whereas the memory clinic is primarily concerned with diagnosis and begins with the subjective complaints of memory impairment, the treatment clinic is primarily concerned with drug intervention and begins with diagnosis of Alzheimer's disease.

The Manchester Memory Clinic introduced a treatment clinic when the first ChEI came on to the market in 1997. The intention was to develop a specialist service through which all prescribing and monitoring of ChEIs in South Manchester could be channelled. Much of the activity in a treatment clinic is nurse-led and alongside the management of the clinic, the nurse has specific responsibility for undertaking:

- suitability assessments;
- pre-treatment education;
- assessments of compliance, tolerance and efficacy of pharmacological treatments.

The treatment clinic operates as the mechanism through which the ChEIs can be introduced and subsequently managed. It has four specific functions, namely:

1   to assess suitability for treatment;
2   to initiate prescription of a ChEI;
3   to monitor individual patient's response;
4   to stop treatment when indicated.

Whilst these functions are quite specific, they contain the possibility for memory clinic nurses to become more extensively involved in developing relationships with people who have mild to moderate Alzheimer's disease. Spending time with that person provides an opportunity for nurses to explore with them their understanding of, and reaction to, the diagnosis.

If counselling is primarily about helping people to find and generate their own solutions to problems (Brearley and Birchley 1986), then in post-diagnostic counselling there has to be a dual emphasis upon assisting people to recognize their feelings and helping them to identify their problems, whilst at the same time offering information to assist resolution. This approach makes counselling sessions dynamic and focused around the person's reactions and responses to the provided information.

This approach reflects the foundations of mental health nursing with an emphasis upon using a therapeutic relationship to work in the 'here and now' with that person's immediate problems (Joel and Collins 1978). Also, such nursing activities display a new direction for the role of the memory clinic nurse, moving away from actions intended to help make a medical diagnosis towards helping the person with dementia understand, and cope with, the diagnosis that has been shared.

Whilst the ChEIs are to be welcomed, recognition should be made that these drugs are only the first generation of treatments for Alzheimer's disease. They have only a limited capacity to help, and reported effects are best described as modest (Burns *et al.* 1999). Despite this outcome, the concept of 'treatment' engenders hope in people with dementia and their families. Unfortunately, the development of the new drugs has caused some people to have an overoptimistic and unrealistic expectation about their efficacy. Sometimes people with dementia hope to regain an ability to recommence certain activities, such as driving, or relatives may believe that the medication will return the person to a former self.

Arguably, these high expectations are only natural and part of the human condition. Yet, even with the introduction of a potentially helpful treatment, there remains a certain amount of inevitability about the illness's progression, and if the expectations of the person with dementia and their family remain unrealistic then there will come a time when reality will bite. At such a time, any positivity or hope initially created by earlier expectations may shatter and will be replaced by a negative, or even a catastrophic, reaction.

It is the role of the memory clinic nurse, through the establishment of a therapeutic relationship, to engage in pre-treatment education that will keep expectations to a realistic level. From experience, this is best achieved by being honest with the person with dementia and their family, and by fully discussing the treatment options and their limitations. At present it is simply not possible to promise far-reaching and enduring improvement. A better alternative is a suggestion that a period of stability may be achieved so that expectations can be tied down to a realistic level, whilst also offering some hope for the future.

Effective pre-treatment education also allows the challenging and threatening possibility that the treatment may be stopped, at a future time to be raised. This, again, reflects the clinical reality of treatment and the understanding that the ChEI is not 'for life' and will invariably be stopped as the increasing cholinergic deficit makes it less effective. Again, working from experience, the sharing of such information is best carried out in the context of post-diagnostic work where there is an opportunity to discuss fully the salient issues.

There are various reasons why treatment could be stopped, including poor compliance, poor tolerance, poor efficacy or the changing health status of the person with dementia. Pre-treatment education allows the nurse to raise the patient's awareness of these endpoints and to suggest that they may form a framework for further contact. In the early weeks of treatment, monitoring by the nurse is in essence concerned with compliance and tolerance rather than efficacy, as it is during this period of time that the possibility of side-effects is greatest. The nurse has a responsibility for monitoring and initially responding to reports of side-effects. As such, there is an expectation that the nurse will be familiar with the side-effects of each ChEI and will record an accurate and specific history and also give immediate advice.

The occurrence of side-effects in some people undertaking treatment may be a factor that results in poor compliance. Current recommendations about the use of the ChEIs by the National Institute for Clinical Excellence (2001) states that a mechanism to ensure compliance should be in place before treatment is initiated. The most appropriate compliance mechanism is the permanent presence of a cohabitee, usually spouse or child, who is prepared to accept responsibility for supervising treatment from day to day. Where this is not possible, usually because the person lives alone, then compliance becomes more problematic.

The nurse should also identify potential difficulties associated with compliance as part of the initial suitability assessments when action may then be taken to resolve the situation. Common actions organized to ensure compliance include introducing weekly deliveries of medication in dosette boxes and arranging daily visits from support workers, carers or district nurses in areas where such services are available. Where compliance with treatment occurs and the person with Alzheimer's disease tolerates medication at an effective dose, most treatment clinics would request the GP to take over prescription (Page 2001). The focus of the nurse's role then changes to monitoring the efficacy of treatment over time.

One of the controversial issues about treatment has been about when and how to assess whether treatment is working. Early advice from the Standing Medical Advisory Committee (1998) recommended a review after three months, with a decision made after that time about efficacy. The latest guidance from the National Institute for Clinical Excellence (2001) has accepted that three months is too early and recommends a first review once the patient has been on an effective dose for two to four months.

Various writers, including Adams and Page (2000), have discussed efficacy monitoring in some detail and have suggested that treatment response be assessed across four domains, namely:

1   cognitive functioning;

2   participation in activities of daily living;

3   the frequency and severity of psychopathology;

4   a global impression of change.

There is a wide range of assessment scales that are available to memory clinic nurses that will monitor changes in each domain. The use of standardized rating scales administered to either the person with dementia or their family allows a reasonably objective baseline measure to be taken and compared against over the period of treatment. It is, however, fair to say that objectivity is never absolute. Cognitive assessments may give a false impression as they are often tiring and anxiety provoking for the person with dementia. Caregiver administered scales are essentially second-hand accounts and are therefore inherently flawed by responder bias, although an experienced nurse should be able to identify and help to address this issue.

Carrying out repeat assessments allows the memory clinic nurse to regularly spend time with the person with dementia and their family, assessing not only their response to treatment but also their adjustment to the illness as it progresses. Being with the person and sharing their experience strengthens the relationship between the nurse and the person with dementia, creating trust and encouraging openness in discussions about changing symptoms or difficulties with coping. This approach allows a much clearer picture to emerge of the person's response to treatment.

The development of an open relationship between nurse, person with dementia and family members can be sufficient to offset some of the difficulties inherent in efficacy assessment. In so doing, it becomes possible to obtain a fairly reliable picture of a person's response to treatment, the whole purpose of which is to allow the nurse to be able to provide honest feedback and for the treating team to make informed decisions about the treatment's continuation.

Disengagement needs to be a planned activity, and as the evidence builds about the increasing severity of a person's dementia and the diminishing efficacy of their treatment, then further support should be considered. The role of memory clinic nurse is to recognize this event and to discuss it openly with the person with dementia and their family. Other health and social care professionals can then be introduced who continue the relationships necessary for the later stages of dementia care.

Conclusion

In this chapter, I have discussed the role of the memory clinic nurse and their need to establish effective relationships with people referred to the service. These relationships should be used with people with dementia and their families within assessment and treatment. Much of the work of any memory clinic nurse is with people who have dementia, and Burns *et al.* (2001) have alluded to that experience as part of a journey on which the person with dementia is accompanied by fellow travellers for some or part of the way. This approach to dementia care nursing is developed by Adams (in press) who argues that

> The overarching skill of psychiatric nurses to people with dementia is to get alongside people with dementia and their carers and to act as fellow travellers. To do this, psychiatric nurses draw upon skills developed within professional practice and everyday life.

If this is a concise summary, the memory clinic nurse is certainly prepared to travel some considerable distance, but it is in the early part of the journey that the memory clinic nurse can be of the greatest help.

By working in a preventative and therapeutic way, the nurse is filling the 'service void' that often follows the diagnosis, and is aiming to help the person with dementia and their family to adjust at this early stage to a life-changing event and to a new reality. The hope is that we can act to help those people discover some positivity in the shared experience of dementia, and offer an opportunity to be involved as active participants in determining the kind of life they wish to lead and the kind of future they wish to build.

References

Adams, T. (in press) The person with dementia, in P. Barker (ed.) *Psychiatric and Mental Health Nursing: the craft of caring*. London: Hodder Arnold.

Adams, T. and Page, S.C. (2000) New pharmacological treatments for Alzheimer's disease: implications for dementia care nursing, *Journal of Advanced Nursing*, 31(5): 1183–8.

Agrell, B. and Dehlin, O. (1989) The Clock Drawing Test, *Age and Ageing*, 27: 399–403.

Audit Commission (2000) *Forget Me Not*. London: Audit Commission.

Asvall, J.E. (2001) Can we turn the table on depression?, in A. Dawson and A. Tylee (eds) *Depression: Social and Economic Timebomb*. London: BMJ Publishing Group.

Bartus, R.T., Dean, R.L., Beer, B. and Lippa, A.S. (1982) The cholinergic hypothesis of geriatric memory dysfunction, *Science*, 217: 408–17.

Beattie, B.L., Bucks, R.S. and Mathews, J. (1999) Administrative and organizational aspects, in G. Wilcock, R. Bucks and K. Rockwood (eds), *Diagnosis and Management of Dementia: A Manual for Memory Disorders Teams*. Oxford: Oxford University Press.

Brearley, G. and Birchley, P. (1986) *Introducing Counselling Skills and Techniques*. London: Faber & Faber.

Burns, A., Russell, E. and Page, S. (1999) New drugs for Alzheimer's disease, *British Journal of Psychiatry*, 174: 476–9.

Burns, A., Page, S. and Winter, J. (2001) *Alzheimer's Disease and Memory Loss Explained*. Middlesex: Altman Publishing.

Clark, B., Hartmann, K. and Thorardotter, A. (1997) *Triage: Life in the Emergency Room*. Baltimore, MD: University of Maryland.

Department of Health (2001) *National Service Framework for Older People*. London: The Stationery Office.

Folstein, M.F., Folstein, S.E. and McHugh, P.R. (1975) Mini-Mental State: a practical method for grading the cognitive state of patients for the clinician, *Journal of Psychiatric Research*, 12: 189–98.

Fraser, M. (1992) Memory clinics and memory training, in T. Arie (ed.) *Recent Advances in Psychogeriatrics*, Vol. 2. London: Churchill Livingstone.

Hassiotis, A. and Walker, Z. (2001) Setting up a memory clinic, in Z. Walker and R. Butler (eds) *The Memory Clinic Guide*. London: Martin Dunitz.

Joel, L.A. and Collins, D.L. (1978) *Psychiatric Nursing: Theory and Application*. New York: McGraw-Hill.

Keady, J. and Gilliard, J. (1999) The early experience of Alzheimer's disease: implications for partnership and practice, in T. Adams and C. Clarke (eds) *Dementia Care: Developing Partnerships in Practice*. London: Baillière Tindall.

Kendrick, D.C. (1985) *Kendrick Cognitive Tests for the Elderly*. Windsor: Nelson.

Kitwood, T. (1997) *Dementia Reconsidered: The Person Comes First*. Buckingham. Open University Press.

Lindesay, J. and Morris, J.C. (1999) Introduction, in G. Wilcock, R. Bucks and K. Rockwood (eds) *Diagnosis and Management of Dementia: A Manual for Memory Disorders Teams*. Oxford: Oxford University Press.

Luscombe, G., Brodaty, H. and Freeth, S. (1998) Younger people with dementia: diagnostic issues, effects on carers and use of services, *International Journal of Geriatric Psychiatry*, 13: 323–30.

McKenna, P. and Warrington, E. (1983) *Graded Naming Test Manual*. Windsor: Nelson.

National Institute for Clinical Excellence (2001) *Guidance on the Use of Donepezil, Rivastigmine and Galantamine for the Treatment of Alzheimer's Disease*, Technology Appraisal Guidance No. 19. London: NICE.

Page, S.C. (1998) Understanding and developing the role of the clinical research nurse. Unpublished MSc thesis, University of Salford.

Page, S. (2001) Dementia care and cholinesterase inhibitors, *Professional Nurse*, 16(10): 1421–4.

Pitt, B. (2001) The history of memory clinics, in, Z. Walker and R. Butler (eds) *The Memory Clinic Guide*. London: Martin Dunitz.

Robinson, P., Ekman, S.L., Meleis, I., Winblad, B. and Wahlund, L.O. (1997) Suffering in silence: the experience of early memory loss, *Health Care in Later Life*, 2(2): 107–20.

Spreen, O. and Benton, A.L. (1969) *Neurosensory Centre Comprehensive Examination for Aphasia*. Victoria: Neuropsychological Laboratory, University of Victoria.

Standing Medical Advisory Committee (1998) *The Use of Donepezil for Alzheimer's Disease*. London: Department of Health.

Wilkinson, D. (2000) How effective are cholinergic therapies in improving cognition in Alzheimer's disease?, in J. O'Brien, D. Ames and D.A. Burns (eds) *Dementia*, 2nd edn. London: Arnold.

Wright, M. and Lindesay, J. (1995) A survey of memory clinics in the British Isles, *International Journal of Geriatric Psychiatry*, 10: 379–85.

Yesavage, J.A., Brink, T.L., Rose, T.L. *et al.* (1983) Development and validation of a geriatric depression screening scale: a preliminary report, *Journal of Psychiatric Research*, 17: 37–49.

10

The community mental health nurse role in sharing a diagnosis of dementia

Practice approaches from an early intervention study

Chris Clark

Introduction

As an experienced community mental health nurse (CMHN) working in mental health services for older people, the author has become increasingly aware that many referrals for people with dementia are received at a time of crisis or extremes of carer stress. At this point, the potential benefits of early diagnosis, such as access to information, advice, support and the prescription of anti-dementia drugs, are lost.

There would appear to be several reasons why early referral tends not to happen, but perhaps the most significant is highlighted in the Department of Health (1996) report *Assessing Older People with Dementia Living in the Community* which comments on a 'lack of awareness and negative attitudes towards dementia and ageing amongst professionals and the public' (p. 3). Compounding this, the Audit Commission (2000) argue that many practitioners see no point in the early diagnosis of what they view as an untreatable condition. These findings point towards the need for improved education about the diagnosis and management of dementia among general practitioners (GPs).

This chapter aims to look at the CMHN role in sharing a diagnosis of dementia and early stage support. It will include and reflect on observations from an Early Intervention in Dementia study which had a CMHN (the author) as the principal investigator/research nurse. This study aimed to encourage GPs to be more proactive in their response to the signs of memory impairment by referring people with suspected dementia for specialist assessment and subsequent diagnosis, including access to specialist support, earlier in their consultation history. Case illustrations will be used to communicate the CMHN's role in this process. All of the names used in this chapter are fictitious to protect the confidentiality and anonymity of the people whose experiences are described. The chapter includes brief reflections about the nature of the interventions undertaken with carers, and briefly discusses outcomes from an associated GP survey of attitudes towards the condition.

Early intervention and diagnostic sharing: a review of the literature

Few people with dementia independently seek medical advice for their memory loss and often families are reluctant to bother the GP with a problem they see as part of the normal ageing process (O'Connor *et al.* 1993). In the author's experience, those who do present are more likely to be persuaded to attend by family members who suspect the diagnosis. Paradoxically, if a diagnosis of dementia is then made, a significant percentage of families do not want the resulting diagnosis to be disclosed to the person concerned (Drickamer and Lachs 1992). Reluctance to share a diagnosis appears to revolve around fear of the future, a lack of understanding about dementia and the need to protect their loved one from pain and upset. Carers often talk of a fear of their relative 'giving up' if they were made aware of what the future may hold, whilst others see no useful purpose in the person knowing as 'nothing can be done'; some simply deny the reality of the diagnosis. Similar reactions from carers were cited in *The Right To Know* (Fearnley *et al.* 1997), with the report's authors also voicing a concern that the person with dementia may consider suicide as a response to hearing the news.

Diagnosing Alzheimer's disease and other related dementias remains fraught with difficulty. Drickamer and Lachs (1992) suggest this 'diagnostic uncertainty' is a frequent reason for non-disclosure, and if a diagnosis is shared, it is often conveyed as 'probable' or 'possible'. They also suggest that this element of doubt is all some carers, and the person with dementia, need to deny it. From the authors' point of view, families are often able to deny the existence of the condition until the unexpected consequences of the disease begin to appear. It is often at this point that both the person and their carer, usually in crisis, present to specialist services, having missed the opportunity for preparation and future planning.

Caring for Carers (Department of Health 1999: 2) reinforced the view that support for carers was vital and should include 'being prepared for the task that is going to happen and having the right kind of information'. Indeed a family systems approach which recognizes and takes into account the needs and interdependence of people with (suspected) dementia and their families is especially important as services have tended to focus on one of these groups at the expense of the other.

Many carers and professionals believe that not informing a person of their diagnosis is unjustified, both morally and ethically, as it denies the person the opportunity for future planning, preparation and treatment. Inevitably, people with dementia will experience erosion in their capacity to make decisions and their competency will be compromised. Consequently, the ability of a person to understand their diagnosis and prognosis will vary and depend upon how early a diagnosis is made, and how much the person can understand the reality of events. How the person is then helped to accept and live with the diagnosis requires skill and sensitivity; in the author's opinion the same sorts of principle apply to carers. As Fearnley *et al.* (1997) remind us, the person with dementia also has the right *not* to know their diagnosis and the right to withhold this information from their carers.

Literature and research supports the need for early assessment and diagnosis of dementia and reinforces the benefits to both the person and their carer(s).

Early assessment and interventions with appropriately focused education would appear to offer scope for improved outcomes. The *Carers' (Recognition and Services) Act Practice Guide* (Department of Health 1995: 4) advised that services should 'recognise the value of early intervention and on-going support in preventing deterioration in the carer's and user's welfare'. The importance of early identification of symptoms and ensuring access to appropriate specialist services were key themes running throughout the Audit Commission (2000) report *Forget Me Not.* In England this was embedded in the *National Service Framework for Older People* (Department of Health 2001) which set out clear guidelines recommending early recognition of symptoms, access to specialist care and increased support to GPs and members of the primary health care team.

Best practice would indicate that legal and financial matters should be addressed whilst a person has the ability to understand and the capacity to consent (Fazel *et al.* 1999). The law relating to capacity to consent requires the person to understand and retain information, again reinforcing the necessity for early intervention and diagnosis (Mental Health Act 1983; Law Commission 1995). Quite apart from the legal necessities, most of us, given the opportunity and faced with such an uncertain future, would wish to plan and prepare and make our wishes known. *Tell Me The Truth* (Pratt and Wilkinson 2001) details extracts of interviews made with people with dementia about their experience of receiving a diagnosis. There is an overwhelming expression from the person with dementia of their right to know and be told their diagnosis. Indeed, it would appear that diagnosis depends as much on the willingness of the individual to accept the signs, symptoms and seek answers as it does upon the GP's skills of identification.

Unfortunately, research continues to highlight the complexities involved in:

- early identification and recognition of symptoms (Iliffe 1994; Wolfe *et al.* 1995; Hamilton 2001);

- difficulty in making a diagnosis (O'Connor *et al.* 1988);

- attitudes towards sharing the diagnosis (Drickamer and Lachs 1992);

- to whom the diagnosis is told (Vassilas and Donaldson 1998; Clafferty 1999).

Nurses' role in sharing a diagnosis of dementia

Much of the current literature that exists around the role of the CMHN focuses on their role with carers; implicitly this means that a diagnosis has already been reached (Gunstone 1999; Ho 2000). CMHNs would appear to have a clear role in sharing a diagnosis of dementia and helping those concerned to come to terms with such a life-changing event. However, this role has tended to be more closely associated with other specialist nursing roles, such as in the fields of palliative care and chronic medical conditions, such as Parkinson's disease.

Each of these specialist roles have the 'patient' very much at the centre of the treatment cycle, and interventions tend to be incremental and stage specific. For instance, there is an emphasis on developing an understanding of the disease, confirming acceptance of the prognosis and allowing the person to make choices within the confines of their abilities. As yet, this role has not been crafted into community mental health nursing practice in dementia, although the author is familiar with the practicalities of this approach within her own practice.

The nurse consultant in dementia care was a welcome development but, as Packer (2001: 19) describes, her role has been 'to play a lead role in the development and delivery of an individually focussed service to people with dementia', a role which has included giving advice and training to nurses and leading research.

Where the role of the CMHN has been identified as working with people with the early stages of dementia, it has tended to be in relation to the development of early stage support groups. These give opportunity for people to share their experiences of dementia and in so doing to learn to live with the condition (Yale 1998; Hawkins and Eagger 1999; Cheston and Jones 2000). From this review, Fearnley *et al.* (1997) provide one of the few accounts in which early interventions by the CMHN with people with dementia and their support networks are described. Highlighted in this report is the value attached to the CMHN's developing a close relationship with the client in order to ensure that interventions are personalized and effective. Here, interventions are grouped under four main headings: (1) assessment, (2) counselling, information and education, (3) problem solving and (4) stress reduction. These interventions can also be applied to the carer.

Research would indicate that much needs to be done to further clarify the kinds of intervention that take place between the person with dementia and the CMHN, and in particular identifying which kinds of support are most beneficial and most welcomed. First, people with dementia need to be introduced to help at an earlier stage of their illness. In order to help reinforce and encourage early referral, GPs need convincing of the benefits. In general, GPs appear to accept that helping carers of people with dementia is necessary; however, convincing them of the benefit to people with dementia is more difficult. The study design that follows describes the author's work to promote early referral of people with dementia to specialist services in order for both them and their carers to be 'better supported' throughout their journey.

Study design

The study took place in Doncaster, South Yorkshire, an area covering 224 square miles. The Health Improvement Programme 2000–2003 details population projections, and for Doncaster suggests a total population of 290,100 by mid-2001. Older people, i.e. those over 65 years of age, equate to 15.7 per cent of Doncaster's population (Office for National Statistics 1998). The two-year study on which the remainder of the chapter is based commenced in October 1998 in the Doncaster area.

The Early Intervention in Dementia (EID) study concerned people with dementia and their families, with the aim to promote better self-care and improved family care. The study was based on two assumptions. First, that if care programmes began earlier with effective assessment and intervention, people with dementia and their families would be more involved in decisions about their future and many of the problems associated with the needs of family carers could be ameliorated. To challenge the negative attitudes towards early intervention for people with dementia and their carers, the benefits of earlier interventions needed to be identified and communicated to those able to change this existing practice. Secondly, people with dementia and their carers, if informed about what to expect, and given the right 'tools' to face the challenges that would arise, would be more able to face the future with confidence.

Within the study design the support offered to the person with dementia and their carers fell into three broad categories:

1   Emotional support and advice, including preparing for life with dementia.

2   Liaison and networking.

3   Training and information.

Each of these three categories is more roundly illustrated in the case examples later in the chapter.

The study was submitted to the local research ethics committee for approval, and this was granted in January 1999. The committee raised concerns that the study may 'insist' that people received a diagnosis, and they sought clarification about how consent would be obtained. Adjustments were needed to consent forms to ensure consent was obtained individually from both the person with dementia and the carer. Assurances were also included in the information sheets to the effect that the 'patient' could discontinue their involvement in the study without affecting their rights to treatment and ongoing support.

An introductory letter with accompanying information about the study was sent to every GP in the Doncaster area. In total, 54 practices were contacted and 162 GPs received information. Letters were sent via the practice managers and included an open invitation for the research nurse to attend the surgeries to provide any additional information and to answer any questions about the study design.

Over the next 12 months the author, acting as the research nurse, accepted referrals for 68 people with suspected cognitive impairment. All were aware of the reason for referral. All people referred had given their consent to be seen by a CMHN and all were seen at home. Each of them had a thorough initial assessment including routine blood screening to eliminate the possibility of any underlying or contributing illness. Other tests such as CT scans or chest X-rays were requested as clinically indicated. Anyone seen who presented with unusual symptoms, progression of symptoms, or with clearly defined differential diagnosis, were referred to either the psychiatrist or other member of the community mental health team.

Once a diagnosis was made this was shared with the person concerned. Following the study protocol, with consent of the carer, ongoing interventions then commenced, details of which were recorded in the nursing documentation.

The stressful effects of caregiving on carers were monitored and formally assessed using the General Health Questionnaire 28 (Goldberg and Hillier 1979). Assessment of carers included identification of the most effective, most frequently used coping strategies employed by carers. The Carers' Assessment of Management

Index (CAMI) (Nolan *et al.* 1995) was used for this purpose, although usage was confined to ongoing interventions.

As part of the study design, GPs were asked by questionnaire and random selected interviews about their appreciation of early intervention work with people with dementia. This gave an invaluable insight into GPs' awareness and attitudes towards dementia. Owing to limited space, these latter two aspects of the study are not described in detail.

Study findings

Although interventions with carers were a focus of the study, they were not at the expense of time spent with the person with dementia. For example, it was found that people receiving a diagnosis of dementia described a range of feelings and emotions from shock to disbelief and fear, even when the diagnosis had been suspected. Moreover, diagnoses were not always disclosed sensitively. One gentleman recalled being told by his doctor that, 'The good news was that he had the body of a 40-year-old, and the bad news, the brain of an 80-year-old.' The doctor then went on to tell the gentleman that he did not need to see him again as 'he could do nothing to help'. It is difficult to imagine the range of feelings and emotions this man must have felt. Sadly this experience was not an isolated occurrence. The task of helping a person to come to terms with their diagnosis and to learn to live with it requires a great deal of skill, patience, sensitivity and time.

As the study revealed, denial was a common way of coping with the diagnosis, as were anger and blame. For some people with dementia, this was a transient phase, a way of adjusting; for others not so. Those who constantly battled against 'the dementia' found themselves 'captives' of the disease. Those who accepted and learnt to live with the condition could ultimately make choices about their future, plan, prepare and find hope in the future, as this case example illustrates.

Case example 1

Mr S is a fit and active man. He is 66 years old. He presented himself to his GP complaining of poor short-term memory and poor concentration. His mother had lived with Alzheimer's disease and he was concerned that he too was developing early signs of the disease. Detailed and extensive tests resulted in his being given a diagnosis of probable Alzheimer's disease. He chose to share his diagnosis with his family.

Despite expecting the diagnosis, it still came as a shock, and both he and his family trivialized and negated the memory difficulties, holding on to the possibility that the diagnosis was a mistake. Some weeks later the family were willing to accept the help of a CMHN who helped both Mr S and his wife to share their fears for the future. The CMHN worked alongside them both, in a relationship based on mutual respect and trust. Together they shared concerns, tackled problems, addressed practicalities brought about by diagnosis, shared the highs and lows, and laughed.

Mr S was able to take charge of his life. He read books about dementia, sorted his financial affairs, signed an enduring power of attorney and talked to his family. He and his wife said they had 'shared' his diagnosis and were now determined to share the preparations for the future. At one emotional meeting with the CMHN, Mr S chose to discuss the point at which he felt his wife should no longer care for him and should look for alternative care arrangements. He so wanted her to have a life of her own, which could include him but not be 'consumed' by him.

Towards the end of the intervention period, Mr S is now cared for away from the family home. His wife agreed to share her care when her husband's care needs became too challenging for her to manage at home. With the knowledge that they had previously discussed and shared this eventuality, the pain of the decision was lessened a little. Early intervention and early diagnosis enabled this man to take responsibility for his future in a way that would not have been possible if diagnosis and interventions had begun later.

In this case example, the CMHN used a variety of skills and intervention techniques. At first the nurse became 'a friend' and confidante, using her knowledge about dementia to help the family adjust to their new circumstances. The nurse was also able to deliver information by stages in an individualized and accessible way, ensuring that such information was absorbed and understood before introducing new sources.

Written information was not the only form in which information was supplied; the CMHN employed other forms of communication to reinforce needs. Pictures, analogies, comparisons or more formal literature all served to help the person with dementia and their carer understand the complex nature of the condition.

The relationship that develops with the person with dementia and their carer enables the nurse to decide which of these information sources is appropriate to use, at what point and at what level. For example, a direct question about 'what is dementia' may appear to open a door to communication, but the person with dementia may not be asking for a full explanation of the physiological changes in their brain. In this study, it was found that the use of timely, appropriate information delivered in 'person-friendly' language contributed towards the person's ability to accept, and understand, their condition.

Even when a diagnosis is confirmed and accepted there can be a breakdown in communication between the person with dementia and their carer. Often this occurs in the earlier stages of the condition when the person with dementia is still actively contributing to joint decision making. Appreciating the difficulties of living with a poor short-term memory can be easily overlooked by the family, and the CMHN may need to develop a mediator/facilitator role in this instance, as this next case example illustrates.

Case example 2

Mrs B initially presented to her GP with a combination of symptoms, including apathy, lack of motivation and frequently 'forgetting' things, a picture suggestive of depression. Her GP took a detailed history and decided to refer Mrs B to the consultant psychiatrist for older people for further investigations. Mrs B was formally diagnosed with Alzheimer's disease, early onset. This was totally unexpected and no longer a 'problem' that could be solved with a 'pill', but one that her family would have to learn to understand and adjust to. Soon after diagnosis the family were introduced to a CMHN who helped to develop an understanding of the condition and suggested options for treatment.

Determined to continue their lives as normally as possible, the couple went on holiday with friends. Each evening over dinner they would discuss what they would do and where they would go the following day. Every morning Mrs B took longer and longer to get ready, and just as they were about to leave Mrs B would insist on going to the toilet, making them both later still. Mr B was angry and frustrated by her behaviour and was embarrassed that they were holding the other couple back. On their return home, Mr B said they would not go again because of the upset his wife had caused, and a tearful Mrs B was so sorry she had spoilt the holiday.

The CMHN spoke with Mrs B alone. At first she was unable to offer an explanation for her actions. She was aware of feeling 'uncomfortable' but could not understand why. The nurse encouraged her to explore this feeling and Mrs B was able to identify the source of her anxiety. Each morning Mr B would get up and get ready to go out but his wife could not remember where they were going. She did not know what to wear, what to take and, at the last minute, thought she had better visit the toilet just in case there was not another one for a while. As the days passed, her anxieties grew and their relationship grew more and more tense.

The couple's attempts to dismiss the memory problem and carry on as normal actually provoked a great deal of anxiety and upset. With the CMHN's help, Mrs B was able to offer an explanation for her behaviour to her husband. He had been totally unaware of the nature of Mrs B's distress and was critical of himself for not recognizing this. As a result, Mrs B was encouraged to ask for prompts and reminders from her husband and not to be 'ashamed' to admit that she could not remember. The couple decided that from now on they would keep a diary in which they would record significant events in detail. Not only could this be used as an *aide-mémoire* for Mrs B, but it could also be a useful tool for reminiscence. Recently, the couple have begun to put together a memory book borne out of Mrs B's fear that she may forget some of her most precious memories.

This example demonstrates that the early experience of memory impairment can provoke extreme anxiety and fear when a person is faced with a new situation. In Mr B's attempt to normalize their lives he had underestimated how disabling Mrs B's short-term memory was, with the result that he had contributed to her anxiety. Mrs B had also failed to openly acknowledge her need for reassurance. The CMHN was able to encourage such openness between the couple, which in turn developed into a greater understanding and awareness of her world.

In both of the examples discussed, the importance of the relationship that developed between the person with dementia, their families and the CMHN has been an essential ingredient and has enabled openness and honesty. Traditionally, nurses are encouraged to care but not to show emotion, fearing, perhaps, that this could cloud judgement and make them less objective. Barker (1991) reflects on the historical restraints such attitudes imposed on nurses, and suggests that nurses have fostered a belief that they are unique individuals who can surmount the everyday rules of human engagement. He goes on to suggest that in order to help people realize their capacity for choice, and potential for constructive living, we must let go of the psychological defences which restrict our way of experiencing the world around us.

The relationships with people with dementia and their families often develop quite naturally over time and create feelings of genuineness, empathy and an 'intuitive knowing'. This ability to engage with people with dementia encourages a therapeutic relationship that enables interventions to be truly 'person-led'.

The two examples so far have focused on people who have a diagnosis of dementia, but, as often happens, those referred to specialist service for assessment of memory problems are often unclear that the purpose of the referral is to determine a diagnosis. In these instances the CMHNs can use their skills and knowledge to screen whether or not the person is ready to receive the diagnosis. This dilemma is more fully explained in the third case example.

Case example 3

Mr T was encouraged to visit his GP by his wife who was concerned that he was becoming a 'little forgetful' and making 'silly' mistakes. Mr T was asked if he would like to see a doctor at the hospital, but refused, and only reluctantly agreed to see the CMHN. During the initial contact Mr T was unresponsive to efforts to engage him in conversation. However, with time and patience Mr T was encouraged to share his understanding of why the CMHN was seeing him and what he had been told by his GP. From the ensuing conversation it became clear that Mr T had been aware of the effects of his failing memory for some time, but felt he had managed to 'keep it under control' and hidden from his wife. He also said he felt exposed and vulnerable and afraid he was losing his mind. Mr T was angry at both the exposure and the feelings it released. Despite his initial fears, Mr T was agreeable to further visits at home by the CMHN. During the resulting meetings the CMHN was able to explore Mr T's understanding of his 'condition' and challenge his negative assumptions about living with memory failure, one of which being if he had a diagnosis of dementia he would no longer have any control over his life.

When Mr T chose to seek clarification of his symptoms, which ultimately led to a diagnosis of dementia, he did so having explored the negative effects of receiving a diagnosis as well as the beneficial ones. Being prepared for diagnosis enabled Mr T to come to terms with his future. What could have been a devastating experience ultimately became liberating and empowering.

This example highlights yet another 'unseen' role of the CMHN in sharing a diagnosis of dementia, that of preparing the person (and their carers, as necessary) for a life-changing diagnosis, and ensuring that the path leading to diagnosis is fully understood. It would be unwise for the professional to force people into receiving a diagnosis when they are not ready to hear it.

Interventions with carers

Early intervention in dementia not only provides essential 'early' diagnosis and support for the person with the condition, but provides a timely opportunity to work with the family network. Stress and burnout in carers of people with dementia has received a great deal of attention in the literature (see Gilleard *et al.* 1984; Kinney and Parriss-Stephens 1989; Nolan *et al.* 1990), yet what is not always recognized is the high levels of psychological distress being experienced by carers at this early stage of the caring journey. To explore this phenomenon further, carers of people with dementia who took part in the study were asked to complete the General Health Questionnaire 28 (Goldberg and Hillier 1979) in order to capture a picture of their overall well-being.

How carers are affected by caring

Twenty carers agreed to complete the General Health Questionnaire 28 (GHQ). Carers completed the initial GHQ soon after the initial assessment of the client. Two recognized methods of scoring were used allowing for the overall level of distress to be measured and to identify where the symptoms of distress were most likely to impact on the carer's well-being. Fifteen carers (75 per cent) who completed the GHQ had scores suggesting that the overall level of distress was high and the psychological health of the carers sampled was extremely fragile.

The test was repeated after approximately six interventions. The number of retests (15) was slightly less; however, the overall level of psychological distress measured as experienced by carers in the smaller sample dropped significantly from 80 per cent to 40 per cent. Subsections of the GHQ were also analysed. The GHQ indicated that 80 per cent of the sample group experienced high somatic symptoms, reducing to 46 per cent at retest, and 93 per cent of carers reported high levels of anxiety, reducing to 66 per cent at retest.

Carers' comments on completing the GHQ were equally revealing and suggested that they were not used to focusing on the impact that caring had upon their well-being. They commented that it was a cathartic experience and one which, in some instances, was accompanied by tears. Some comments suggested embarrassment at their GHQ scoring and others apologized: 'I know it's not good' – a comment from a carer who was experiencing high levels of distress; 'You'll be seeing me next'; and 'All the answers are the same' from two carers commenting on what they thought were high scores.

Anecdotal evidence from case studies suggests that providing information to carers greatly reduces levels of anxiety, as does confirmation of the problem. Confirmation of the problem and a diagnosis had the most beneficial effect initially.

> We've struggled on for 18 months not really being sure if he had a memory problem or not. Now we know what's wrong I'm sure we can deal with it, at least we know where to start.
>
> (Mrs W)

Confirmation that 'someone' was taking notice and trying to help provide a sense of relief:

> I knew something was happening but wasn't sure why he was behaving like this. I thought I was imaging the problem with his memory and his mood. I thought I was to blame in some way.
>
> (Mrs W)

Information, written, verbal and sources of information were highly valued. Most carers asked about the illness and its effects, the prognosis and who can help. Once again this underlines the importance of the temporal dimensions in family care, i.e. people usually want to know what the future holds for them in order that they can plan, anticipate, stop worrying unnecessarily, deal with things with greater certitude and knowing that their efforts are recognized and supported by others. This finding is consistent with other research on ways of working with older people with mental health problems or those with dementia and their carers, which stresses the importance of temporality or caregiving stages which are commonly experienced (see, for example, Kobayashi *et al.* 1993; Nolan *et al.* 1996; Ferguson and Keady 2001). Some family carers, on the other hand, only wanted information about the here and now and did not want to look too far ahead.

Carers of people with dementia are highly valued and are the 'backbone' of care in the community. They carry out their case activities under considerable stress and personal hardship and can lose their identity, health and hope for the future. The study demonstrated that psychological distress exists, as much in 'new' carers as in those for whom caring has become a part of their lives. Given the tools to cope, education, support and the most precious commodity of all, time, their psychological distress can be reduced and their feelings of well-being increased. Ultimately their quality of life and that of the person they care for is likely to be enhanced.

Conclusion

The aim of this chapter was not to issue a guide to how to inform someone of a diagnosis of dementia, but to look at how promoting and encouraging early interventions, which could lead to early diagnosis, could ultimately help both the person themself and their carers to accept, adjust and most importantly learn to live with dementia.

The chapter began by introducing the concept of early interventions before looking at the existing literature supporting the need to be more proactive with this client group. There is a paucity of literature around the nurse's role in sharing diagnosis of dementia with the person who has dementia. More research in this area is needed, especially around identification of the process involved and defining the relationships.

The EID study was designed to gain an understanding and gauge the appreciation of the benefits of early interventions, a road that led to working alongside people at the very beginning of their journeys. The chapter highlighted a few examples of where the specialized skills and knowledge of the CMHN were felt to be essential to ensure that process of acceptance and adjustment. Being able to 'share' a diagnosis has far-reaching consequences for the person with dementia and for everyone involved in their life. The examples in this chapter clearly reinforce the need to promote and encourage early identification and earlier interventions, promoting a realistic awareness of a deteriorating condition and the new challenges that this may now raise. Given this knowledge, people with early dementia and their carers have the opportunity to be more involved in decision making and planning for the future, as Drickamer and Lachs (1992: 950) remind us:

> Just as patients with cancer are often afraid of extreme pain near the end of life, many persons with a dementing condition in the early stages have a sense of 'losing their minds' and seek to express their thoughts before losing capacity. Unless they are informed about what is happening to them and are given a chance to express themselves, they will lose that opportunity for ever.

Current practice often results in support being offered at a relatively late stage of the person's condition and with a tendency to be more reactive and 'problem solving' it is often too late to consider some preventative or education-orientated interventions.

The Human Rights Act 1998 sets out standards to ensure that anyone, or anything, that denies or compromises basic human rights can be challenged. Arguably, denying a person the right to diagnosis and treatment is a fundamental breach of this Act, although we have yet to see such a premise tested in court. Until then it is up to the professionals to guide and advocate on behalf of this group, and to value their interventions as much as they are valued by those who receive them.

References

Audit Commission (2000) *Forget Me Not: Mental Health Services for Older People*. London: Audit Commission.

Barker, P. (1991) Finding common ground, *Nursing Times*, 87(2): 37–8.

Cheston, R. and Jones, K. (2000) A place to work it out together, *Journal of Dementia Care*, Nov/Dec: 22–4.

Clafferty, R. (1999) Alzheimer's disease – telling patients their diagnosis, *Progress in Neurology and Psychiatry*, 3: 63–9.

Department of Health (1995) *The Carers' (Recognition and Services) Act. Practice Guide*. London: The Stationery Office.

Department of Health (1996) *Assessing Older People with Dementia Living in the Community: Practical Issues for Social and Health Services*. London: The Stationery Office.

Department of Health (1999) *Caring for Carers: A National Strategy for Carers*. London: The Stationery Office.

Department of Health (2001) *National Service Framework for Older People.* London: The Stationery Office.

Drickamer, M.A. and Lachs, M.S. (1992) Should patients with Alzheimer's disease be told their diagnosis?, *New England Journal of Medicine*, 26(14): 947–51.

Fazel, S., Hope, T. and Jacoby, R. (1999) Assessment of competence to complete advanced directives: validation of a patient centred approach, *British Medical Journal*, 318: 493–7.

Fearnley, K., McLennan, J. and Weaks, D. (1997) *The Right to Know? Sharing the Diagnosis of Dementia.* Edinburgh: Alzheimer's Scotland – Action on Dementia.

Ferguson, C. and Keady, J. (2001) The mental health needs of older people and their carers: exploring tensions and new directions, in M. Nolan, S. Davies and G. Grant (eds) *Working with Older People and their Families: Key Issues in Policy and Practice.* Buckingham, Open University Press.

Gilleard, C.J., Belford, H., Gilleard, E., Whittick, J.E. and Gledhill, K. (1984). Emotional distress amongst the supporters of the elderly mentally infirm, *British Journal of Psychiatry*, 145: 172–7.

Goldberg, D.P. and Hillier, V.F. (1979). A scaled version of the General Health Questionnaire, *Psychological Medicine*, 9: 139–45.

Gunstone, S. (1999) Expert practice: the interventions used by a community mental health nurse with carers of dementia sufferers, *Journal of Psychiatric and Mental Health Nursing*, 6: 21–7.

Hamilton, L. (2001) Dementia: early diagnosis is vital for best care, *Nursing Times*, 97(9): 41–2.

Hawkins, D. and Eagger, S. (1999) Group therapy, sharing the pain of diagnosis, *Journal of Dementia Care*, 7(5): 12–13.

Ho, D. (2000) Role of community mental health nurses for people with dementia, *British Journal of Nursing*, 9(15): 986–91.

Iliffe, S. (1994) Why GPs have a bad reputation, *Journal of Dementia Care*, Nov/Dec: 24–5.

Kinney, J.M. and Parriss-Stephens, M. (1989) Caregiving Hassles Scale: assessing the daily hassles of caring for a family member with dementia, *The Gerontologist*, 29(3): 328–32.

Kobayashi, S., Masaki, H. and Noguchi, M. (1993) Developmental process: family caregivers of demented Japanese, *Journal of Gerontological Nursing*, 19(10): 7–12.

Law Commission (1995) *Mental Incapacity*, Report No. 231. London: The Stationery Office.

Mental Health Act (1983). London: The Stationery Office.

Nolan, M.R., Grant, G. and Ellis, N.C. (1990) Stress is in the eye of the beholder: reconceptualising the measurement of carer burden, *Journal of Advanced Nursing*, 15: 544–55.

Nolan, M., Keady, J. and Grant, G. (1995) CAMI: a basis for assessment and support with family carers, *British Journal of Nursing*, 14(14): 822–6.

Nolan, M., Grant, G. and Keady, J. (1996) *Understanding Family Care – A Multi-dimensional Model of Caring and Coping.* Buckingham: Open University Press.

O'Connor, D.W., Pollitt, P.A., Hyde, J.B. *et al.* (1988) Do general practitioners miss dementia in elderly patients?, *British Medical Journal*, 297: 1107–10.

O'Connor, D.W., Fertig, A., Grande, J. *et al.*(1993) Dementia in general practice: the practical consequences of a more positive approach to diagnosis, *British Journal of General Practice*, 43: 185–8.

Office for National Statistics (1998) cited in *Health Improvement Plan for Doncaster 2000–2003*, p. 88: 2.6.

Packer, T. (2001) A nurse consultant in dementia care, *Signpost to Older People and Mental Health Matters*, 15(3): 19–23.

Pratt, R. and Wilkinson, H. (2001) *'Tell Me The Truth': The Effect of Being Told the Diagnosis of Dementia from the Perspective of the Person with Dementia.* London: Mental Health Foundation.

Vassilas, C.A. and Donaldson, J. (1998) Telling the truth: what do general practitioners say to patients with dementia or terminal cancer?, *British Journal of General Practice*, 48: 1081–2.

Wolfe, L.E., Woods, J.P. and Reid, J. (1995) Do general practitioners and old age psychiatrists differ in their attitudes to dementia?, *International Journal of Geriatric Psychiatry*, 10: 63–9.

Yale, R. (1998) *Developing Support Groups For Individuals With Early-stage Alzheimer's Disease*. Maryland: Health Professions Press.

11

Group therapy
The double bonus effect of intervention for people with dementia and their carers

Kath Lowery and Michelle Murray

Introduction

Group interventions are heralded as a constructive means of working with people with the potential to address the psychosocial and cognitive domains (Jones *et al.* 2002). Over the past few decades, adopting this therapeutic approach has increasingly become an established and acceptable way of offering interventions for people with dementia and their carers. In addition to addressing therapeutic need, it has the potential to reverse the social exclusion that people with dementia and their carers may encounter.

There are a number of key issues around establishing these groups, which include its composition, who leads the group and the nature of the intervention. Driving the composition of the group is the purpose and objective of the group. The group could be composed of people with dementia themselves, their family members or a mix of both. For example, in a family therapy approach in a clinical setting, this would include the person with dementia as well as immediate family members, whereas Corbeil *et al.* (1999) worked in dyads in a group setting with the person with dementia and their key carer.

The purpose and membership of the group underpin decisions about the type of intervention used. There is a wide range of interventions available and well established with people with dementia that can be managed through group activity. These include reminiscence therapy, reality orientation, drama, art and music therapy. Interestingly, a more structured psychotherapeutic approach is gaining credibility, which is perhaps as a result of earlier diagnoses, a more person-centred approach to dementia care and a shift away from the legacy of Freud who considered psychotherapy unsuitable for older people. Hausman (1992) illustrates a psychodynamic approach for people with dementia, whilst Teri and Gallagher-Thompson (1991) take a more behaviouralist approach, both of which encompass the psychological needs that occur in dementia. Equally, there is an array of interventions that are appropriate for group work with carers, including psychosocial support, educational, psychotherapeutic and cognitive behaviour therapy. These examples given for both carers and people with dementia are not exhaustive but merely illustrate the diversity and wealth of strategies available in the field of dementia care.

Important consideration needs to be given to who will lead the groups, and if it is to be a professional then it is necessary to ensure that they are equipped to fulfil the role. More important than any specific disciplinary background, is that they have confidence in their skill and expertise to manage and facilitate the nature of the intervention and the membership of the group. A carer or person with dementia may be the most appropriate person to take the lead if this is in keeping with the nature of the intervention and group composition. In a culture of both self-help and service user involvement, reliance on personal expertise and experience may enhance therapeutic processes within the group. Appropriate training, support and supervision are critical to attain both quality and enrichment for the group and its leader, irrespective of their lay or professional position.

In group therapy environments for people with dementia and carers, a social milieu may be achieved alongside the opportunity to enhance personal or cognitive skills and or addressing psychological needs. Jones *et al.* (2002: 22) describe a group for people with dementia as

> . . . a place where members open up, share their experiences, and learn coping strategies from one another. Furthermore, a group can be somewhere which allows the person with dementia to let go and to begin to learn to adjust and participate in the grieving process.

This chapter describes examples of group therapy in the community with two discrete groups: one with carers applying principles of cognitive behavioural therapy and the other exemplifying support groups for younger people with early onset dementia that encompass activity and family therapies.

Cognitive behaviour therapy as a group intervention for carers of people with dementia

Carers, who may be either family or close friends, are frequently fundamental to the care of the person with dementia, often delaying, or in some cases preventing, the need for institutional care. Their activity has long since been recognized as the cornerstone of care in the community providing support to the five out of six people with dementia living at home (Gilhooly 1986). Importantly, it has also been established that this caring role is generally taken on by either a spouse or a child (Parker and Lawton 1994), and consequently may be borne alone and with little perceived support. Not surprisingly, carers have received much attention from both the academic research arena and clinical staff who seek both to understand the impact of this role and to learn how carers can best be supported. Such is the acknowledgement that carers have their own distinct needs and may require support, that they have a right to their own individual assessment that is reinforced with the Carers (Recognition and Services) Act 1995. Current and projected demographic trends evidence a growing older population with an exponential rise in the number of people with dementia and a corresponding demand for an increased number of carers. Within the clinical practice role of community mental health nurses (CMHNs) there is a need to be equipped to offer proactive evidence-based interventions and strategies to minimize the potential negative effects of the caring role.

Evidencing carer distress/burden/impact on well-being and outcome

Current descriptions of outcomes for carers of people with dementia predominately lie within the psychological domain, with recognition of consequent impact on social, financial and physical health. The 36 Hour Day (Mace *et al.* 1999) comprehensively portrays the demanding role of the carer, leaving little doubt about the burden or stress that may be incurred. A survey by the Alzheimer's Disease Society (1993) provided worrying evidence of the extent of the detrimental impact of caring, with 97 per cent of carers who responded having physical complaints or psychological distress. The gravity of the psychological disturbance may be diverse, varying from stress and tiredness to depression. Manifestation of depression has been identified in numerous studies, with prevalence rates most commonly between 25 per cent and 50 per cent (Williamson and Shultz 1993; Coope *et al.* 1995; Lowery *et al.* 2000).

Clarifying the scope of effects on carers cannot be considered in isolation and it is important to elicit the factors in the trajectory of the experience of caring that have been identified as predicating burden, distress and depression. These include one or more of the following:

- Lack of informal support (Zarit *et al.* 1980).

- Behavioural and/or psychological symptoms of the person with dementia. These include withdrawal and apathetic inactivity (Greene *et al.* 1982; Logiudice *et al.* 1995), mood disturbance (Donaldson *et al.* 1998), restlessness (Gallagher-Thompson *et al.* 1992), psychosis (Donaldson *et al.* 1998) and aggression (Gilleard *et al.* 1982).

- Multiple care needs and restriction of carer opportunities (Gilleard *et al.* 1984).

- The relationship between the carer and the person with dementia. These include age, coping styles and gender (Saad *et al.* 1995; Yee and Schulz 2000).

Cumulatively this knowledge has underpinned the development of interventions for carers, and continues to do so.

Group interventions with carers

Perhaps the most commonly used group intervention with carers has been that of an initial series of meetings sharing information followed on with regular meetings for informal support. The information meetings may involve invited speakers to talk to carers on a range of issues including: 'dementia', 'coping/dealing with problem behaviour', 'benefits' and 'taking care of yourself'. The premise behind this is that giving the information will enable the carer to have better information and understanding whilst simultaneously offering a degree of support from both the professionals running the group and the other carers. A less common, but more measurably successful, approach to education, was that of Brodaty and Gresham (1989) involving a ten-day training programme for carers in the hospital setting. Whilst these groups have their place, they have not consistently been found to impact significantly on the depression, stress and burden that carers frequently experience (Brodaty *et al.* 1994).

Oswald *et al.* (1999) reported promising outcomes from their psycho-educational research, which involved a number of workshops with specific skills training for carers about the person they were caring for, for example memory work and problem solving, information on the dementia disease process. The authors acknowledge the design had limitations and further work is needed to add clarity to questions raised in the study, not least the delayed effect or response to the intervention.

Cognitive behaviour therapy as an intervention for carers of people with dementia

Of the many changes that can occur when caring for someone with dementia who is experiencing diminishing cognitive capacity, there can be a changing psychological and behavioural profile in addition to declining functional abilities. This places practical, tangible demands on the carer that combine with the unpredictability and uncertainty of changes and challenges that occur throughout the progression of dementia. The coping strategies and attribution style of carers (Saad *et al.* 1995; Donaldson *et al.* 1998) are important indicators of carer susceptibility to negative outcomes or increased burden as a result of their caring role.

All this indicates that there may be potential value in working with carers to facilitate application of more positive coping strategies and attribution style, cognitive behaviour therapy (CBT) promising one such approach. Previous CBT intervention with carers, in a one-to-one partnership with a psychologist, provided evidence of positive outcomes for the carers (Marriot *et al.* 2000), reinforcing the potential utility of CBT for carers of people with dementia. The costly nature of one-to-one therapy with a specialized practitioner is unlikely to be practical and it may be more prudent to offer this as a group intervention. That said, the more generic application of CBT is developed further by Peter Ashton in Chapter 7 of this book.

The Newcastle CBT intervention

In Newcastle-upon-Tyne, a project was developed with the local mental health trust and the local branch of the Alzheimer's Society to develop a CBT group for carers. The focus of the group was educational for the carers and provided an opportunity for collaborative working across agencies and with carers. An experienced nurse trained in CBT methods delivered the sessions to the group with supervision from a senior specialist therapist. An Alzheimer's Society staff member also attended to gain experiential learning in this technique.

Recruitment to the group was through both self-referral to the local Alzheimer's Society and professionals, for example CMHNs and day hospital staff. Twenty carers were invited to attend one of two groups for eight one-and-a-half hour sessions one evening per week. The group was also invited to 'booster' sessions at six-monthly intervals to review progress, revise and reinforce techniques. One person dropped out after attending one session.

To support the carers, attendance arrangements were made with the Alzheimer's Society for care support at home and, where necessary, transport was also provided. The Alzheimer's Society provided the venue, and relatives who accompanied a carer were able to access a day care place at the venue for the duration of the CBT session.

A manual was produced to standardize the intervention and included the following topic area information on dementia: the illness; common problems/changes in behaviour; taking care of yourself. The contents of the sessions were focused on teaching carers to understand the link between an action or event leading to biased or negative thinking and the resultant damaging emotions, and, importantly, how to break these links. For example, the person with dementia may exhibit unwanted or difficult behaviour triggering carers' thoughts and biases (for instance, 'they know what they're doing') leading to detrimental consequences of being a carer and an impact on the carer's emotions (for instance, self-doubt, distress). Carers were taught to keep diaries to identify their emotions and responses about specific situations and the contributing biased thinking that fed the negative emotions. The knowledge that they gained in relation to the process of dementia enabled them to replace biased thinking with evidence. A theoretical example is outlined below.

Mr X (person with dementia) always has the same clothes on and looks dishevelled. Carer A may frequently tell Mr X to change or buy new clothes with no result, leading to thoughts and biases which may include:

- Feeling ashamed or 'shown up'.
- He's getting lazy, he just neglects himself.
- He just wants me to do everything for him.
- He doesn't appreciate me, he's doing it deliberately to have a go at upsetting and annoying me.

During these thoughts, carer A may feel burdened and responsible, with no personal time. This results in stress and distress and may lead to feelings of guilt about not being a 'good' carer. Being informed about the dementia process allows a different set of knowledge-based thoughts to be added to the repertoire, for example:

- He might not remember that he's worn the clothes or realize the ones he has got on are dirty. If he knew he would be so ashamed.
- He might not recognize the new clothes that I've bought him as his.
- He might be depressed.

These latter thoughts are based on evidence, are explanatory and are less blame-centred, leading to recognition that there is a difficulty which may benefit from an active or different approach. Developing a strategy to this situation may include involving Mr X and carer A in selecting clean clothes together the night before or in the morning, or, if Mr X, has paid carers reviewing their input to support hygiene and changes of clothing.

Within dementia, care problems are unlikely to resolve. They may change as the illness progresses, but it is important to respond in the here and now for both carers and the person with dementia. In the situation described above, it is the carer's way of thinking and emotional response that shifts, but there is the opportunity to rethink and respond to the event to further maximize care for the person with dementia. Although dishevelled clothing is not an obvious 'risk' in terms of health care, to the carer it may reflect an external measure of their own competency.

In the CBT session, carers were able to work through similar problems, developing their skills in recognizing bias thinking and challenging their responses to situations. As part of the process, carers were encouraged to use their diaries between sessions to test the techniques and review them at the following session. Attendees at the group were not pre-screened to assess their ability to assimilate this approach, which purist therapists would perhaps advocate, and generally this did not appear to adversely affect the group or their perceived benefits.

Anecdotally the group was successful, with carers able both to demonstrate their application of CBT and to comment on overall improvement in their feeling of well-being. Commonly those who attended identified how they were able to cope better, felt less pent up and were able to keep things in perspective. Additionally, the group continued to meet long after its planned duration at the request of the members: itself evidence of its success.

Developing the role of CBT

Using CBT as a group intervention with carers of people with dementia is in its infancy. There is a paucity of literature surrounding its effectiveness, but that should not detract from the evidence to support developing CBT as a group intervention for carers. James *et al.* (2001), who provided the clinical expertise to the Newcastle CBT group, succinctly describe the value of CBT as 'distinguishing fact from fiction', so enabling the carer to deal with actual events. Intentionally challenging biased thinking allows for attribution shift and healthier coping styles.

Support groups for carers are a frequent and established way of working with carers. Group CBT does not supersede these groups but offers a strategy and technique for carers to cope with the difficulties that often accompany their role. Within the theoretical evidence base of knowledge about the stress and burden of the caring role, the CBT group addressed important issues. Contributing factors such as lack of knowledge and information, behavioural and psychological disturbances were addressed through the educational aspect of the group. Lack of an informal support network and peer support was remedied through the connections made between group members, although this was secondary to the key agenda of the group.

To date, there is no consistent evidence that group interventions are effective for carers, one exception being Brodaty's training intervention and group therapy (Brodaty *et al.* 1994; Seymour 1999). Seymour (1999) reported positive outcomes for carers, particularly offspring of people with dementia, using a family support model drawing on attachment and loss. One of the important and perhaps unique aspects of this study was that carers were recruited within six months of the person they were caring for being diagnosed with dementia. Early stages of dementia can be particularly stressful for both carers and the individual as it is a time of great change and adjustment. With the advent of memory clinics and a drive for earlier diagnosis, carers are likely to be met much earlier in the disease process than previously. It would seem wise to equip carers as early as possible to use positive methods to overcome the difficulties encountered as a carer.

Evidencing clinical practice with carers carries many methodological challenges. It is perhaps wise to remember the old adage 'one man's meat is another man's poison'. Carers are individuals with unique needs, and interventions are likely to be more successful if they are tailored to each carer's needs at that point in time. Further clarity is required around those interventions that have a delayed response to outcomes: Do we need to question the selection of outcomes? Do new strategies of problem-solving skills acquired through CBT take time to be integrated into a carer's knowledge before they are applied? What is the process of carer adaptation? A further positive aspect of CBT is that it can be applied outside the caring role so that people are being prepared with life skills not just ones that relate to caring.

Groups for younger people with dementia

A pioneer in support groups for people with dementia, Robyn Yale, opens her book *Developing Support Groups for Individuals with Early-stage Alzheimer's Disease* (Yale 1998) with a quotation:

> It helps to know you aren't alone – listening to how others deal with similar problems . . . It makes me feel much better to know there are people like me.

Although much of the research on dementia has been focused upon the carer (stress levels and the impact of caring) and the person with dementia (symptomatology and neurophysiology), there is little research seeking to understand the perceptions, views and experiences of those people with a diagnosis of dementia. When people have received a diagnosis of dementia they can often be viewed as different from the person they were previously. The role of the person changes, as do their abilities. The younger person with a diagnosis of dementia often no longer performs many of the tasks we take for granted in our everyday lives. For most people, the ability to drive, cook, mind the children, budget our finances is just an everyday occurrence that we think little about. Asen (1995) suggests that daily life is full of routines, many of which are comforting and reassuring. When a person has an impairment of their memory they are often no longer able to participate in their routines and doomed to fail at obstacles set before them. This can be applied to many aspects of an individual's life, such as family, social and work life.

The concept of personhood introduced in the early 1990s by Kitwood and Bredin (1992) acknowledged the importance of listening to and communicating with people with dementia, creating environments that promote personhood, enabling individuals to make informed choices and involving them in decisions concerning their needs and care. As Packer outlined in Chapter 8, it is an approach that has allowed services to overcome some of the more dismissive aspects of understanding dementia as solely a physiological experience. Group settings offer a social context to therapeutic interventions with people with dementia and so respect wider dimensions of living with dementia.

Group work can take many forms, and this section describes three ways of working with the younger person with dementia. As described earlier, it is essential to determine what you are setting out to do, for instance a family therapy approach may have different theoretical frameworks to draw upon and different structures, some working as a multi-disciplinary team whereas other clinicians choose to work alone (Marriott 2000).

The Manchester support groups

Manchester's service for younger people with dementia is multi-agency and the team recognizes how people value sharing their experiences with each other. The openness and frankness of the discussions that take place have often surprised carers. This openness has always been encouraged, although on occasions some service users cannot always participate appropriately. They may be disinhibited or have little or no insight into their condition. The ability to share experiences and the value of this is reiterated in the work of Yale (described in Cox and Keady 1999). Yale recognizes that 'they are primarily relieved to meet one another . . . as they forge a common bond in facing and coping with AD'. Yale goes on to suggest that 'people often have similar feelings, concerns and experiences to share regardless of how old they are when they develop dementia'.

In Manchester, the group focused initially on those with Alzheimer's disease, so that there were similarities between group members. People with a multi-infarct dementia often have marked difficulties with motivation and lethargy although fine motor movement and visuo-spatial awareness are rarely affected. The person with an alcohol-related dementia might have very poor short-term memory problems and poor motivation. Both of these groups have very different needs that would require attention in a support group.

Group 1

The first support group to run was facilitated by a CMHN and a speech and language therapist, each with experience of working with people with a young onset dementia and their families. The series of sessions was run for a group of four people who had a diagnosis of Alzheimer's disease who appeared to have developed a common bond whilst receiving day care. Offering a more formalized session provided the group with confidentiality and support. The individuals that were chosen were all able to give their consent to participate and it was made clear that if an individual felt uncomfortable at any point they could withdraw immediately.

Within the facility used for day care there was a video link. For the purpose of evaluation, all group members and their carers were asked to sign a video consent form and each session was video recorded. The sessions were run once a week, with different topics explored at each session. The topics were identified in the first session by the group members and were as follows:

- Group and individual goal setting
- Anxiety, confidence and coping strategies
- Communication in different situations and with different people
- Positive thinking and taking each day as it comes
- Difficult situations
- Evaluation – setting new objectives.

Group 2: the activity group

This group was introduced to evaluate the person with dementia in an informal setting. It is available one session a week and is facilitated by an occupational therapy technician. The benefits of such groups are to experience a feeling of achievement and working towards a goal.

It is essential to identify and plan each process so that individual needs can be taken into account. Some individuals need assistance with complex tasks whereas others may need verbal prompting only. Two members of staff run the group. Where possible it is useful for the planners to stay involved throughout the duration of each project to promote a feeling of ownership and commitment to and for the younger person with dementia.

The main aims of activity groups are:

- *Social.* For many people life is hectic and lacks the scope to explore non-work-related activities. The group is designed to give the younger person with a dementia an opportunity to participate in or develop hobbies that they may not have previously had time to do. It is also a useful way to assess an individual's ability to communicate and interact with others. It offers positive rewards and an end product.
- *Psychological.* In particular the activity group sought to affect mood and behaviour, self-esteem, levels of anxiety and concentration.
- *Neurological.* The activity group provides the opportunity for people to relearn and maintain skills around hand–eye coordination, short-term memory and recall (for example, following instructions), fine motor movements and visuo-spatial awareness.

Some examples of activity groups run include: mosaics, horticulture, seasonal activities, for example Christmas decorations, silkscreen paintings, woodwork, painting, pottery and stained glass painting.

Group 3: the family therapy group

Marriott (2000) recognizes that family relationships are important, and family therapy approaches recognize this by working with the individual and their family system rather than working with the individual alone. The family team that was established in 1990 has experience of working with adults over the age of 65 with a mental health issue. In 1998 the team also began to see people with a young onset dementia. There are many different family teams, each often working very differently. The Manchester team has a multi-disciplinary membership consisting of a consultant old age psychiatrist, psychologists, social workers and nurses. To date, 11 people with a young onset dementia have been referred to the family clinic. The reasons for this have been: family conflict following change of role, life events, caring responsibilities; marital difficulties; bereavement; adjusting to illness; drug and alcohol problems; and stresses and strains of caring.

Marriott (2000) describes the roles of family team members as two members of the team – co-therapists – who meet with the family in one room, and the remaining team members who constitute a support team. The support team sits in a separate room and is connected by a video and telephone link. One of the members of the support team has the role of peer consultant whose responsibilities are to coordinate the session, to write letters to referring and other agencies, and to pass messages using the telephone link from the support team to the therapists during the family meeting. The team aims to offer a unified approach, where the service complements that offered by other parts of the mental health service. Other agencies are often invited to observe or participate in sessions where it is deemed helpful.

Conclusion

The boundaries of dementia care are widening, with an emphasis on hearing the voices of those with dementia and their carers. It is no longer acceptable to dismiss dementia as a disease where little or nothing can be done. With the growing acceptance of social psychology and person-centred care, CMHNs have the opportunity to enable people with dementia and their carers to engage in a range of therapeutic activities which may be either to resolve specific problems or to enhance their sense of well-being through social participation. Group work as a vehicle to deliver therapeutic intervention offers the potential to achieve both, a double bonus in a world where there are perhaps few positives. Undoubtedly, some people with dementia may reach a stage where conventional or adapted group methods may no longer be appropriate, but for those for whom they are, we should be making every effort to discover what works and integrating this into routine clinical practice.

References

Alzheimer's Disease Society (1993) *Deprivation and Dementia*. London: Alzheimer's Disease Society.

Asen, E. (1995) *Family Therapy for Everyone. How to get involved*. London: BBC Books.

Brodaty, H. and Gresham, M. (1989) Effect of a training programme to reduce stress in carers of patients with dementia, *British Medical Journal*, 299: 1375–9.

Brodaty, H., Roberts, K. and Peters, K. (1994) Quasi-experimental evaluation of and educational model for dementia caregivers, *International Journal of Geriatric Psychiatry*, 9: 195–204.

Coope, B., Ballard, C.G., Saad, K. *et al.* (1995) The prevalence of depression in the carers of dementia suffers, *International Journal of Geriatric Psychiatry*, 10: 237–42.

Corbeil, R.C., Quayhagen, M.P. and Quayhagen, M. (1999) Intervention effects on dementia caregiving interaction: a stress adaptation modelling approach, *Journal of Aging and Health*, 11(1): 79–95.

Cox, S. and Keady, J. (eds) (1999) *Younger People with Dementia: Planning, Practice and Development*. London: Jessica Kingsley.

Donaldson, C., Tarrier, N. and Burns, A. (1998) Determinants of carer stress in Alzheimer's disease, *International Geriatric Psychiatry*, 13: 248–56.

Gallagher-Thompson, D., Brookes, J.O., Bliwise, D. *et al.* (1992) The relations among caregiver stress, 'sundowning' symptoms, and cognitive decline in Alzheimer's disease, *Journal of American Geriatric Society*, 40: 807–10.

Gilhooly, M.L.M (1986) Senile dementia: factors associated with caregiver's preference for institutional care, *British Journal of Medical Psychology*, 56: 165–71.

Gilleard, C.J., Boyd, W.D. and Watt, G. (1982) Problems for caring for the elderly mentally infirm at home, *Archives of Gerontology Geriatrics*, 1: 151–7.

Gilleard, C.J., Gilleard, E., Gledhill, K. and Whittick, J. (1984) Caring for the elderly mentally infirm at home: a survey of the supporters, *Journal of Epidemiology and Community Health*, 38: 319–25.

Greene, J.G., Smith, R., Gardiner, M. and Timbury, G.C. (1982) Measuring behavioural disturbance of elderly demented patients in the community and its effect on relatives: a factor analytic study, *Age and Ageing*, 11: 121–6.

Hausman, C. (1992) Dynamic psychotherapy with elderly demented patients, in G. Jones and B.M.L. Miesen (eds) *Care-giving in Dementia,* Vol. 1. London: Routledge.

James, I., Powell, I. and Reichelt, K. (2001) Cognitive therapy for carers: distinguishing fact from fiction, *Journal of Dementia Care*, 9(6): 24–6.

Jones, K., Cheston, R. and Gilliard, J. (2002) Sharing problems through group psychotherapy, *Journal of Dementia Care*, 10(3): 22–3.

Kitwood, T. and Bredin, K. (1992) Towards a theory of dementia care: personhood and well-being, *Ageing and Society*, 12: 269–87.

Logiudice, D., Waltrowicz, W. and McKenzie, S. (1995) Prevalence of dementia among patients referred to an aged assessment team and associated stress in their carers, *Australian Journal of Public Health*, 19: 275–9.

Lowery, K., Mynt, P., Aisbett, J. *et al.* (2000) Depression in the carers of dementia sufferers: a comparison of the carers of patients suffering from dementia with Lewy bodies and the carers of patients with Alzheimer's disease, *Journal of Affective Disorders*, 59: 61–5.

Mace, N.L., Rabins, P.V. and McHugh, P.R. (1999) *The 36-Hour Day: A Family Guide to Caring for Persons with Alzheimer's Disease, Related Dementing Illnesses and Memory Loss in Later Life*, 3rd edn. Baltimore, MD: Johns Hopkins University Press.

Marriott, A. (2000) *Family Therapy with Older Adults and their Families*. Bicester: Winslow Press.

Marriot, A., Donaldson, C., Tarrier, N. and Burns, A. (2000) Effectiveness of cognitive-behavioural family interventions in reducing burden of carers in care of patients with Alzheimer's disease, *British Journal of Psychiatry*, 176: 557–62.

Oswald, S.K., Hepburn, K.W., Caron, W. *et al.* (1999) Reducing caregiver burden: a randomised psychoeducational intervention for caregivers of persons with dementia, *The Gerontologist*, 39(3): 299–303.

Parker, G. and Lawton, D. (1994) *Different Types of Care, Different Types of Carer: Evidence from the General Household Survey*. London: The Stationery Office.

Saad, K., Hartman, J., Ballard, C. *et al.* (1995) Coping by the carers of dementia suffered, *Age and Ageing*, 24: 495–8.

Seymour, J. (1999) *Caring and Coping with Loss in Dementia: A Support Training Package for Carers*, Abstract. Newcastle: United Kingdom Dementia Research Group.

Teri, L. and Gallagher-Thompson, D. (1991) Cognitive-behavioural interventions for treatment of depression in Alzheimer's patients, *The. Gerontologist*, 31(3): 413–16.

Williamson, G.M. and Schulz, R. (1993) Coping with specific stresses in Alzheimer's disease caregiving, *The Gerontologist*, 33: 747–55.

Yale, R. (1998) *Developing Support Groups for Individuals with Early-stage Alzheimer's Disease*. Maryland: Health Professions Press.

Yee, J. and Schulz, R. (2000) Gender differences in psychiatric morbidity among family caregivers: a review and analysis, *The Gerontologist*, 40(2): 147–64.

Zarit, S.H., Reever, K. and Bach-Peterson, J. (1980) Relatives of the impaired elderly: correlates of feelings of burden, *The Gerontologist*, 20: 649–55.

12

Psychosocial interventions with family carers of people with dementia

Helen Pusey

Introduction

The term 'psychosocial interventions' has been attached to a myriad of activities throughout health care literature. The purpose of this chapter is to unravel the concept of psychosocial interventions and explore the possibilities of utilizing a specific component, family intervention, to reduce carer stress and improve the quality of life for people with dementia.

The impact of caring for someone with dementia has been well documented. There are numerous reports of high levels of strain, distress and depression among carers (Knight *et al.* 1993). It is more stressful than providing physical care alone (Davis 1992) and those caring for someone with dementia experience higher rates of depression and poorer physical health than population norms (Schulz *et al.* 1990). Carers are often overwhelmed by the enormity of their role and the non-cognitive features of dementia such as psychotic symptoms, depression and behaviour disturbance are the most demanding to deal with (Donaldson *et al.* 1998).

Historically there has been little specialized support for carers, with the responsibility resting predominantly with the community mental health nurse (CMHN) allocated to the care of the person with dementia. However, there appears to be no clear theoretical model used by CMHNs providing support for carers (Carradice 1999). Although there is an absence of a framework in nursing, there have been numerous attempts to develop strategies to support carers of people with dementia. These have been undertaken by a range of health and social care practitioners utilizing a range of interventions. The earliest models were support groups that focused on general education (Bourgeois *et al.* 1996), but this has expanded to include a broad range of approaches including stress management, enhancing social networks and emotional support. These interventions have been delivered in both group and individual formats. Despite this substantial amount of research activity, a model widely accepted and applied by nurses is still lacking. This means that CMHNs are likely to be utilizing any number of different approaches, many of which may lack a research evidence base. This position is cause for concern and clearly contradicts the notion of clinical governance that states that mental health professionals adopt practice that is underpinned by an evidence base (Department of Health 1998). Clinical governance requires practitioners to demonstrate they are using the most clinically effective treatment strategies for service users. In addition, carers have the right to expect access to professionals who will deliver the most effective interventions to alleviate their stress.

CMHN interventions

There has been little published work that has assessed the efficacy of mental health nursing in any speciality. This question was considered by Carradice (1999) in her qualitative study of CMHNs in dementia care. She explored the evidence of mental health nurses' efficacy and found it to be limited. Outcome studies have shown mental health nurses to be less effective than social workers (Sheppard 1991) and there has also been concern expressed about mental health nurses using interventions shown to be ineffective, for example client-centred counselling and relaxation training for agoraphobia (Gournay *et al.* 1993). Within dementia care the picture is similarly bleak. Matthew (1990) found that CMHNs had no systematic plan of action for treatment and carers' needs were considered only when a crisis arose. Furthermore the nurses had only a minimal effect on enabling carers to receive information and the carers themselves had little confidence in their nurses.

Carradice (1999) suggests that the lack of a theoretical model is a possible explanation for the dearth of demonstrable effectiveness of mental health nurses. Within dementia care this has been explored by Adams (1999) who observed the practice of four nurses in dementia care. He concluded that the nurses were not using any specific theoretical framework. Carradice (1999) went on to study eight nurses using interpretative phenomenological analysis to explore their theoretical models. She concluded that although the model used was comparable to the stress process model, the nurses did not have a sophisticated understanding of its constructs or the links between them. The actual model used by the nurses was seen as a pragmatic one drawn from their experience rather than theoretical knowledge. She concluded that the lack of training in the use of theoretical models would jeopardize the efficacy of any interventions (Carradice 1999).

However, the Admiral Nurse service may challenge this position and a more detailed appraisal of their role and evidence base is provided by Soliman in the next chapter. However, briefly, Admiral Nurses work primarily with the carer and continue to do so for as long as is appropriate even after the person with dementia has moved into residential care or died. Their role encompasses the provision of emotional support, the provision of information and skills for carers and the provision of consultancy, training and education for other professionals. The Admiral Nurse service is unusual in that it articulates and utilizes a specific model for practice. This model was developed from a stress management model devised by Zarit *et al.* (1985) and identifies the unmet needs as the cause of stress. Admiral Nurses use a 19-item assessment schedule to identify and quantify those needs. Their interventions are then based around the provision of education, emotional support and the skills needed to deal with the symptoms of dementia.

There has been only one study of the effectiveness of Admiral Nurses. A controlled trial without randomization was carried out in London to compare Admiral Nurse service teams with community mental health teams (Woods *et al.* 1999). The results showed little difference between the groups apart from a greater reduction for anxiety on the GHQ (General Health Questionnaire) for the Admiral Nurse service. Given the lack of evidence of effectiveness for mental health nurses in general, these results suggest that the use of a theoretical framework for assessment is not sufficient to make a significant difference. Although providing a model for assessment, perhaps the theoretical framework used by Admiral Nurses gives insufficient guidance for the actual interventions. For example, among the strategies for meeting the needs associated with emotional support, the Admiral Nurse literature states the provision of 'counselling'. This generic term, in common with many mental health nursing 'interventions', lacks any indication of what the nurse will actually be doing.

This paucity of articulated skills and evidence of effectiveness has been embraced in other areas of mental health, with the most notable example coming from the care of people with psychosis. Following a number of concerns raised that the skills of mental health nurses do not meet the needs of their clients (Pratt 1997), there has been a revolution in the care for people with psychotic illnesses and their carers. The change in skill acquisition and care delivery began to take shape in 1992 with the development of two Thorn courses. These courses were based on the work of Brooker *et al.* (1994) who demonstrated the effectiveness of a range of psychological and social interventions that improved outcomes for people with a psychotic illness and enabled their carers to cope more effectively. This approach to care provision became known as psychosocial interventions (PSI). Brooker *et al.* (1994) also demonstrated that CMHNs can be taught to use PSI approaches in their routine clinical work. Research has continued and there is a clear evidence base demonstrating the effectiveness of PSI in reducing relapse rates in schizophrenia and improving social and clinical outcomes. Crucially, these improvements are not limited to the person with schizophrenia, but have also been shown to improve outcomes for carers (Mari and Streiner 1994). The demand for PSI-trained professionals has been so great that provision has now grown to the point where there are around 40 courses nationwide offering multi-disciplinary preparation for PSI.

Within the field of care for psychosis, the term 'psychosocial intervention' has attracted many different definitions. One that captures the essence describes it as a range of problem-solving activities, delivered by individuals and services involving the user and their carer, with the aim of improving the health and quality of life of people with a serious mental illness and their carers (Baguley and Baguley 1999). In the context of psychosis, this model is based around three elements: the concept of expressed emotion, the stress vulnerability model, and cognitive behavioural approaches to mental health problems. Although all the components of PSI are important and provide substance to the theoretical model, it is the inclusion of the latter, cognitive behavioural approaches, that perhaps begins to illuminate how PSI fills the skills void in mental health nursing.

A specific feature of PSI, incorporating all the above elements, is known as family intervention. The aim of family intervention is to educate and support families, assisting them to acquire a range of coping skills to help them deal with the difficulties they face (Fadden 1998). This reduces stress in families and can have an impact on the course of the psychotic illness. Although caring for someone with dementia is very different from caring for someone with schizophrenia, it seemed likely that there may be similarities in the clinical approach required to reducing stress.

The evidence base for PSI in dementia care

Many studies concerned with reducing carer stress utilize strategies that could be recognized as components of the PSI model of family intervention and a systematic review was carried out to assess the effectiveness of the current evidence base in dementia care (Pusey and Richards 2001). This review examined the evidence from studies where the intervention was concerned with the provision of information, education or emotional support. Outcomes of interest were psychological health, physical health and quality of life. As the aim was to assess evidence of effectiveness, the inclusion criteria for study design were randomized controlled trials or controlled trials without randomization. Thirty studies met the inclusion criteria and these were assessed for quality. Overall the methodological quality was poor with notable weaknesses in sample size and randomization. In part, this resulted in a paucity of strong evidence to support a definitive approach to supporting carers. The 'strongest' evidence came from Mittleman *et al.* (1995) who reduced carer depression with individual and family counselling. This was followed by Teri *et al.* (1997) who demonstrated lower levels of depression in both carers and the individual with dementia using behavioural techniques.

Despite the methodological weakness across all the studies, there were conclusions that could be drawn. The best evidence was for individual interventions rather than groups. This supported earlier findings by Knight *et al.* (1993). In addition, although there was often scant details of the theoretical framework used to underpin the intervention, the strongest evidence arose from those that had a behavioural component focusing on problem solving and strategies for behaviour management. These elements feature prominently in PSI and so it was concluded that developing PSI with carers of people with dementia was an avenue worth investigating (Pusey and Richards 2001).

Since that systematic review was undertaken, a study has been published that lends even greater weight to that argument. Marriott *et al.* (2000) adapted cognitive-behavioural family intervention for carers of people with dementia and undertook a prospective single-blind randomized controlled trial delivered by a psychologist. Carers who scored 5 or above on the GHQ were allocated one of three groups. The intervention group received family intervention and a modified version of the Camberwell Family Interview (CFI). The CFI is an in-depth interview designed to elicit a rating of expressed emotion. In this study it represented an opportunity for carers to talk and express feelings. The two control groups consisted of an information-only group and a group who were also given the CFI. The results of this trial demonstrated that those carers who received family intervention had significant reductions in distress and depression both at post-treatment and at the three-month follow-up. In addition there were significant reductions in behavioural disturbance at post-treatment and increased activity in the person with dementia at follow-up. There was little effect from delivering the CFI alone, and delivering information alone had no impact on burden. Additionally, an important finding was that family intervention was an acceptable strategy to carers.

Developing PSI in dementia care

PSI can be thought of as a range of interventions, a collection of strategies addressing the needs of the individual with the illness and their carer. Family intervention forms a cornerstone of PSI and in schizophrenia the main aim is to reduce relapse and enhance coping strategies. In dementia, the aim is to reduce carer stress as opposed to altering the disease process (Marriott *et al.* 2000). However, as the results from Marriott and her colleagues demonstrate, a reduction in carer stress appears to have an impact on quality of life for the person with dementia.

Stress vulnerability model

In trying to explore how the PSI model of family intervention relates to dementia, the first issue that should be considered is the underpinning theoretical framework. When the stress vulnerability model is referred to in PSI it usually relates to Zubin and Spring's (1977) model of schizophrenia. This model argues that schizophrenia is episodic and stress related where an individual may have an intrinsic vulnerability but the development of acute symptoms will relate to the individual's coping strategies, resources and perceived stress. In family interventions, this model dovetails with the stress vulnerability model of family coping (Falloon *et al.* 1993). In dementia care, although it could be argued that a stress vulnerability model has relevance for the progression of dementia, the stress vulnerability model of family coping is the central tenet. This model conceptualizes stress as an individual's response to threat. This response can be manifested as a physical, behavioural or psychological response or a mixture of all three. Every individual will respond in a unique way to stress, and this response will be influenced by factors such as bio-genetics, personality and previous experience. An individual will have their own threshold for stress, which if exceeded can put them at risk of developing physical or psychological health problems. The type of problem developed will be determined by their specific vulnerability. This may be due to biological factors, previous history or present poor health (Falloon *et al.* 1993).

The model categorizes stress into two types. Ambient stress is the stress associated with everyday living. It is the accumulated stress we experience from being part of a household, from having personal and social relationships, from the pursuit of leisure or work activities and from the environment in general. The other type of stress is the stress arising from discrete life events such as the breakdown of a relationship, the loss of a job, or the development of a mental health problem in a family member. Stress from any source can be responsible for levels exceeding the threshold, and the longer this level is maintained the higher the risk of health problems.

However, stress levels can be mediated by individual coping behaviour. This behaviour will include not only the individual's response to the source of stress, but also their attempts to resolve associated problems and the responses and attempts at resolution of those in their social and family network (Falloon *et al.* 1993). Facilitating effective coping strategies is a primary function of family intervention.

Expressed emotion

The second building block of PSI is expressed emotion (EE). EE can be described as the measure of verbal report and tone of voice (Barrowclough and Tarrier 1992). Environments are considered high EE where there is a high level of emotional over-involvement, hostility and criticism. It is a factor considered important for both professional and family care environments. Although the constituents of high EE, for example overinvolvement, have negative connotations in families, it is important to stress that high EE should be viewed as an ordinary family response to difficult and demanding circumstances. It is recognized that high levels of EE are associated with quicker relapse in schizophrenia (Baguley and Baguley 1999) and poorer outcome in a number of other client groups, including those with depression, anorexia and learning disabilities (Fearon *et al.* 1998). Although the evidence base in dementia care is less well developed, it has been shown that among carers there is a positive relationship between high levels of strain and distress and high EE (Bledin *et al.* 1990). However, the relationship between EE and stress should not be simplified. There have been attempts to understand high EE as a reaction to charac-teristics in the client (Hooley and Richters 1995), or as an inherent characteristic of the relative, but evidence does not support these models (Fearon *et al.* 1998). Within dementia care there have been efforts to explore EE as a facet of the interpersonal relationship between the carer and the individual with dementia (Fearon *et al.* 1998). Here, high EE is associated with problems in that relationship and studies have shown that a poor pre-morbid relationship predicts more critical and hostile com-ments (Gilhooly and Whittick 1989), and low current intimacy is associated with high EE (Fearon *et al.* 1998).

Given this evidence of a relationship between stress and EE, it seems appro-priate to suggest that expressed emotion is a suitable theoretical concept for CMHNs to consider in their interventions. However, this suggestion is not new. Adams (1996) has already argued this point, but it does not appear to have been considered by researchers, educators or practitioners as an important theory for nurses.

Cognitive and behavioural approaches

The third element of PSI is cognitive behaviour therapy (CBT) approaches. The PSI model in psychosis utilizes cognitive-behavioural approaches on two fronts. They have been shown to be effective for modifying symptoms such as delusions and hallucinations. They are also an effective needs-led and goal-defined strategy for the family intervention component. CBT is a widely used intervention based on the theory that thoughts will influence behaviour and feelings; a position developed by Peter Ashton in Chapter 7 of this book. Although there are numerous variants of CBT, the central proposition is that psychological problems arise as a result of certain patterns of thinking and behaviour (Enright 1997). It suggests that negative patterns of thinking tend to be automatic and pervasive and will influence the individual's perception of the world around them and this in turn affects mood and self-esteem. Beck (1976) suggested that negative thinking originates from attitudes and assumptions. If an individual is depressed, they become entrapped in a cognitive triad comprising negative views of self, current experience and the future. The person's behaviour will also be affected; for example, activity outside the home is reduced, leading to less stimulation and an exacerbation of the depression (Enright 1997). Although initially focused on depression, the efficacy of CBT is well documented and utilized in a range of problems, including pain, medically unexplained symptoms and anxiety (Enright 1997). The CBT intervention focuses on symptoms and thought processes and encourages a sense of self-control and self-responsibility. Self-monitoring and patient involvement is central to the intervention. Thus it is very much a collaborative process where professional and patient are partners rather than being an intervention that is done to the patient.

In dementia, the CBT approaches have been adapted by Marriott (in press) but are similar to those used in family intervention in schizophrenia. The starting point should be a comprehensive assessment using a specific, validated tool. The Relative Assessment Interview (Barrowclough and Tarrier 1992) could be used to identify a number of key features. It will determine the carer's understanding of dementia, the amount and type of distress experienced by the carer, the coping strategies the carer currently adopts, the impact of dementia on the carer, the quality of the relationship with the person with dementia, and areas of strength. This assessment provides an overview of the carer's needs and considers relevant EE components. As there are high levels of psychological morbidity among carers, this assessment tool might be accompanied by others such as the General Health Questionnaire (Goldberg and Hillier 1978).

Following a thorough assessment, the next stage would be the collaborative identification of problems and the arrangement of a hierarchy of priorities. The strategies systematically adopted to help carers can be divided into three categories; education, stress management and enhancing coping skills (Barrowclough and Tarrier 1992; Marriott *et al.* 2000). All components of the intervention and the order in which they are delivered should be tailored to the specific needs of the carer, but the logical starting point is education. The foundation of the intervention is to assist carers to perceive dementia in a way that will result in less stress for themselves and a less stressful environment for the person with dementia. It also helps to develop a relationship where the nurse is immediately offering something to the carer (Falloon *et al.* 1993). Hence education is often the first focus of the intervention but will feature throughout care delivery. Education will cover a wide range of issues about dementia and will include carer reactions. For example, if the carer believes that difficult behaviour exhibited by the person with dementia is a deliberate attempt to upset them, this will increase their distress.

As mentioned earlier, stress is manifested physically, behaviourally and psychologically (Falloon *et al.* 1993). These symptoms of stress could appear as muscle tension or excess stomach acid (physical), avoiding situations or curtailing non-caring activity (behavioural), and always expecting the worst or feeling out of control (psychological). Thus the stress management intervention will address these areas as appropriate. A feature of using abbreviated CBT approaches will involve the carer recording and monitoring their own stress. This aids the recognition of the carer as an active participant in the intervention and helps them to recognize the progress they make (Enright 1997). Any physical stress that the carer is experiencing should be addressed immediately as symptoms such as increased hormone levels and excessive gastrointestinal activity can lead to serious disorders (Falloon *et al.* 1993). Examples of relaxation training could include progressive muscle relaxation or imagery techniques.

Helping carers to manage their psychological responses to stress should start with educating the carer about the relationship between thinking and feeling. The goal is to enable the carer to recognize and challenge negative, irrational thoughts and maladaptive underlying assumptions. Examples of thinking errors are: all-or-nothing thinking, overgeneralization, catastrophizing, ignoring the positive, jumping to conclusions, and unrealistic expectations of self. Examples of maladaptive underlying assumptions include: 'I must be liked by people at all times' and 'If I make a mistake as carer I am incompetent'.

Marriott (in press) has outlined the relationship between caring and stress. The demands of caring can often lead to increased isolation and reduced contact with support networks (Gilhooly 1987). This makes them particularly vulnerable to stress (Zarit *et al.* 1980). Unfortunately stress can make a situation more demanding than it actually is, resulting in behavioural responses to that stress. This can lead to the abandonment of all other activity, overprotection, excessive self-sacrificing or emotional overinvolvement (Seymour 1991). Carers are encouraged to identify alternative ways of coping, to look after their own needs and to develop social support networks. Examples could include enlisting help from other members of the family and introducing pleasurable activities into their day.

Two skills in the achievement of reducing all types of stress reactions are goal setting and six-step problem solving. These skills provide a specific and structured approach and, because this process is done collaboratively, reinforce carer strengths and resources. Goal setting could be utilized in a number of components of family intervention; for example, increasing social contact could be addressed with goal setting. The principles of goal setting (Falloon *et al.* 1993) are:

1   Choose readily attainable targets.
2   Prioritize goals that will enhance quality of life most easily.
3   Break ambitious goals down into attainable steps.

4   State goal in terms that describe the activity exactly: specify all actions, where, when, with whom, how often, for how long and so on.

Goals should be specific, thus the example above, increasing social contact, should be expressed as 'meeting a friend for a leisurely activity once a fortnight'. If a carer had difficulty achieving this goal, a problem-solving strategy could be employed to facilitate the activity.

Problem solving is often referred to but it is sometimes difficult to identify what exactly is meant by this approach. The components of problem solving are probably found among the strategies of many people but often not in a consistent and organized fashion. The six-step approach offers a specific and focused strategy and is an alternative to maladaptive strategies often adopted such as avoiding the issue, denying a problem, resignation to fate, and 'roll of the dice' random selection of solutions. The six steps in problem solving (Falloon *et al.* 1993) are:

1   Pinpoint the problem.
2   Generate a list of all possible solutions/ideas.
3   Evaluate each solution/idea.
4   Choose the 'best' solution.
5   Plan and implement the solution.
6   Review results.

As with goal setting, the key to successful problem solving lies in the specificity of the problem identification. In addition, success will be dependent upon the correct identification of the problem.

Conclusion

The family intervention component of PSI has been shown to be effective when delivered by a psychologist (Marriott *et al.* 2000). However, given that nurses have been trained to utilize this approach in psychosis, coupled with a finite source of psychology provision, it is, arguably, time to consider widening the delivery to all members of the multi-disciplinary team involved in community dementia care. This corresponds with calls by Gournay *et al.* (2000) to train CMHNs from all fields in abbreviated cognitive behaviour therapy. In addition, within dementia care specifically, Adams (1996) suggested that nurses should develop a wider range of therapeutic approaches including cognitive therapy. The author is currently evaluating the effectiveness of training the nursing members of a community mental health team to deliver family intervention. Early indications from a small pilot study show that family intervention delivered by nurses could have an impact on carers' psychological morbidity. It appears to challenge traditional practice, highlighting previously unrecognized need and provides a framework for intervention (Pusey 2001). Supporting carers effectively requires specific skills, and it appears unreasonable and immoral that those skills are now routinely afforded to the carers of those with other severe and enduring mental illnesses but not to those caring for someone with dementia.

References

Adams, T. (1996) Informal family caregiving to older people with dementia: research priorities for community psychiatric nursing, *Journal of Advanced Nursing*, 24(4): 703–10.

Adams, T. (1999) Developing partnership in the work of community psychiatric nurses with older people with dementia, in T. Adams and C. Clarke (eds) *Dementia Care: Developing Partnerships in Practice*. London: Baillière Tindall.

Beck, A.T. (1976) *Cognitive Therapy and the Emotional Disorders*. London: Penguin.

Baguley, I. and Baguley, C. (1999) Psychosocial interventions in the treatment of psychosis, *Mental Health Care*, 2(9): 314–17.

Barrowclough, C. and Tarrier, N. (1992) 'Interventions with Families', in M. Birchwood and N. Tarrier (eds) *Innovations in the Psychological Management of Schizophrenia*. Chichester: Wiley.

Bledin, K., Kuipers, L., MacCarthy, B. and Woods, R. (1990) Daughters of people with dementia: expressed emotion, strain and coping, *British Journal of Psychiatry*, 157: 221–7.

Bourgeois, M., Schulz, R. and Burgio, L. (1996) Interventions for caregivers of patients with Alzheimer's disease: a review and analysis of content, process and outcomes, *International Journal of Ageing and Human Development*, 43(1): 35–92.

Brooker, C., Falloon, I., Butterworth, C. *et al.* (1994) The outcome of training community psychiatric nurses to deliver psychosocial intervention, *British Journal of Psychiatry*, 160: 834–44.

Carradice, A. (1999) A qualitative study of the theoretical models used by mental health nurses to guide their assessments of family care givers for people with dementia. D.Clin.Psy. thesis, University of Sheffield.

Davis, L. (1992) Building a science of caring for family caregivers, *Family and Community Health*, 15: 1–9.

Department of Health (1998) *A First Class Service*. London: The Stationery Office.

Donaldson, C., Tarrier, N. and Burns, A. (1998) Determinants of carer stress in Alzheimer's disease, *International Journal of Geriatric Psychiatry*, 13: 248–56.

Enright, S.J. (1997) Cognitive behaviour therapy: clinical applications, *British Medical Journal*, 314: 1811.

Fadden, G. (1998) Family intervention in psychosis, *Journal of Mental Health*, 7(2): 115–22.

Falloon, I.R.H., Laporta, M., Fadden, G. and Graham-Hole, V. (1993) *Managing Stress in Families: Cognitive and Behavioural Strategies for Enhancing Coping Skills*. London: Routledge.

Fearon, M., Donaldson, C., Burns, A. and Tarrier, N. (1998) Intimacy as a determinant of expressed emotion in carers of people with Alzheimer's disease. *Psychological Medicine*, 28(5): 1085–90.

Gilhooly, M.L.M. (1987) in J. Orford (ed.) *Coping with Disorder in the Family*. London: Croom Helm. Chapter 7, Senile Dementia and the Family.

Gilhooly, M.L.M. and Whittick, J.E. (1989) Expressed emotion in caregivers of the dementing elderly, *British Journal of Medical Psychology*, 62: 265–72.

Goldberg, D.P. and Hillier, V.F. (1978) A scaled version of the General Health Questionnaire, *Psychological Medicine*, 9: 139–45.

Gourney, K., Devilly, G. and Brooker, C. (1993) The CPN in primary care: a pilot study of the process of assessment, in C. Brooker and E. White (eds) *Community Psychiatric Nursing: A Research Perspective*, Vol. 2. Melbourne: Chapman & Hall.

Gourney, K., Denford, L., Parr, A. and Newell, R. (2000) British nurses in behavioural psychotherapy: a 25 year follow-up, *Journal of Advanced Nursing*, 32(2): 343–51.

Hooley, J.M. and Richters, J.E. (1995) Expressed emotion: a developmental perspective, in D. Cicchetti and S.L. Toth, *Rochester Symposium of Developmental Psychology. Vol. 6, Emotion, Cognition and Representation*, New York: University of Rochester Press.

Knight, B.G., Lutzky, S.M. and Macofsky-Urban, F. (1993) A meta-analytic review of intervention for caregiver distress: recommendations for future research, *The Gerontologist*, 33(2): 240–7.

Mari, J.D. and Streiner, D.L. (1994) An overview of family interventions and relapse on schizophrenia: meta-analysis of research findings, *Psychological Medicine*, 24: 565–78.

Marriott, A. (in press) Helping families cope with dementia in T. Adams and I. Manthorpe (eds) *Dementia Care*. London: Arnold.

Marriott, A., Donaldson, C., Tarrier, N. and Burns, A. (2000) The effectiveness of a cognitive-behavioural intervention for reducing the burden of care in carers of patients with Alzheimer's disease, *British Journal of Psychiatry*, 176(6): 557–62.

Matthew, L. (1990) A role for the CPN in supporting the carer of clients with dementia, in C. Brooker (ed.) *Community Psychiatric Nursing: A Research Perspective*. London: Chapman & Hall.

Mittleman, M.S., Ferris, S.H., Shulman, E. *et al.* (1995) A comprehensive support program: effect on depression in spouse-caregivers of AD patients, *The Gerontologist*, 35: 792–802.

Pratt, P. (1997) *Pulling Together*. London: Sainsbury Centre.

Pusey, H. (2001) An evaluation of a training program in family intervention for a community mental health team for older people. Unpublished report.

Pusey, H. and Richards, D. (2001) A systematic review of the effectiveness of psychosocial interventions for carers of people with dementia, *Aging and Mental Health*, 5(2): 107–19.

Schulz, R., Visintainer, P. and Williamson, G.M. (1990) Psychiatric and physical morbidity effects of caregiving, *Journals of Gerontology: Physical Sciences*, 45: 181–91.

Seymour, J. (1991) Pathological caring: a long-term problem that must be solved, *Geriatric Medicine*, 21: 17.

Sheppard, M. (1991) *Mental Health Work in the Community: Theory and Practice in Social Work and Community Psychiatric Nursing*. London: Falmer Press.

Teri, L., Logsdon, R.G., Uomoto, J. and McCurry, S.M. (1997) Behavioural treatment of depression in dementia patients: a controlled clinical trial, *Journals of Gerontology, Series B, Psychological Sciences and Social Sciences*, 52: 159–66.

Woods, B., Willis, W. and Higginson, I. (1999) An evaluation of the Admiral Nurse service: an innovative service for the carers of people with dementia. Unpublished report, North Thames R&D Directorate.

Zarit, S.H., Reever, K.E. and Bach-Peterson, J. (1980) Relatives of the impaired elderly: correlates of feelings of burden, *The Gerontologist*, 20: 649–55.

Zarit, S., Orr, N.K. and Zarit, J.M. (1985) *The Hidden Victims of Alzheimer's Disease: Families under Stress*. New York: New York University Press.

Zubin, J. and Spring, B. (1977) Vulnerability: a new view of schizophrenia, *Journal of Abnormal Psychology*, 86: 103–26.

13

Admiral Nurses
A model of family assessment and intervention

Alison Soliman

Introduction

One family's experience of caring in the mid-1980s for husband and father Joseph Levy, who had a vascular dementia, became the catalyst for the development of the Admiral Nurse Project. Although the family had sufficient money to buy in the care Mr Levy needed, the other members of the family felt that there was little support available to them as carers. Accordingly, in 1990 a proposal for an Alzheimer's specialist nurse was worked up by a group of carers and professionals into the Admiral Nurse Pilot Project. The nurses were named after Mr Levy, a keen amateur yachtsman, who enjoyed the nickname 'Admiral Joe'.

As this initiative implies, this chapter describes the work of Admiral Nurses who provide a specialist intervention to support carers of people with dementia. Within the text the origins and philosophy of the service are explored, as well as the evidence base upon which it was established. A detailed explanation of the assessment tools used by Admiral Nurses is followed by examples of casework in the form of extracts from two anonymized case studies. The case studies are used with the permission of each Admiral Nurse and their carer as client. The chapter concludes with an attempt to assess the service's practice efficacy and with a review of future challenges.

The origins and philosophy of the Admiral Nurse service

Originally, the vision of the Admiral Nurse service was to fund a pilot project, which, if it could be demonstrated to be successful, would develop into a national service for carers of people with dementia, along similar lines to the Macmillan Nursing Service. Part of the pilot project, therefore, involved an evaluation, which was initially conducted by Silvester and McCarthy (1992a), to measure the effectiveness of Admiral Nurse interventions. This evaluation was designed to look at changes in need over time as measured by the (at the time) newly developed Admiral Nurse Assessment Schedule (ANAS, introduced later in the chapter). Following this approach, 20 carers were rated at initial face-to-face contact and after three months; for 80 per cent of the sample, 'need' scores at three-month follow-up had reduced, indicating a reduction in stress/burden experienced by carers. In the 20 per cent of cases where need scores increased, the increases were generally small and had reduced by the time of the next interview (Silvester and McCarthy 1992a). However, the study design did not allow a conclusion to be drawn that the Admiral Nurses were responsible for the positive change that occurred, only that carer needs, as defined by the ANAS, were met during the period of assessment. Therefore, to improve the robustness of the study design, another approach to evaluating the pilot project was adopted. This was undertaken in the same year (1992) and conducted by former carers. The primary aim of this study was to elicit the carers' point of view to service intervention and involved carrying out semi-structured interviews with 20 carers receiving the Admiral Nurse service. On analysis, most comments were shown to be positive with an 'overwhelming appreciation of the service from those who have used it' (Jarvis *et al.* 1992: 20).

Despite the limited nature of these evaluations, the pilot project was extended on a permanent basis and services developed initially in central London. There are, in 2003, 15 Admiral Nurse teams in total, spread over London, Kent and the north-west of England, with new developments taking place in the West Midlands and the South East. To provide an operational framework for this development, in 1994 the Dementia Relief Trust, now "for dementia", was established with a remit to improve clinical practice, enhance the evidence base of the service and provide ongoing support for Admiral Nurses. The Admiral Nurse service operates as a partnership between "for dementia" and a host NHS provider agency, which carries responsibility for employing the Admiral Nurses.

Admiral Nurses' workload consists of a balance between casework and consultancy. The consultancy role includes:

- advice on casework;
- education and training;
- promoting high standards of care for people with dementia and their carers at a local or strategic level.

In contrast, casework involves Admiral Nurses working in the community with people of all ages with dementia and carers, provided a diagnosis of dementia has been, or is likely to be, made, and the person with dementia lives within the Admiral Nurse 'catchment area'. However, the primary focus of the Admiral Nurse is on the carer as client. The Admiral Nurse works with carers throughout the duration of the condition and beyond, and interventions can range from providing information around the time of diagnosis, through to support following the person with dementia's admission into residential care, or death. Consequently, levels of carer need may vary, peaking around times of change and transition. By intervening at an early stage and playing a preventative role, the primary intention is to preserve the physical and mental health of the carer, which, in turn, can be of benefit to the person with dementia.

Focusing on the carer as client can include direct work with the person with dementia and addressing the relationship between the person with dementia and the carer. Alternatively, the Admiral Nurse may refer to other services where their input is assessed as being needed.

The evidence base of the Admiral Nurse service

The research findings described in this section constitute the evidence base of the Admiral Nurse service.

1. Dementia can have a significant effect on the family unit

Most people with dementia live in the community, with about half being cared for at home by their family and friends, with responsibility for care usually resting on one individual, usually a spouse or adult child (Keady 1996). The average age of carers is between 60 and 65 years, and many are much older (Levin 1997). Nolan *et al.* (1996) distinguish between stress affecting an individual carer and that affecting the wider family unit.

2. Caring is stressful

Opie (1994) believes that stress is an inevitable part of caring, as it is of life in general, but others (Boss 1988; Benner and Wruebel 1989) point out that it can be positive and provide opportunities for growth and challenge. Nevertheless, many studies have shown that caring can adversely affect carers' emotional and physical well-being (Zarit *et al.* 1985; for reviews see: Keady 1996; Briggs and Askham 1999).

3. Caregiving changes over time

Aneshensel *et al.* (1995) describe caregiving as a career with different stages, each presenting distinctive sources of stress. First, there is the preparation for, and acquisition of, the carer role; secondly, the carrying out of care-related tasks and responsibilities within the home and possibly within an institution; and thirdly, disengagement from caring, which often entails bereavement, recovery and social reintegration.

4. Carers have difficulty accessing services and articulating their needs

Briggs and Askham (1999) suggest that one of the difficulties carers can face when having their needs assessed is that they do not have enough information about services available to make an informed choice. Briggs and Askham cite research by Connell *et al.* (1994) showing that carers often receive a 'fragmented' service delivery, with those from ethnic minority communities facing additional barriers to service provision. Several studies (Haffenden 1991; Philp *et al.* 1995; Askham 1997) have shown that both knowledge and uptake of services are poor among people with dementia and their carers.

5. *Carers are not homogenous*

The dynamic and multi-dimensional nature of caring produces a diversity of responses (Morris *et al.* 1988; Keady and Nolan 1996). Carers adapt quite differently to similar situations (Zarit and Edwards 1996), and theories of stress and adaptation (see, for example, Lazarus and Folkman 1984) can help to explain these different responses. For example, stress can be deemed a subjective experience that occurs when there is a perceived mismatch between the nature of the demand and the person's ability to respond to it (Lazarus and Folkman 1984; Nolan *et al.* 1996). The theoretical model of objective and subjective burden, where objective burden relates to the frequency of dementia-related 'problems' (i.e. severity of dementia) and subjective burden is the carer's interpretation of how stressful they find coping with each problem, helps to understand differences in carer experience. In such a way the severity of the dementia does not necessarily correspond to carer burden: some carers can cope well with many problems, whereas others may find one or two problems burdensome and a rationale for giving up the caregiving role. Thus coping is one construct that has been identified as explaining why carers in similar circumstances show variability in dealing with exhibited stress (Pearlin *et al.* 1990). Nolan *et al.* (1996: 68) suggest that to help carers increase their coping skills, a 'comprehensive assessment' of each carer's unique circumstances needs to be undertaken which looks at the types of stressor they face, what coping strategies they use and how effective they feel they are.

The evidence base for Admiral Nurse interventions

Building on the demonstrated rationale for involvement with family carers of people with dementia, the Admiral Nurse service has integrated several theoretical frameworks into its practice in order to generate an approach to intervention and assist in an evaluation of its efficacy. The main tenets of this approach are outlined below.

The use of Zarit et al.'s *(1985) stress management model*

Admiral Nurse interventions reflect the work of Zarit *et al.* (1985) who describe three factors that impact on the degree of burden experienced by carers: the symptoms of dementia and how the carer responds to them; the social support available; and the quality of the prior relationship between carer and person with dementia (p. 73). The stress management model Zarit and his colleagues developed had three components: (the input) information, (the process) problem solving, and (the output or goals) managing problem behaviour and increasing social support. Individual counselling, family meetings and support groups may be ways of working to achieve such goals.

The problem-solving process is seen as having several stages:

1 Identifying the problem, the trigger factors and the consequences. Asking the carer to keep a daily record may be seen as helpful strategies to pinpoint such issues.

2 Thinking of as many alternative solutions as possible. This might include reframing the 'problem behaviour' and trying to understand it from the perspective of the person with dementia.

3 Exploring the advantages and disadvantages of each solution and choosing one.

4 Cognitive rehearsal, i.e. encouraging the carer to carry out the steps mentally, and anticipate any problems.

5 Carrying out the plan.

6 Evaluating the outcome. In particular, it is important to establish whether or not the 'problem behaviour' has been reduced or if there is a need to find an alternative solution.

Some carers readily accept the need to 'problem solve' as they may have already tried alternative solutions or have used this approach in other areas of their lives. For other carers, problem solving may be more difficult as they may feel 'overwhelmed' by the situation or they may have difficulty in facing up to the permanence of the diagnosis. Each situation presents its own unique challenge, although the bedrock of the Admiral Nurses' approach to assessment is contained in the Admiral Nurse Assessment Schedule.

Background to the Admiral Nurse Assessment Schedule

Zarit *et al.*'s (1985) work provided the original impetus for the development of the ANAS (see Figure 13.1), which is an adaptation of the Support Team Assessment Schedule developed for clinical audit in the context of palliative care (Higginson and

1. Person with dementia's generic health needs
2. Person with dementia's mental health needs
3. Carer's generic health needs
4. Carer's mental health needs
5. Need for advice about medication
6. Need for insight into the disease and prognosis
7. Understanding the symptoms of dementia
8. Skills in responding to the behaviour of the person with dementia
9. Communication between carer and other support services
10. Appropriate accommodation
11. Financial needs
12. Practical aids
13. Practical support
14. Carer's need for support in organizing regular time away
15. Carer's need for support in organizing long-term relief
16. Carer's need for bereavement support
17. Carer's need for improved informal support
18. Carer's need for support in recognizing own needs
19. Carer's need for support in relinquishing role

Figure 13.1 Admiral Nurse Assessment Schedule

McCarthy 1993). The ANAS consists of 19 items, which were created during the pilot project after observation of Admiral Nurse practice, discussion with the pilot team and a comprehensive literature review, which is detailed below. A rating scale was added to the schedule, with scores ranging from 0 to 4, to reflect the level of need and intervention required: (0 = no intervention required, and 4 = immediate action necessary).

What the ANAS covers

The first nine items are concerned with the health needs of the person with dementia and their carer and the difficulties that might arise in caring at home. Items 10 to 15 are concerned with the more social and practical supports needed, the provision of services and communication, financial, accommodation and respite needs. The last four items relate to bereavement and personal needs.

The evidence base of the ANAS

The research evidence that was available at the time, and upon which the ANAS was based (Silvester and McCarthy 1992b), is outlined below:

- The physical and mental health needs of the person with dementia were considered key areas as they addressed the person with dementia's health status and need to minimize dependency (Twigg *et al.* 1990).

- The health care needs of the carer are also vital as carers may be frail and have psychological problems of their own (George and Gwyther 1986; Levin *et al.* 1989).

- Carers need to recognize the likely course of the condition, and seek advice at an early stage if possible (National Consumer Council 1990; Social Services Inspectorate 1991a).

- Support by welfare services and informal networks are a protection against stress (Levin *et al.* 1989).

- Service providers must communicate effectively (Social Services Inspectorate 1991a,b).

- Practical aids are needed and greatly valued (Gilleard *et al.* 1984; Ferris *et al.* 1987; Social Services Inspectorate 1991b).

- There may be financial problems and need for respite care (Whatmore and Mira-Smith 1991).

- Carers also need to anticipate death and bereavement and be supported in discussing their feelings about relinquishing care (Bass and Bowman 1990).

An example of scoring

The following case vignette is used to illustrate the scoring system of the ANAS with regard to one item, 'Behaviour of the person with dementia' (see Figure 13.2), where the care objective is to provide the carer with the support and skills necessary to adjust to the behaviour of the person with dementia.

ITEM 8 **Behaviour of the person with dementia – skills**

Carer's need for skills in responding to the behaviour of the person with dementia. Rating the skill of the carer should be based on the Admiral Nurse's judgement of the carer's response and not simply derived from the carer's view of their ability to deal with the behaviour.

0 = **No support needed.** Carer has skills appropriate to deal with the behaviour of the person with dementia.

1 = Carer has skills appropriate to deal with behaviour problems most of the time. **Would benefit from further support/reinforcement.**

2 = Carer has some skills but **support needed to develop** them/or others effectively. E.g. often finds person with dementia's behaviour problematic/is embarrassed by it.

3 = Carer frequently finds person with dementia's behaviour problematic. Has few skills. Carer and person with dementia suffering as a result. **Considerable support needed.**

4 = Carer has no skills; does not cope effectively with person with dementia's behaviour. Carer often responds inappropriately. **Immediate need for intervention/support.**

Figure 13.2 Item 8 of the Admiral Nurse Assessment Schedule

Case vignette

In this scenario a 70-year-old woman cares for her 87-year-old aunt who has Alzheimer's disease. The carer finds that on the mornings her aunt is due to attend the day centre, she gets out of bed only after a great deal of cajoling and assistance. Dressing and getting the aunt ready for the day causes her to become more agitated, and frequently angry and abusive. For the carer these occasions are extremely distressing and lead her to worry that day centre attendance must end. The carer also reports that she experiences a lot of stress because of her aunt's repeated attempts to telephone her dead mother, and continuous requests to be taken home.

The use of the ANAS in practice

In Item 8 of the ANAS (see Figure 13.2), this item was rated 3, reflecting the carer's need for advice about possible strategies to confront and overcome these difficulties. The behaviour of the person with dementia was frequently seen as problematic, and given that the carer was initially unable to limit the upset, both were experiencing some degree of distress. The item could not have been rated 2 as the carer exhibited 'no skills' in dealing with her aunt's behaviour and her reaction to the event was more than simply 'embarrassment'. Equally, the response did not merit a 4 rating as the carer did not cope effectively and her response, in becoming angry and upset, might be considered appropriate. In other words, her previous coping pattern was not abusive or violent (Silvester and McCarthy 1992b: 8–9).

As can be seen in this illustration, assessment is an ongoing process although a baseline measure needs to be established so that change can be instigated and monitored over time. Accordingly, Admiral Nurses may take up to three visits before completing the baseline assessment. Further assessments are then carried out after three months (maximum) and then every six months, or more frequently if necessary.

All assessments and interventions are recorded in a specially developed database named AMANDA (Activity Monitoring Admiral Nurse Database), in compliance with local policies and the terms of the Data Protection Act 1998. This database prompts the Admiral Nurse to carry out assessment reviews at the agreed intervals. The database also acts as a case management tool as, in addition to providing demographic information on clients, three levels of work are recorded: intensive, holding and maintenance. This form of case weighting helps to make sense of case-load numbers. Anonymized data are drawn from the database to report to the Admiral Nurse Service Advisory Committee every six months. Information on individual teams, such as the number of referrals received in the period, both appropriate and inappropriate, their source and ethnicity, is presented at a quarterly steering group meetings in the newer services.

At present, a number of nurses are piloting the use of the Carers' Checklist as an adjunct to the ANAS. The Carers' Checklist (Hodgson *et al.* 1998) is based on the theoretical model of objective and subjective burden, which has been described previously. The checklist consists of 26 behaviours, and carers are asked to rate how frequently these occur and how stressful they find them. The checklist concludes with sections on services and how much overall burden carers perceive there to be.

All newly appointed Admiral Nurses receive training on the use of the ANAS as part of their induction programme. To develop greater consistency in its use, periodic inter-rater reliability exercises are held with the nurses, using role-played carer/nurse interviews on video, during which scores are discussed and consensus ratings are agreed. These exercises serve to establish more objective means for identifying carer needs.

Developing therapeutic interventions

Adams (1994) argues that CMHNs in dementia care need to bring a wide range of psychotherapeutic approaches to their role. In the experience of Admiral Nurses, the first step along this road is to establish a trusting and therapeutic relationship. Admiral Nurse, Madeline Armstrong, writes that, in her practice, forming a therapeutic relationship with the person with dementia and the carer at the assessment stage underpins all future care. Gaining this trust may involve the nurse's therapeutic use of self and awareness of body language, facial expression and tone of voice (Armstrong 1998). According to Zarit *et al.* (1985), information giving is also crucial as it helps to establish the practitioner's credibility as someone who understands the problem; it can also help to alleviate a sense of crisis brought about by the family's uncertainty of the future and to put problems in a workable perspective. The importance of problem solving has already been discussed and Zarit *et al.* (1985) believe that it is important for practitioners to explore fully each problem with the carer, showing that one can have a non-judgemental response. The stress that the carer experiences over the problem may mean that they can see no logical and obvious solution to the dilemma. An appraisal of such issues follows in the two reported case studies.

Before this is addressed, however, one example of a therapeutic intervention that has helped to enlarge the 'intervention toolbox' from which Admiral Nurses can draw is solution-focused brief therapy (George *et al.* 2000). The essence of this therapy is to:

- work with the person rather than the problem;
- look for resources rather than deficits;
- explore possible and preferred futures;
- explore what is already contributing to those possible futures;
- treat clients as the experts in all aspects of their lives.

A group of Admiral Nurses is also investigating the usefulness and transfer-ability of a cognitive behavioural family intervention, as described by Marriott *et al.* (2000). This intervention protocol covers:

- stress management, including challenging negative thoughts and teaching relaxation techniques;
- understanding dementia, including looking at the family's perception of the main difficulties, their strengths and needs, and their perceptions of what helps and what does not;
- strengths and needs: further work on identifying difficulties which have a practical solution and those which require a changed family/carer approach;
- problem solving;
- managing behavioural responses: increasing social contact, encouraging time out and respite.

The following two case studies illustrate the use of both the ANAS and the range of interventions carried out by Admiral Nurses. The case studies describe the need for clinical supervision, which is facilitated for dementia, as the organiza-tion believes that effective clinical supervision is central to the success of the work of Admiral Nurses. The first case study[1] explores issues arising from the nature of the previous relationship and how this impacts on future care. One of the interesting features of the second case study[2] is an illustration of how the Admiral Nurse went about establishing a therapeutic relationship with the carer, and the importance of this as the care needs unfolded.

Case study 1

Jenny had been caring for her mother, Rose, and father, Bob, for many years. Rose was diagnosed with Alzheimer's disease and Parkinson's disease, and after Bob's death Jenny gave up work and moved her mother into her own house to care for her.

Rose would constantly ask her daughter about her husband and would become inconsolable, devastated and tearful as she grieved all over again. It would take Jenny hours to settle her mother down at night. Rose does sometimes have lucid moments when she is aware of Bob's death.

Jenny, an only child, was very close to her father, but not to her mother. She described Rose as 'a cold person, not interested in me'. Jenny expresses ambivalent feelings about her caring role. She often feels distressed and resents her mother when she has to talk daily about her father's death. Jenny feels she did not grieve adequately because of her mother's behaviour. Jenny's retired husband is supportive, but he also feels awkward with Rose's repetitive questions.

Using the Admiral Nurse Assessment Schedule, two of the needs identified were around understanding the symptoms of dementia and the skills needed by the carer to deal with the behaviour of the person with dementia.

I discussed this case in individual clinical supervision and was directed to Miesen's work on 'parent fixation', i.e. the person with dementia's insistence that their parents are still alive, which Miesen attributed to the emotional insight of the person with dementia regarding their own losses and experience of bereavement. He concluded that the dementing process fosters feelings of fear and insecurities and the resulting calling out of parent fixation could be interpreted as a cry for comfort and reassurance – an expression of need, not simply a sign of confusion (Holden and Woods 1995: 36).

Although Rose is calling for her husband, these theories help to promote some insight into the anxiety she may be experiencing. She has lost her partner of 63 years; she has physical and cognitive limitations, which possibly render her frightened and dependent; she has moved from a familiar environment to live with her daughter; and their previous relationship was somewhat strained.

I was able to discuss some of these theoretical ideas in a simplified way with Jenny. She seemed keen to understand and learn but said she had tried everything and so was a little sceptical. Rose's belief that her husband is alive possibly helps her to feel safe. By correcting her behaviour, which Jenny often does, she experiences the bereavement again and her need for security increases, thus causing her to call for her husband even more.

I suggested to Jenny that when her mother has lucid periods she should encourage her to talk about her feelings (validation), her loss and past memories. This approach may enable Rose's husband to 'become a living reality in her memory' (Miesen 1992: 41).

I discussed with Jenny the use of touch as a means of reassurance, but she said she would not feel at ease holding Rose's hand and 'she would not let me either'. We were able to talk about the closeness she had had with her father since early childhood. She said that Rose had not been a tactile person except with her husband, and even now she would not accept a hug from her daughter.

I discussed some of the issues in this case in peer group supervision. I found this very useful as consultation with Admiral Nurse colleagues enabled me to explore aspects of care from different perspectives.

Case study 2

Julia Fry was referred by the carers' worker from the local carers support project, who had been visiting her for some time dealing with practical issues, like claiming attendance allowance and council tax benefit. However, she felt she was no longer fulfilling the need for support that Mrs Fry required.

Mrs Fry has been caring for her 75-year-old husband, Stan, over a number of years. She cannot remember a significant time when her caring role began, but thinks his memory problems probably started with changes to his personality up to 10 or 15 years ago. His decline has been slow, and in this time she has gradually done more in the house and now for him personally.

I visited Mrs Fry for the first time at their bungalow. She had asked me to call whilst Mr Fry was out so that we could talk privately. Mrs Fry said it was the first time since she had been caring for Mr Fry that someone had visited her solely to talk about her needs.

Using the Admiral Nurse Assessment Schedule some of the urgent needs I identified were around the carer's mental and physical health, need for insight into the disease, and support in relinquishing the caring role.

I was concerned about Mrs Fry's own physical and mental health. Her anxious behaviour, complaints of poor short-term memory and limited concentration, and weight loss made me think she was depressed. This was confirmed after an assessment by the psychogeriatrician, which included a cognitive assessment by the team psychologist. All members of the multi-disciplinary team agreed that Mrs Fry was becoming overwhelmed by the job of caring for her husband and it was having serious implications for her own health. As the Frys already had an extensive care package, it was felt Mrs Fry needed considerable support and advice in how to relinquish her caring role. Mrs Fry said she would like to continue to see me and it was agreed that I should continue to work with her to guide her through this period of transition.

The next time I visited I gave Mrs Fry some information about dementia and answered some of her questions. I also talked about activities she could do with her husband that they would both find enjoyable. I spoke to her about diet, showed her a pamphlet and encouraged her to ask questions. I monitored her weight to make sure the weight loss did not continue.

On the next visit we went together to do some personal shopping for her. The shopping trip gave me an opportunity to assess Mrs Fry away from home in a non-caring environment. She visibly relaxed as we started to select a new outfit for her. I felt that the trip was very worthwhile in giving us time to build on our relationship. Mrs Fry said she had enjoyed the morning and she decided that next time we should go and look at a nursing home with a view to permanent placement for Mr Fry. After visiting the home together Mrs Fry decided to place Mr Fry on the waiting list for a room.

Although initially relieved at making the decision, Mrs Fry subsequently became very anxious about all the arrangements for the placement and her decision to relinquish care hit her hard. Her feelings of guilt and loss needed to be expressed and I was able to help her with this. She asked that we both talk to Mr Fry about the placement, as she felt a tremendous guilt about not including him in the decision. It was a time of sadness for them both.

I encouraged them to sit together and hug each other to offer the reassurance of their long relationship. It was a difficult meeting and I was grateful that I had the benefit of peer group supervision.

Admiral Nurse service: assessing practice efficacy

As the number of teams has grown, local evaluations have supported the ongoing development of the Admiral Nurse service (see, for example, Foley and Allen 1996). In 1998 the NHS Executive North Thames Region commissioned a larger, multi-site outcome study (Woods *et al.* 1998). This study compared four Admiral Nurse teams with conventional services located within mental health services for older people. Outcomes for both carers and people with dementia were examined.

The study demonstrated that there was a significant reduction in carers' needs for both groups; this was greater for the Admiral Nurse sample. Both samples showed areas of reduced need and no differences in outcome for the person with dementia. The conclusions drawn from the study were that active engagement with the carer beyond a baseline assessment is associated with reduced carer stress, although carers receiving an Admiral Nurse service showed a significantly greater decline in anxiety. A primary focus on carers appears to be associated with greater met need for carers; and the exclusive focus on dementia by Admiral Nurses may well equip them to better meet carers' needs for information and education. In comparison with current models of service provision where the focus is primarily on the person with dementia, there appears to be little lost by working primarily with the carer. However, it was suggested that the Admiral Nurse model might need to be reassessed to address working through the carer to modify behaviour and mood of the person with dementia (Teri *et al.* 1997) and one of the drawbacks of the study, as Keady and Adams (2001) point out, is that an eight-month follow-up period is short.

Future challenges

It may seem a paradox that Admiral Nurses are described as dementia specialists yet they work predominantly with carers. This raises the questions of whether this focus on the carer marginalizes the person with dementia, and to what extent the Admiral Nurse should work with the person with dementia. There is much debate both within and outside the service on this issue. In practice, the degree of direct involvement of the Admiral Nurse with the person with dementia varies from one nurse to another, and according to local circumstances and resources. For example, if the carer does not live with the person with dementia, the Admiral Nurse may or may not see the person with dementia. If Admiral Nurses work in an area where there are specialist dementia teams, or CMHNs, this has a bearing on the extent to which they work with the person with dementia. The complexity of this aspect of the work, where a balance needs to be struck between the needs of the carer and the person with dementia, is captured in the Admiral Nurse Competency Framework which has been developed with the Royal College of Nursing and is reported more fully in Chapter 18.

Another ever-present tension lies in maintaining a balance between the case-work and the consultancy aspects of the Admiral Nurse role. All nurses spend much time in direct casework activity. However, there usually comes a point when demand outstrips the capacity to meet it. One of the key features of the service is the open referral system, and the benefit of this system could disappear if those referred have to go on a waiting list.

Finally, there is the challenge in today's health care climate of being able to demonstrate that a service is evidence based, provides value for money and achieves the desired health outcomes. For the Admiral Nurse service this will primarily be addressed by the deployment of an evaluative framework using data gathered from the AMANDA database. However, this is a challenge faced by all CMHNs working with people with dementia and their carers and we all need to meet this challenge head on.

Notes

1   Case study 1 is extracted from a case study by Admiral Nurse Susan Drayton for the ENB N11 at Middlesex University, July 2000. Reported with permission of the author.
2   Case Study 2 is extracted from a case study by Admiral Nurse Penny Hibberd for the ENB N11 at Middlesex University, January 2000. Reported with the permission of the author.

References

Adams, T. (1994) The emotional experience of caregivers to relatives who are chronically confused – implications for community mental health nursing, *International Journal of Nursing Studies*, 31(6): 545–53.

Aneshensel, C.S., Pearlin, L.I., Mullan, J.T., Zarit, S.H. and Whitlatch, C.J. (1995) *Profiles in Caregiving: The Unexpected Career*. London: Academic Press.

Armstrong, M. (1998) Mental health assessment for older people, *Elderly Care*, 10(4): 41–2.

Askham, J. (1997) Supporting elderly people and informal carers at home, in I. Norman and S. Redfern (eds) *Mental Health Care for Elderly People*. London: Churchill Livingstone.

Bass, D.M. and Bowman, K. (1990) The transition from caregiving to bereavement: the relationship of carer-related strain and adjustment to death, *The Gerontologist*, 30: 35–42.

Benner, P. and Wruebel, J. (1989) *The Primacy of Caring: Stress and Coping in Health and Illness*. Menlo Park, CA: Addison-Wesley.

Boss, P. (1988) *Family Stress Management*. Newbury Park, CA: Sage.

Briggs, K. and Askham, J. (1999) *The Needs of People with Dementia and Those who Care for Them: A Review of the Literature*. London: Alzheimer's Society.

Connell, C., Kole, S., Benedict, C.J. *et al.* (1994) Increasing coordination of the dementia service delivery network: planning for the community outreach education program, *The Gerontologist*. 34(5): 700–6.

Ferris, S., Steinberg, G., Stulman, E., Kahn, R. and Reisberg, B. (1987) Institutionalisation of Alzheimer's disease patients: reducing precipitating factors through family counselling, *Home Health Care Quarterly*, 10(1): 23–51.

Foley, B. and Allen, H. (1996) The need for and nature and utility of the Admiral Nurse service: a preliminary report. Unpublished report, Riverside Mental Health Trust.

George, L.K. and Gwyther, L.P. (1986) Caregiver well-being: a multidimensional examination of family caregivers of demented adults, *The Gerontologist*, 26: 253–9.

George, E., Iveson, C. and Ratner, H. (2000) *Solution Focussed Brief Therapy: Course Notes*. London: Brief Therapy Practice.

Gilleard, C.J., Gledhill, K. and Whittick, J.E. (1984) Caring for the elderly mentally infirm at home: a survey of the supporters, *Journal of Epidemiology and Community Health*, 38: 319–23.

Haffenden, S. (1991) *Getting it Right for Carers. Setting up Services for Carers: A Guide for Practitioners*. London: Social Services Inspectorate.

Higginson, I.J. and McCarthy, M. (1993) Validity of the support team assessment schedule: do staff's ratings reflect those made by patients and their families?, *Palliative Medicine*, 7: 219–28.

Hodgson, C., Higginson, I. and Jefferys, P. (1998) *Carers' Checklist: An Outcome Measure for People with Dementia and their Carers*. London: Mental Health Foundation.

Holden, U. and Woods, R.T. (1995) *Positive Approaches to Dementia Care*, Edinburgh: Churchill Livingstone.

Jarvis, J., Jason, J. and Butterworth, M. (1992) *'The Carers' Critique'. The Admiral Nurse Project: A Service for Carers of People with a Dementing Illness – A Critical Appraisal of the Clinical Service from the Carers' Point of View*. London: Dementia Relief Trust.

Keady, J. (1996) The experience of dementia: a review of the literature and implications for nursing practice, *Journal of Clinical Nursing*, 5: 275–88.

Keady, J. and Adams, T. (2001) Community mental health nurses in dementia care: their role and future, *Journal of Dementia Care*, 9(2): 33–7.

Keady, J. and Nolan, M. (1996) Behavioural and instrumental stressors in dementia (BISID): refocusing the assessment of caregiver need in dementia, *Journal of Psychiatric and Mental Health Nursing*, 3: 163–72.

Lazarus, R.S. and Folkman, S. (1984) *Stress, Appraisal and Coping*. New York: Springer.

Levin, E. (1997) Carers – problems, strains, and services, in R. Jacoby and C. Oppenhiemer (eds) *Psychiatry in the Elderly*. Oxford: Oxford University Press.

Levin, E., Sinclair, I. and Gorbach, P. (1989) *Families, Services and Confusion in Old Age*. Aldershot: Avebury.

Marriott, A., Donaldson, C., Tarrier, N. and Burns, A. (2000) Effectiveness of cognitive behavioural family intervention in reducing the burden of care in carers of patients with Alzheimer's disease, *British Journal of Psychiatry*, 176: 557–62.

Miesen, B. (1992) Attachment theory and dementia, in G. Jones and B.M.L. Miesen (eds) *Care-giving in Dementia: Research and Applications*. London: Routledge.

Morris, R.G., Morris, L.W. and Britton, P.G. (1988) Factors affecting the emotional well-being of the caregivers of dementia sufferers, *British Journal of Psychiatry*, 153: 147–56.

National Consumer Council (1990) *Consulting Consumers in the NHS: A Guideline Study. Services for Elderly People with Dementia Living at Home*. London: National Consumer Council.

Nolan, M., Grant, G. and Keady, J. (1996) *Understanding Family Care*. Buckingham: Open University Press.

Opie, A. (1994) The instability of the caring body: gender and caregivers of confused older people, *Qualitative Health Research*, 4(1): 31–50.

Pearlin, L.I., Mullan, J.T., Semple, S.J. and Skaff, M.M. (1990) Caregiving and the stress process: an overview of concepts and their measures, *The Gerontologist*, 30(5): 583–91.

Philp, I., McKee, K., Meldrum, P. *et al.* (1995) Community care for demented and non-demented elderly people: a comparison study of financial burden, service use and unmet needs in family supporters, *British Medical Journal*, 310: 1503–6.

Silvester, S. and McCarthy, M. (1992a) Evaluating a community nursing service for supporters of elderly people with dementia. Unpublished. University College London.

Silvester, S. and McCarthy, M. (1992b) Evaluation of the Admiral Project: a community nursing service for carers of people with dementia. Unpublished. University College London.

Social Services Inspectorate (1991a) *Carer Support in the Community*. London: The Stationery Office.

Social Services Inspectorate (1991b) *Getting It Right for Carers*. London: The Stationery Office.

Teri, L., Logsdon, R.G., Uomoto, J. and McCurry, S.M. (1997) Behavioural treatment of depression in dementia patients: a controlled clinical trial, *Journal of Gerontology*, 52(4): 159–66.

Twigg, J., Atkin, K. and Perring, C. (1990) *Carers and Services: A Review of Research*. London: The Stationery Office.

Whatmore, K. and Mira-Smith, C. (1991) *Eldercare in the 1990s*. Mitcham: Age Concern.

Woods, B., Wills, W. and Higginson, I. (1998) *An Evaluation of the Admiral Nurse Service: An Innovative Service for the Carers of People with Dementia*, Final report to NHS Executive North Thames R&D Directorate. London: Dementia Relief Trust.

Zarit, S.H. and Edwards, A.B. (1996) Family caregiving: research and clinical intervention, in R.T. Woods (ed.) *Handbook of the Clinical Psychology of Ageing*. Chichester: Wiley.

Zarit, S., Orr, N.K. and Zarit, J.M. (1985) *The Hidden Victims of Alzheimer's Disease: Families under Stress*. New York: New York University Press.

14

Normalization as a philosophy of dementia care

Experiences and practice illustrations from a dedicated community mental health nursing team

Dot Weaks and Gill Boardman

Introduction

This chapter aims to describe the philosophy and practice approach that has been developed in one community mental health nursing team for people with dementia in mid-Scotland. The goal of the service is to enable people with dementia and their carers to live a meaningful life, which is of value to them, where, and how, they choose to live it. It is not the intention to give a detailed account of all aspects of our work; instead the focus is on the theory, values and practice of some of our more specialist functions.

Fundamental to the way that the service works is the philosophy of normalization, which is rooted in the discipline of learning disability. Barker and Baldwin (1991) describe an aspect of this philosophical approach as being where caring staff work with people with learning difficulties to enable them to have as normal an experience of living as possible given their limitations.

Our philosophy of dementia care has developed in response to our strongly held belief that people with dementia and their family carers have the right to access care that enables them to continue to live their lives as fully as possible. In other words, we are practising within a philosophy of normalization. The difference between our approach and that of the field of learning disability is that we are trying to preserve, rather than create, the 'normal' aspects of the life of the person with dementia and their family. This philosophy is endorsed by Clarke (1997: 300) who challenges the profession:

> ... to refocus dementia care management on its interpersonal dimensions. To achieve this may mean letting go of some aspects of current professional thought and practice. There is a need to question the use of healthcare interventions that reinforce the abnormality of caregiving and the pathology of dementia.

This challenge affirmed our intuitive approach, which merged with Clarke's (1997) research findings, and which had developed over the previous ten years. Our practice was built firmly on our belief that the therapeutic relationship we engaged in with the person with dementia and the family carer was of paramount importance in enabling and encouraging continuance of their own unique relationship with each other. This philosophical approach was embedded in our belief that the needs of people with dementia and their family carers were met within a family system. In order that this might be achieved, the aim of the community mental health nurse (CMHN) is to become an integral part of that system.

These beliefs initially arose from a process of experiential learning, spending time with people with dementia and their families and listening to their narrative, rather than emerging from an awareness of any theoretical stance or political dictate. Reflecting on our experience, along with taking cognizance of the views of the recipients of our care, enabled us to continually develop and refine our practice. In turn, this constant reflection and critical appraisal of our practice enabled us to create and define our approach to care. There is a special quality to this approach, which marries practice, research and theory. However, in the first instance, our practice was driven by intuition which freed us to be creative in our caregiving.

Developing community mental health nursing practice

In the 1980s, one of the authors (DW) was sister in charge of a day hospital for people with dementia. Whilst working in this position it became obvious that, in order for the person with dementia to maintain as normal a lifestyle as possible, they needed the help and understanding of their family carer. Whilst family support groups were set up within the day hospital, there were no specialist services that embraced the family ethos of care available within the community setting. From evidence gathered within the day hospital setting, it was clear that this was a gap in service provision, and the setting up of a specialist community nursing service proved to be a natural progression as a health care professional.

In 1987, DW became the first CMHN to provide a dedicated service for people with dementia and their family carers within Perthshire, Scotland. Perthshire is one of the largest counties in Scotland covering 2000 square miles comprising both urban and rural localities. The population is 130,000, of whom approximately 25 per cent are over 65 years of age. This high percentage of older people reflects the desirability of the area as an 'ideal place to retire'.

Within one year of establishing the service, it was clear that there were limitations to what one practitioner could achieve trying to serve such a large area. When the co-author (GB) joined the service, the CMHN Dementia Team was formed. Since its inception, the team has evolved to include, by 2002, nine specialist practitioners working in a community setting.

The CMHN Dementia Team

The team is unique in Scotland in that it concentrates on working with people with dementia and their families regardless of age, whereas the traditional service would often be based on the over-65s regardless of their diagnosis. The team is centrally located within Murray Royal Hospital, Perth, and has an open referral system. The majority of our referrals come from medical colleagues – three consultants in old age psychiatry, and the 118 general practitioners (GPs) in the area. Increasingly, referrals are being made by social work colleagues, individuals and their relatives who are concerned about their memory. The CMHNs are assigned to one of the five localities within the county, and work closely with the practices, primary care and social work staff. In the course of a year, the team has a corporate caseload of around 300 patients and families. The more senior team members also take on many different roles, for example teaching, contributing to publications, research, and providing advice to national advisory committees. There are strong links with Alzheimer's Scotland – Action on Dementia, the Dementia Services Development Centre and the Centre for Social Research in Dementia, the latter two situated in Stirling University. We act as a resource for other professionals and are involved in raising public and professional awareness.

What the CMHN Dementia Team does

Planning Signposts for Dementia Care Services (Alzheimer's Scotland – Action on Dementia 2000) draws on the best evidence available on what should be provided as core services for people with dementia. These five services are:

- diagnostic and assessment services;
- early stage responses:
    - therapeutic;
    - support and education;
- community care responses;
- long-term care responses;
- palliative care responses.

What the team offers is as follows:

- A model of assessment and intervention that is focused on the person with dementia in relation to their family situation.
- Increasing involvement in the identification and screening of people with early cognitive impairment.
- Psycho-educational counselling, with one of the senior members of the team having a formal counselling training to MSc level.

- Facilitation of five family support groups run in conjunction with Alzheimer' Scotland – Action on Dementia throughout Perthshire.

- An intent to provide a long-term therapeutic relationship with families throughout the course of the illness; at times it may be enough to provide a telephone counselling service.

There is a need for an inter-disciplinary approach to provide a comprehensive range of services, however *Planning Signposts for Dementia Care Services* emphasizes that early access to these services can have a positive impact on the 'wellbeing of the person with dementia and his or her carer and how they both experience and cope with the illness as it progresses' (p. 15).

The CMHN Dementia Team is involved to varying degrees in all of the five core services identified in *Planning Signposts for Dementia Care Services*, and most of its interventions are carried out within the individual's own home. Wherever possible, the team member tries to include the families or chosen significant others of the person with dementia, whether they live within the immediate environs or at a distance. A considerable proportion of the team's time is spent in telephone counselling and it is making increased use of technology to maintain e-mail contact with many of the family carers.

Theoretical base

Whilst its initial approach to dementia care was intuitive, it was essential to explore theories that would underpin the team's practice. The influential literature at that time was the work of Zarit *et al.* (1985), Adams (1987) and Peplau (1990). Zarit *et al.* (1985) emphasized the importance of stress reduction using psycho-educational counselling with both patient and family; an approach to practice also found influential to the Admiral Nursing service in England (see Chapter 13 for further information about the service). Adams (1987: 9) promoted the use of a counselling approach to people with dementia and their families:

> The literature on the subject is meagre, but in time through research and learning from health visiting and social work, community nurses may develop a knowledge base for the rapidly expanding area of the elderly mentally ill.

Peplau (1990: 38) emphasized nursing as a 'significant therapeutic interpersonal process which functions cooperatively with other human processes that make health possible for individuals'. This emphasis on the relationship between people was significant for team members as CMHNs. The distinct contribution of nursing to health care was also identified by Peplau at this time.

The writings of the authors of the three works cited above continue to be an ongoing influence, and their work validated the team's thinking that it was vital to focus not only on the person with dementia, but also on family and associate carers. Over time it has become clear that by far the most important aspect of the team's work is establishing and maintaining a therapeutic relationship. Kitwood and Bredin (1992) suggested that the lived experience of dementia and its pathology do not match. They also believed that professionals continuing to work within the framework of a medical model do so at the expense of neglecting the importance of family relationships and the personhood of the person with dementia. In a subsequent publication, Kitwood (1997: 19) acknowledges that 'maintaining personhood is both a psychological and neurological task'. We believe that the process of normalization identifies the need of people with dementia and their family carers, at times, to medicalize the changes that dementia brings to their lives in order to make meaning of their own unique experience.

Therefore, a CMHN with the knowledge of dementia as a pathological process and a commitment to the importance of both the therapeutic and family relationship has much to offer the person with dementia and their family. A framework embracing these two components was adopted as the foundation of a model of care that the CMHNs within the team have continued to practise and develop.

The team sees its development as very much part of the culture that Kitwood (1997: 2) promoted when he stressed the need to provide an approach to care that:

> . . . looks far more to human than to medical solutions. Many people have found their way intuitively to such an approach and a new culture of dementia care is slowly coming into being.

The relationship

> The relationship is the first condition of being human. It circumscribes two or more individuals and creates a bond in the space between them which is more than the sum of the parts.
>
> (Clarkson 1995: 4)

Many authors emphasize the importance of the therapeutic relationship within the field of dementia care. However, few highlight the qualities and components of this relationship. In the team's experience and the experience of those for whom it cares, there are many key elements to this relationship. The complexities of elucidating these elements should not be underestimated. In preparation for this chapter, and in order to help clarify what is important from the consumers' perspective, we invited comments about this therapeutic relationship from people with dementia and their family carers. We asked a wide spectrum of patients and carers for their thoughts about the relationship they had with their CMHN. Everyone participating was aware of the purpose of this exercise and consented to be involved. The question was posed in various group settings so that people's 'real' thoughts and feelings could be represented in this chapter. All names appearing in the text have been changed to preserve anonymity. Anecdotal evidence, gleaned from letters received from carers, also highlights the centrality and importance of this therapeutic relationship. For example, one 40-year-old carer wrote about her therapeutic relationship with her CMHN:

> I have had great benefits from my time with her, she is a good listener, non-judgemental, and the trust I feel is enormous, she is a very natural woman . . .

gives just the right amount of support, I talk all the time and things pour forth. I feel a sense of freedom, . . . a sense of knowing myself better and growing . . . and the CMHN has been instrumental in all of that . . . hearing her say it is OK to feel a particular way at times and the guilt to be taken away is wonderful . . . but also to know that she has not taken anything away from my shoulders and placed them on her own.

(Mary, caring for her mother)

Other comments from caregivers were:

The CMHN left us to make our own rules within the context of what was possible. The CMHN did not get between her as the carer and her sister [the person with dementia] which was vital. Lots of helping professionals come into the home and tell me what to do and this undermined my confidence as carer and also affected my relationship with my sister. One of the things the CMHN helped me to do was to preserve our normality for as long as possible. It felt like I was always having to move the goalposts [of the relationship] and the CMHN helped me make these adjustments.

(Sarah, caring for her sister)

You don't come in with a lot of jargon or rules, you provide truthful answers to sometimes some very difficult questions but you never took away the hope.

(Helen, caring for her parents)

Practical advice and information coupled with honest feedback engendered great confidence in me as a carer. Through the CMHN I was able to have access to the possibility of making new relationships [within the context of the carers' support group] which enabled me to have a social life that I thought for me was over. This was one of the many positive aspects of being a carer.

(Charlie, caring for wife)

Matthew wrote retrospectively about the three-year period that the CMHN was involved with his parents:

Even more clearly than at the time I can see how your intervention, with all the support service to which you gave access, allowed them to share a far longer time together at home than would otherwise have been possible . . . It is almost a year since my father died and my mother is only now ready to learn a bit more about Alzheimer's . . . She says that she recognizes that she simply could not take in anything about it while she was looking after father, but is now ready to do so, so the copies of the material which you gave me, I am getting back from my daughter so that mother can now read it . . . Thank you for the way in which you made so many things possible for them.

(Matthew, caring for his parents)

From the above comments and the team's experience of working with people with dementia and their families, it is evident that the important components and qualities of this therapeutic relationship are characterized by the following, and these frame the type of therapeutic relationship in which the team practices:

- Trust
- Non-judgemental attitude
- Respect
- Honesty
- Support
- Autonomy
- Enabling
- Empowering
- Encouraging interdependence
- Promotion of self-worth
- Engendering a warm, empathic understanding.

Clarke's (1997) research identifies three strategies adopted by family carers to help them maintain a normalized relationship with the person with dementia. First, the strategy of pacing was identified. This allows the person with dementia and their family carer to disengage and distance themselves from the physical and psychological demands of caring. This strategy was also found in our survey:

> When day care was suggested, I was not too keen . . . after all it is my duty to care for my husband . . . However with a little encouragement from my CMHN, I now use day care for him and this lets me have some time for myself.
>
> (Jean, who is 61 years old, caring for her husband)

The second strategy identified by Clarke (1997) is that of confiding, where the carer is encouraged and enabled to unburden the stress they feel in their caregiving role. Problem solving is part of this process, as we also found:

> It seemed very disloyal at first talking about my wife and my problems with coping, but now I look forward to my CMHN coming so that I can get things off my chest.
>
> (Willie, who is 77 years old, caring for his wife)

Thirdly, Clarke (1997) identifies how carers use rationalizing to 'cognitively manage' caring for the person with dementia. This strategy involves the carer in acknowledging the changes in the person they are caring for which can be attributable to the disease process. This can then help to normalize the relationship with the person with dementia:

> When I talk to people in the carers group, I count my blessings . . . sometimes I feel I should not be in the group because my problems don't seem so bad.
>
> (Sally, who is 48 years old, caring for her mother)

These three normalizing strategies are facilitated and supported by the team's clinical practice. Much of its work is centred around the use of the CMHN's therapeutic relationship and use of counselling to facilitate and encourage expressions of grief and loss. This is evident for both the person with dementia and their carers who both have individual and shared losses to come to terms with. This bereavement process is ongoing throughout the illness and the team aspires to continuity in having the same team member involved in this process whenever possible until a negotiated point of closure. This practice is also recommended by Clarke (1997: 300), who states:

> Continuity of carer allows the professional carer access to the knowledge base of the family and the person with dementia, and thus allows care to move away from the pessimism of continual decline in dementia to the optimism of sustained family relationships which promote the wellbeing of the person with dementia.

The team's clinical practice

The team's clinical practice has evolved by encouraging team members to become both reflective and reflexive practitioners. Over the years, the team's nursing focus has shifted from being carer orientated and embracing stress management and problem-solving approaches, to seeking genuine partnerships with the person with dementia and their immediate carers. One of the catalysts for change has been due to the fact that, in partnership with consultant colleagues in old age psychiatry, the team has encouraged GPs in the area to identify, and refer to the service, people who have early memory problems. Listening to people with dementia and their families over many years has brought many challenges to the team members, and has fuelled a commitment to early diagnosis. One person with dementia (aged 52), spoke at a national conference about her diagnosis, saying:

> I am the only one who knows what is going on in my mind. Your imagination is far worse than anything you can actually tell. I read a lot and came across what was happening to me in reading. It came as a relief when I was told, or when I told the doctor. Then she told me that I was not going to die in the next two years and that I can make the most of my life. I was already depressed before being diagnosed but when I got over the initial 'I'm very sorry for myself' I felt better . . . I was desperate to know my diagnosis . . . I have never been an ostrich.
> (cited in Fearnley *et al.* 1997: 4)

It is not appropriate to explore here the complexities of the right to know a diagnosis of dementia, but this area is well summarized by Fearnley *et al.* (1997: 36)

> It is the right of the person with dementia to be given an early and accurate diagnosis, if he or she wishes, and information about the condition. Where there is an early diagnosis and both the person with dementia and the carer have the information they need, they are able to work together to deal with both the practical and emotional problems the illness brings. Access to the continuing support of an appropriate, skilled, professional practitioner is vital in allowing the whole family to find positive ways of living with dementia.
> (p. 36)

One of the advantages of early diagnoses is the opportunity that this gives practitioners to form a therapeutic alliance with the person with dementia and/or family carers, allowing that relationship to reach a potential that may not otherwise have been possible. The team is therefore able to explore the use of Clarke's (1997) three normalizing strategies in a way that embraces the caring partnership so that it involves more fully the person with dementia. The person with dementia then becomes the person who genuinely has the lead role in the plan of care, thus encouraging the strategy of 'pacing'.

The forming of such an early therapeutic alliance supports an environment in which the person with dementia and/or their carers can feel able to confide as much or as little as they choose. Psycho-educational counselling facilitates the category of rationalization when it becomes possible for the person with dementia and their carer to select the information they wish to assimilate in order to normalize the changing relationship in the light of the disease process.

What has early diagnosis meant for practice?

Cheston (1997), whilst reviewing the literature on psychotherapeutic work with people with dementia, states 'the earlier in the progression of the disease that the intervention begins, then the more chance there is that the therapeutic intervention will achieve its goals'. When the team started to work with people with an early diagnosis (around 1992), there was very little in the literature that gave the practitioners any guidance about how to 'help' people come to terms with a diagnosis of dementia. Furthermore, the team was working against the professional nihilism that prevailed concerning pre-cholinesterase inhibitor treatments. The fear and anxieties that being so exposed to the person in the 'front line', rather than working one step removed with the carers, highlighted team members' own discomfort and vulnerability to feelings of being impotent and inadequate both personally and professionally. Now, ten years on, seeing people at this early stage of their illness and accompanying them on their pathway through dementia is the accepted norm within the team. Cheston (1997) helps us to make sense of these feelings and enables us to place them in context:

> When we engage in psychotherapeutic work with people with dementia, then we are listening to people talking about a pain that may well one day be our own or that of our husbands, wives, fathers and mothers. We cannot make this future 'better' in the sense of taking this pain away, we can only try and listen and to help the person feel that they have been heard.

These feelings of anxiety and fear were revisited, however, when three of the team members set up a self-help group for people with dementia. This was uncharted territory for those practitioners, and although there was some literature which gave an insight into such groups, the 'felt experience' was very different. The reasons behind the setting up of this group again came from the people with dementia who wanted to meet others in similar circumstances. Cheston (1997) provides insights into how interventions that:

... aim to increase levels of insight must proceed with caution and with an awareness of the social dynamics surrounding the person with dementia. Not only may increases in insight lead, at least initially, to an intensification of emotional reactions, but without support from the other important people in their life, the person with dementia is unlikely to be able to maintain any progress that has been made.

The people attending this group were all well known to the author (DW), as were their families, and much preparatory work had been done with them prior to this group meeting. It was of paramount importance that the group members dictated the content, the structure and pace of each session and took ownership of this. At the end of the group programme a summary of the content was written up and given to each member so that they could refer to it and share it with their family members. This is comparable to the carers' rationalization strategy where they compare and contrast their own specific circumstances with those of others.

The group gave an opportunity for people with dementia to tell their own story and listen to the narrative of others faced with similar difficulties. Some comments from the group members were:

> Most interesting to know that other people have similar feelings with the same problems as myself. Good to have a blether [chat] with them.
>
> (John, 70 years)

> I thought a bad memory was just a bad memory . . . but now I am not so sure. I hadn't realized what it was developing into and the strain that it was putting on to my wife. It has given me much cause to think.
>
> (Ron, 72 years)

> Loss of memory can be very embarrassing and one can become quickly exiled. I think a great deal can be learnt from other members' experiences on how to overcome this unpleasant situation.
>
> (Alan, 87 years)

> I was quite apprehensive and embarrassed, but when the group was finished I was much wiser as regards knowledge of the subject and that I was not alone.
>
> (Anne, 63 years)

All of the people attending the group enjoyed meeting other people in similar circumstances to themselves, and friendships developed as a result of this. One member was keen to know more about the cause and effects of dementia. These statements reflect the comments of the evaluation of the first memory class held in the area and highlights an area of working in true partnership.

This has meant the team's becoming more integrative and flexible in its approach to care. It has moved on from its original ethos of trying to manage the situation in which people with dementia and their families find themselves, and is now adopting a more collaborative approach. In becoming true partners in care, as in all partnerships, the power balance rotates and revolves. For example, the setting of the consultation may influence who feels they have the power in the relationship. In a clinic setting it is usual to assume that the professional has more power than the person with dementia. In past times, it would have been the norm to assume that the professional had more information about the disease than the person with dementia and their family carers. However, in these days of early diagnosis and easier access to sources of information (for example, through the internet), it may be that the greater knowledge base lies within the family. The concept of true partnership is indeed a complex one where the dynamics in the relationships are constantly changing, but the team strives to attain an equal power base.

In summary, the ultimate goal of the team's clinical practice is to enable the person with dementia and their carers to live meaningful lives which are of value to them, wherever and however they choose to live it.

Reflections

The past 15 years of practice as specialist CMHNs in dementia care have witnessed many changes that have influenced the team's practice, and yet there has been a certain stability within the team. For instance, only one member of the team has left over this time, and all members of the team have opted to remain focused in dementia care. The length of time that team members have worked together parallels many patient/carer long-term relationships. As the team has developed, so too have team members developed a deeper understanding of their practice and of each other. They have also attempted to improve the integration between the team and available theory/practice advancements as well as becoming more self-aware. Accordingly, clinical supervision is essential as it generates a focus for self-examination as practitioners – a point Kitwood (1997: 16) would seem to support:

> Thus we are invited to look carefully at ourselves and ponder on how we have developed as persons: where we are indeed strong and capable, but also where we are damaged and deficient. In particular, we might reflect on our own experiential resources for us to be able to help other people in their need.

Weaks (2002) suggests that the relationship needs to be central to make supervision a meaningful activity. There are indeed many parallels between the core conditions described in the supervisory relationship and those pertinent to other meaningful relationships. These three core conditions are that of safety, equality and challenge, and Weaks (2002) suggests that each of these three components needs to be present in equal measure for the relationship to function at its optimum level. Supervision also enhances the ability to learn good psychological care – a point that is reinforced by Carradice, Keady and Hahn later in this book (Chapter 16). We have learnt that there is a fine balance between a neurological stance and a social-psychological stance, and that both have an influence on the process of dementia and that of normalization. Conversely, the same fine balance comes between the needs of the person with dementia and the family carer. This produces not only ethical dilemmas, but also, at times, conflict of interest, and we need to be prepared to roll up our sleeves and get on with the task of conflict resolution. It would be naive not to recognize the tension this can cause the team member. This is a time that informal supervision can be of benefit.

Another positive aspect of supervision is in the defining of acceptable risk. In promoting normalization, we have a responsibility to explore what level of risk is acceptable as normal within that family setting. Scotland is fortunate to have the Adults with Incapacity (Scotland) Act 2000 to help put into place welfare interventions that would benefit the person when they are no longer able to act on their own behalf. The appointing and instructing of a welfare attorney prior to incapacity can ensure the continuance of personal control.

Policy changes, both in local and central government, have and will impinge on the organizations in which we work. We are in the early stages of an amalgamation of health and social work services, and this will undoubtedly present opportunities and threats to the CMHN Dementia Team and to the way in which it conducts practice. One of the biggest problems is the constant under-resourcing of community services in general and in particular for people with dementia. Despite the rhetoric of dementia being a National Health Service funding priority for the 1980s and 1990s (National Health Service 1980, 1988), there remains little in the way of evidence that suggests this was so.

A common humanity is needed to help move us forward. However, when we reflect on this statement we have come to recognize that it was this common humanity that gave the team members the impetus to create and develop this specialist service. The writing of this chapter has enabled us to realize the way in which we continually strive to listen to the people with dementia and their families, and it is this simple action that has stood us in good stead to help meet their needs.

Moving forward – the future

In preparation for joint working we need look no further than this quote from Clarke (1999: 360):

> Realise and value the impact that all health and social care professionals can have in return on people with dementia and their families. The rest, the development of partnerships in practice, will, I think, follow as sure as day follows night.

There arises a huge challenge to social and health care services about how they can provide care that reflects a philosophy of normalization. The person with dementia and their carers are the experts on themselves, and professionals would do well to recognize this and act accordingly. Adopting a philosophy of normalization has allowed us to influence the way in which people with dementia and their families have coped:

> It takes no great philosopher, no expert practitioner, no outstanding researcher, to work alongside people in a way that values them as an individual.

(Clarke 1999: 363)

References

Adams, T. (1987) Dementia is a family affair, *Community Outlook*, February: 7–9.

Alzheimer's Scotland – Action on Dementia (2000) *Planning Signposts for Dementia Care Services*. Edinburgh: Alzheimer's Scotland – Action on Dementia.

Barker, P.J. and Baldwin, S. (1991) *Ethical Issues in Mental Health*. Cheltenham: Stanley Thornes.

Cheston, R. (1997) Psychotherapeutic work with people with dementia: a review of the literature, at http://www.bath.ac.uk/~hssr1lc/psychdm2.htm (accessed 10 October 2001).

Clarke, C.L. (1997) In sickness and in health: remembering the relationship in family caregiving for people with dementia, in M. Marshall (ed.) *The State of the Art in Dementia Care*. London: Centre for Policy on Ageing.

Clarke, C.L. (1999) Taking partnership in dementia care forward, in T. Adams and C.L. Clarke (eds) *Dementia Care: Developing Partnerships in Practice*. London: Ballière Tindall.

Clarkson, P. (1995) *The Therapeutic Relationship*. London: Whurr.

Fearnley, K., McLennan, J. and Weaks, D. (1997) *The Right to Know? Sharing the Diagnosis of Dementia*. Edinburgh: Alzheimer's Scotland – Action on Dementia.

Kitwood, T. (1997) *Dementia Reconsidered: The Person Comes First*. Buckingham: Open University Press.

Kitwood, T. and Bredin, K. (1992) Towards a theory of dementia care: personhood and well-being, *Aging and Society*, 12: 269–87.

National Health Service (1980) Scottish Health Authorities: Priorities for the Eighties. ISBN: 0114916896.

National Health Service (1988) Scottish Health Authorities Review of the Priorities for the Eighties and Nineties. ISBN: 0114934037.

Peplau, H. (1990) Peplau's development model, *Nursing Times*, 86(2): 38–40.

Weaks, D.A. (2002) Unlocking the secrets of good supervision: a phenomenological exploration of experienced counsellors' perceptions of good supervision, *Counselling and Psychotherapy Research*, 2(1): 33–9.

Zarit, S.H., Orr, N.K. and Zarit, J.M. (1985) *The Hidden Victims of Alzheimer's Disease*. New York: New York University Press.

15

Assessing and responding to challenging behaviour in dementia

A focus for community mental health nursing practice

Marilla Pugh and John Keady

Introduction

From the time when Alois Alzheimer first documented his 'unusual illness of the cerebral cortex' (see Stelzmann *et al.* 1995), the more challenging attributes of dementia, such as wandering and aggression have come to define, in the public, professional and, arguably, the academic imagination, the characteristics of dementia. For researchers in the field it was this construction of dementia that led to the plethora of research studies in the 1980s and early 1990s that explored the nature of carer stress, constructed numerous 'caregiver burden scales' and ultimately identified the person with dementia and their unpredictable behaviour as the root cause of 'the problem'.

As time has moved on, the notion of what constitutes challenging behaviour in the field of dementia care, and whose constructions take precedence in formulating its meaning, has become clouded. Many of the preheld assumptions have come under increasing scrutiny and criticism (Kitwood 1997). For instance, we know from subjective accounts from carers that the time spent at the onset of the person's (undiagnosed) dementia, and the subsequent diagnostic quest, are among the most stressful experiences in the entire caregiving trajectory (Kuhlman *et al.* 1991). Similarly, for people with dementia, coping with the demands of living alone is seen to be challenging, with continual adjustment and imaginative coping efforts necessary to maintain activities of living within 'safe' limits and boundaries (Alzheimer's Society 1994). As such, it is becoming increasingly necessary to understand the context/environment for the exhibited behaviour and what its purpose represents. Just who is it that is being challenged?

To begin to address this changing face of dementia care, and to take a more egalitarian view of what constitutes challenging behaviour, and professional assessment of need, this chapter divides into three distinct sections. First, the current literature on the nature of challenging behaviour will be more fully developed. The historical perspectives of dementia are briefly explored, together with more (professionally driven) definitions of what denotes challenging behaviour and how it can be measured. Secondly, the chapter presents three (anonymized) case studies drawn from the current practice of one of the authors (MP) to outline some of the issues noted to be challenging when faced by the community mental health nurse (CMHN) in their daily practice. These case studies cover three care settings, namely: a younger person with dementia with disinhibited behaviour; working with a person with dementia and staff in residential care who have conflicting interpretations of attention-seeking behaviour; and balancing a person with dementia's right to live alone with dementia against protection from the consequences of their actions. Finally, the chapter presents a discussion on the preceding text and points a way forward for community mental health nursing practice in dementia care in working with challenging behaviour.

Challenging behaviour: inner meaning and observed reality

Stelzmann *et al.*'s (1995) English translation of Alzheimer's 1907 article in which he (Alzheimer) described the 'unusual illness' of Auguste D, a 51-year-old woman admitted to the Frankfurt insane asylum in Germany, is an intriguing read for a number of reasons. For one, it contains a personal history of Auguste D that brings us closer to her as a person and then documents the post-mortem changes in her 'evenly atrophic brain' (Stelzmann *et al.* 1995: 430) after her death – Auguste D was to spend some four-and-a-half years in the asylum. Read in conjunction with the English translation of the later discovery of the case file of Auguste D (Maurer *et al.* 1997), a case file that also contained a photograph of her taken in 1902, it is an enduring legacy of the impact of the condition on people and their families. Moreover, Alzheimer's case description of Auguste D became the blueprint for 'Alzheimer's disease' and the ensuing medical discourse that surrounded the experience of dementia for much of the twentieth century.

By studying Stelzmann *et al.*'s (1995) translation of Alzheimer's 1907 article, the reader is immediately struck by the recognizable traits in Auguste D's behaviour and the asylum staff's struggle to interpret the meanings behind her actions. For example, prior to her admission to the asylum in 1901, Auguste D is reported by Dr Alzheimer as showing evidence of: jealousy towards her husband; a rapid loss of memory; carrying things from place to place and hiding them; believing that someone was trying to kill her; crying loudly. On admission from home to the asylum, the translation reveals the following telling observation:

> She [Auguste D] is completely delirious, drags around her bedding, calls her husband and daughter and seems to suffer from auditory hallucinations. Often she screamed for many hours. Unable to understand the situation, she starts screaming as soon as an attempt is made to examine her.
>
> (Stelzmann *et al.* 1995: 429)

Behaviours that we would, today, record as challenging. Indeed, 'challenging behaviour' is a term that has its roots in the field of learning disability (Emerson

1995) and, as stated earlier, has come to define the 'disruptive' behaviours exhibited by people with dementia in both the community (Keady and Nolan 1996; Hawranik and Strain 2001) and residential care (Moniz-Cook *et al.* 2001) environments. For instance, Holm *et al.* (1999) stress that, over the course of dementia, 'impairments' are found in cognitive, non-cognitive and behavioural functions that encompass agitation, irritability, mood liability, verbally disruptive behaviour and physical aggression. Transference of such behaviours into the formation of assessment tools for use in care homes, for instance, has become commonplace. The recently published Challenging Behaviour Scale (CBS) for older people living in care homes (Moniz-Cook *et al.* 2001) lists 25 such behaviours ranging from 'physical aggression' (operationalized as hits, kicks, scratches, grabbing), to 'spitting', 'faecal smearing' and on to 'demands attention'. Whilst it may be possible to then list the frequency of the behaviour, rate its difficulty and the amount of 'challenge' it presents to staff, the compilation of such a list interprets challenging behaviour from a purely professional perspective. Arguably, such scales, as well intentioned as they are, also run the risk of separating the person from the nature, context and meaning of their actions and label the person according to their presented behaviour.

Continuing to build on this professional construction of challenging behaviour, both Swearer *et al.* (1988) and Burns *et al.* (1990) suggest that around 80 per cent of people with dementia display one or more 'troublesome behaviours'. Previously, clinical management of such behaviours has been by drug prescription, usually low-dose antipsychotics, in order to limit the distress to the person with dementia and, it must be said, to those in close contact with the individual. However, it is vital that antipsychotic medication is not seen as the first port of call in managing such 'troublesome behaviours', as the evidence clearly states that overuse of such drugs can lead to a worsening of the dementia, oversedation, falls and tardive dyskinesia (American Psychiatric Association 1994). Moreover, there is the thorny issue of ensuring the person with dementia's consent to take such medication and the legal role of practitioners in assisting in such processes (Jones 2001). Recent guidance by the Royal College of Psychiatrists (see Palmer 1999) has also suggested that clinical management should exclude any underlying causes of the 'behavioural disorder' by searching for evidence of an 'acute physical illness, environmental distress or physical discomfort' (p. 39).

The shift in the literature now appears to be that 'challenging behaviour' in a person with dementia is indicative of inner meaning. It is not merely 'challenging' but also a way for the person to get their message across, having lost the skills to communicate their needs and wants in the usual ways (Killick and Allan 2001). Drawing on the work at the Bradford Dementia Group in the UK, Innes and Jacques (1998) cogently argue that the person-centred approach provides the framework and value-laden philosophy necessary to look beyond the presented behaviour to the message of communication it entails. If we hold this paradigm as a truism, then in order to find a more meaningful definition of challenging behaviour we must begin to look at how those living (and working) with the condition both understand and construct 'the challenge'.

Challenging behaviour and community mental health nursing practice

From the authors' collective practice experience, the CMHN role in responding to the challenging behaviour of the person with dementia is multi-faceted, not least because each client is referred to the service at different times and at different points in their journey through dementia. Similarly, there may not always be a shared understanding behind the initial referral, with the carer seeking confirmation that 'something is wrong', whilst the person with (undiagnosed) dementia may not believe that there is anything untoward happening. As such, the CMHN has to tread a fine line between understanding the nature of the referral and responding to the conflict in understanding that might be present in the family situation.

In routine practice, a referral to the CMHN has usually been made because of some kind of challenging behaviour that has been brought to the attention of the general practitioner (GP) by the family and/or person with dementia themself. At this time, the CMHN has the opportunity to befriend the family and the person with dementia. Notwithstanding other constraints, the more time invested with the family at the beginning of a relationship to build up a feeling of trust and professional competence in their actions, the more effective the CMHN appears to be in being able to maintain the relationship with the family and 'stay involved'. As one of the authors (MP) has found over the years, going to a client's home clutching a host of behavioural and stress-rating scales can be counterproductive and the first visit is best constructed as a 'fact-finding mission' in order to allow the person with dementia (at times undiagnosed) and the family a chance to 'tell it as it is'. It would usually be at this initial, or follow-up, visit that the carer, or person with dementia, or both, would mention the nature and context of the challenging behaviour.

In MP's experience, there are many behaviours that people with dementia display that are not seen as challenging by their family carer, but that could be categorized as such in textbooks, as these two case vignettes illustrate.

Case vignette 1

Hour after hour, Mrs Jones (the person with dementia) constantly followed her husband around the house. The greatest concern of the CMHN was that this was stressful for Mr Jones as he could not possibly endure the restrictions on his time and social activities that such actions engendered. However, on discussion with Mr Jones he saw this behaviour as 'helpful' as it allowed him to 'keep an eye' on his wife without compromising her independence. It was, after all, his wife's decision to follow him around the house. This interpretation of events and the meanings Mr Jones attached to them served as an important lesson to the CMHN in that it was important not to use a professional lens to view such behaviour and constructions of stress. Equally, it served as an important reminder for the CMHN to listen and get to know the person with dementia, their family and biography as much as possible before being tempted to give advice.

Case vignette 2

Mrs Saunders looks after her husband, ex Wing Commander Graham Saunders. In the evening, Mrs Saunders found it difficult to persuade her husband to take off his clothes and put on his pyjamas ready for bed. Mrs Saunders became upset and distressed when her husband refused to comply with this simple request, and he, in turn became, angry and intimidating towards his wife. It was a cycle of discontent that was proving distressing for the couple. After discussing this issue with the CMHN, Mrs Saunders agreed to try to leave Mr Saunders in his own clothes and allow him to 'sleep in them'. Mr Saunders could then have his regular shower and put on his clean clothes in the morning. This strategy worked well and, on reflection, Mrs Saunders confided to the CMHN that she just needed 'permission from someone in authority' to say that it was all right to let her husband sleep in his clothes and that it was not 'dirty' to do this. Providing legitimacy to carers' decision making is an important, yet invisible, aspect of community mental health nursing practice and one that needs to be articulated in a variety of ways, including through documentation.

However, there are often other forms of challenging behaviour facing family carers and people with dementia that cannot be so easily solved, as these more detailed case studies illustrate.

Case study 1: client whose behaviour challenged the abilities of the family

Mrs James was diagnosed with fronto-temporal lobe dementia in 1997. She was 51 years old at the time. The CMHN became involved from the point of diagnosis and discovered from Mr James that he had noticed changes in his wife's memory as far back as 1994. A significant event that stands out in his mind was the morning of their daughter's graduation. Mrs James knew there was something important happening that day, but could not remember what it was.

Mrs James was referred to the CMHN by the GP because he felt that Mr James needed to have a break from caring for his wife. Following an initial assessment of the domestic situation, it was apparent that Mr James was extremely tired and worried about the future. He was attempting to hold down a full-time job and look after his wife with no help at all from outside agencies. It was becoming obvious to him that his wife could be left alone only for shorter and shorter periods. He would rush home from work at lunchtime to check on his wife, and arrive home at 5.00 pm wondering what he would find. Due to Mrs James having a fronto-temporal lobe dementia, she displayed many obsessional traits that, interestingly enough, worked to the carer's advantage. For example, every Thursday, without fail, Mrs James would take exactly the same route to the local shop to buy 'word search' magazines. She would return and spend the whole morning at the kitchen table attempting to complete them. This meant that Mr James could relax a little knowing his wife was safe and occupied. The most worrying feature of her condition for him was her habit of walking up quietly behind him, and then either grabbing his waist or tapping him on the top of his head as a joke. This was regardless of the task he was performing, whether it was carrying a pan of boiling water from the cooker or stirring food on the hob. Also, immediately after Mrs James had done this, she would forget and do it again a few minutes later. As Mr James explained to the CMHN: 'It wasn't funny the first time, so on the eighteenth time you wanted to scream at her.' For Mr James, this repetitive behaviour was almost too much to bear on a daily basis.

To alleviate the situation, the CMHN arranged for Mrs James, with her permission, to attend a specialist dementia day centre. This day centre had the capacity to give one-to-one attention so that Mrs James could be constantly occupied in order to minimize upset to others and herself. The nurses at the day centre undertook non-verbal communication techniques to help cope with the behaviour and ensure that Mrs James did not feel excluded in any way. Staff also made sure that they never turned their back on Mrs James, although Mrs James adapted her behaviour by attempting to kiss staff on the lips.

Mrs James also took to pacing in a repetitive fashion and, after excluding any other physical cause for the behaviour, the consultant psychiatrist prescribed a trial of low-dose antidepressant medication to help stem her obsessional movement. Unfortunately, this approach did not help, as the repetitive behaviour continued to such an extent that Mr James asked the advice of the CMHN about retiring early from his work. He was advised to discuss his pension rights with his firm's financial department since the company already knew of his home situation. Once Mr James had all the financial information to hand, he decided that he had both the necessary financial security to retire early and the altruistic motives to care for his wife. To continue to support the couple, the CMHN then arranged for a trained home care worker to visit Mrs James at home for two afternoons a week. The home care worker also visited the day centre to see how the nurses worked with Mrs James's behaviour, building on a plan initiated by the CMHN. This helped a great deal and the home care worker was soon able to take Mrs James shopping. This, at first, was challenging to the home care worker as Mrs James would attempt to kiss strangers in the supermarket. However, with the CMHN assessment and intervention on the next few visits to the supermarket, it was found that if Mrs James was kept constantly occupied with pushing the trolley and organizing the groceries in it, the behaviour diminished.

Slowly, over the months and years, the strong relationship forged between Mr James, his wife and the CMHN helped to overcome other obstacles in their relationship. Mr James was able to take comfort in the fact that no problem was insurmountable if help was sought and preventative measures put in place. Mr James continues to attend the carers' support group once a month and gathers strength from the friends he has made. The CMHN has also continued to have regular clinical supervision and has kept a detailed record of the behavioural and cognitive interventions that have helped to keep the couple together for the past five years.

Community mental health nursing activity in residential care

There have been many studies looking at the person with dementia's behaviour in residential care homes and various methods of behaviour modification have been postulated. Some go as far as to suggest the provision of behavioural intensive care units (Mintzer *et al.* 1993), where it is advocated that a client with a particular challenging behaviour, for example agitation or repetitive behaviour, would benefit from being admitted for a limited period. In such a setting it is suggested that the person with dementia can be monitored more closely so that the primary cause of their behaviour can be assessed and modified. Contemporaneously, the person's home can be adapted and their family re-educated in preparation for their relative's return home.

In contrast, other articles suggest methods of measuring behaviour using various rating scales to give parameters to the behaviour and its negative impact on the person/family. Examples of these scales include:

- Cohen-Mansfield Agitation Inventory (Cohen-Mansfield 1986).
- Staff Observation and Assessment Scale (Palmsteirna and Wistedt 1987).
- Disruptive Behaviour Rating Scales (Mungas *et al.* 1989).
- Rating Scale for Aggressive Behaviour in the Elderly (RAGE) (Patel and Hope 1992).
- Brief Agitation Rating Scale (Finkel *et al.* 1993).
- Disruptive Behaviour Scale (Beck *et al.* 1997).
- Perceived Difficulty in Managing Challenging Behaviour: The Challenging Behaviour Vignettes (Silver 1998).
- Challenging Behaviour Scale (Moniz-Cook *et al.* 2001).

The careful measurement and monitoring of challenging behaviour suggests that the behaviour can in some way be changed or modified. In a study by Allen-Burge *et al.* (1999) it is argued that, once a behaviour has been identified as challenging, various approaches and interventions can be used to reduce the behaviour, for example through the use of tactile stimulation, including the playing of gentle music and recounting cherished memories. Consequently, addressing and responding to challenging behaviour in a residential care setting requires a different approach by the CMHN from that encountered in the home situation. However, many lessons can be learnt and transferred from one environment to the other. Firstly, and most importantly, each person with dementia should be treated as an individual and not labelled the same as their 'behaviour', as this can lead to increased levels of conflict and upset (Johnson 1996). In the community, the person with dementia's family continue to possess significant knowledge about the person's biography, and in working in a residential setting this also must be gathered and collated. Secondly, it is essential that a good relationship is built up between the residential home staff, the family carer(s) and the CMHN. If care staff have a good understanding of the person's biography, their likes and dislikes and so forth, then the meaning of presented challenging behaviour may be easier to identify and, better still, understood. This issue is further explored in the next case study.

Case study 2: client in residential care

Mrs Turner had been admitted to Fairhaven Residential Home in early 1999 following a fall at her home and a short spell in the local general hospital. Her family (daughter and son-in-law) had noticed that she had become increasingly forgetful and unsteady on her feet. So, when the hospital social worker suggested that residential care 'might be a good option for all concerned', they decided that this was the best alternative in order to keep Mrs Turner 'safe and sound'. The family looked carefully at numerous places and finally decided upon Fairhaven Residential Home as a friend had recommended it having visited an aunt there in the past. Also, the staff appeared friendly whenever they were shown around, and the residents seemed happy in their surroundings. Mrs Turner duly moved into the home in February 1999, taking residence in her own room. Many of her personal belongings and possessions were brought with her, such as pictures, ornaments and a quilt cover.

This peaceful transition was soon to be disturbed. In May 1999 the CMHN (MP) was telephoned by the officer-in-charge of Fairhaven Residential Home asking for advice on how to look after Mrs Turner. The officer-in-charge explained that Mrs Turner, who had initially 'settled in very well', had changed character and was now 'very difficult to manage'. By further exploring these issues it appeared that Mrs Turner was taking up too much of the carer workers' time whenever they went into her room. If a care worker tried to make an excuse and leave, Mrs Turner would use all manner of means to keep them in the room. If the carer workers avoided going into Mrs Turner's room, she would simply put herself on the floor, or feign being unable to get up from the toilet so that they would have to attend to her. The officer-in-charge wondered if this behaviour was due to Mrs Turner's 'dementing illness'.

Within a few days the CMHN visited the home and was able to talk with the officer-in-charge, Mrs Turner and her daughter. Mrs Turner's daughter explained that before her mother had been admitted to hospital, she had been living alone in a remote area of North Wales that was difficult to access. She had visited her mother two or three times a week, but her mother had been resistive to any other offers of help. Her daughter had wanted to get services involved but Mrs Turner declined all offers. Therefore, an admission to hospital, coupled with the hospital social worker's suggestion of a residential home placement, had been seen by the daughter as an ideal opportunity to solve this dilemma and assuage her mother's loneliness. More concerningly, it transpired from the conversation that neither her daughter nor the social worker had sought Mrs Turner's opinion on the desirability of the move prior to its occurrence. The officer-in-charge also informed the CMHN that Mrs Turner could not be persuaded to leave her room to socialize with other residents even for meals.

As an initial response, the CMHN talked with Mrs Turner in private and it soon became apparent that she was very unhappy. Is seems that she resented being in Fairhaven Residential Home even though the staff were 'nice to her', and the thought of mixing with a number of strangers in a communal lounge was 'terrifying'. It also transpired that Mrs Turner had lived alone since the late 1960s when her husband, Harry, had passed away, and she had learnt to enjoy her own company. As Mrs Turner had become frailer, both cognitively and physically, her daughter had begun to visit more frequently and Mrs Turner started to look forward to these visits more and more.

By building a detailed profile over a number of visits, it appeared that the reawakened social side of Mrs Turner was being integrated into her present actions whereby she looked forward to the care workers coming into her room 'to talk', but she felt she must keep them there in case they 'did not return for a long time'. Moreover, Mrs Turner understood her daughter's reasons for wanting her to live in Fairhaven Residential Home, but this coincided with a reduction in the visits of her daughter to see her; her daughter believing that her mother did not need to see her as often. The most upsetting thing for Mrs Turner was her belief that she had been abandoned.

The CMHN had discussions with staff and Mrs Turner's daughter, and a behavioural approach was decided upon. The main body of the programme involved reassuring Mrs Turner that when a member of staff was leaving her room she was given a time that the staff member would return. The importance of sticking to this time and not missing it was reiterated to the staff. Another part of the programme involved Mrs Turner's daughter's visits. As her daughter worked in the town close to Fairhaven Residential Home, it was agreed that she would visit for an hour after work, three days a week instead of spending the whole of Wednesday afternoon visiting her mother. The programme and the reasons for it were explained to Mrs Turner so that her cooperation and consent could be gained. This was duly given and Mrs Turner said that she would look forward to her daughter's more frequent visiting.

It was explained to the care staff the possible reasons for Mrs Turner's behaviour and the fact that her capacity to remember time may be diminishing. A series of cards prompting Mrs Turner to remember when a member of staff would come back to her was made. The CMHN monitored the programme weekly. The first week was quite disappointing in that the staff had found it difficult to adhere to the programme because of the demands on their time, but with encouragement they persevered and towards the end of the second week, when Fairhaven Residential Home had more staff available, there was a marked difference in Mrs Turner's behaviour. By the end of the third week there had been no more incidents of Mrs Turner putting herself on the floor, and only on one occasion had she got herself to the toilet and remained there. Over the following weeks it was noticed that her relationship with her daughter had changed dramatically and her daughter felt more relaxed and 'less guilty' over her role in placing her mother in care.

This case study illustrates the importance of all parties working together to understand the context and meaning of the exhibited behaviour. The behaviour programme and its evaluation simply directed the care programme to a more person-centred framework and allowed Mrs Turner to articulate her needs and desires within achievable goals. The case study further illustrates the need to see challenging behaviour as a form of communication and not simply as a problem that needs managing.

Living alone with dementia

Whilst an under-researched area of dementia care, the available literature has consistently demonstrated both the difficulties in reaching this population and, once detected in the community, the adverse risks that are associated with living alone with the condition. For example, the Alzheimer's Society (1994) report *Home Alone* found that those people living alone with dementia were at an increased risk of financial abuse, neglect and self-injurious behaviour. Similarly, the legal protection afforded to practitioners involved in the care of those living alone with dementia, and the need to balance personal freedom of the person with dementia against acceptable levels of risk, is fraught with difficulties (Jones 2001). The following practice dilemma illustrates this point.

Case study 3: client living alone

Mrs Davies is 97 years old and lives alone in a large terraced house with her little dog Del. She has lived alone for 30 years since her husband's death. According to her GP, Mrs Davies had been diagnosed with dementia since approximately 1992. Mrs Davies has two nieces and a nephew, all of whom live at least 10 to 20 miles away. However, a niece and nephew each visit once a week.

Mrs Davies was referred to the community mental health nursing service in 1999 and MP has been her CMHN since this time. Mrs Davies is a fiercely independent woman who does not believe that there is anything wrong with her. Previously, MP has managed to persuade Mrs Davies to accept home care (although she refuses to pay for it), and this has increased to three times a day, seven days a week. After many false starts, Mrs Davies also attends the local day centre for people with dementia, mostly three times a week. Sometimes she flatly refuses to go, saying she is 'far too busy'. Mrs Davies leads a very active life, most days walking into town with her dog for meat, bread and her pension. She has, so far, always managed to find her way back home.

MP has built up a good relationship with her family and the GP, and this has helped in times of crisis. For instance, on one occasion Mrs Davies took herself on the bus to her previous home some 35 miles away, forgetting that she had moved to her current address 30 years ago. Her old house is now an Oxfam shop in a busy high street, and the police were called because she was verbally abusing the staff, demanding that they leave her house and 'take their junk with them'. MP rose to this challenge by calling a meeting with Mrs Davies's family and her GP to discuss her future needs. All parties agreed that, apart from the obvious risk of her repeating the incident, Mrs Davies was not actually a danger to herself and that she should remain at home.

The situation remained the same until early 2001 when MP received a telephone call from the local police to say that Mrs Davies was calling them frequently using the 999 service. The officer explained that she had telephoned 57 times in two months and the content of the calls was always about 'someone stealing her property'. At another time, the CMHN called to find black smoke billowing out of the kitchen. Mrs Davies seemed unperturbed by this and happily allowed the nurse to investigate. It appeared that she had attempted to grill frozen, oven-bake fish and chips in the polystyrene container. She had then gone into the next room and forgotten about them.

Such challenges require imaginative solutions. After dealing with any immediate dangers, the CMHN arranged for the home carer to visit half an hour earlier each day in order that the care worker and Mrs Davies could prepare Mrs Davies's lunch together. This plan failed, as Mrs Davies did not want any help in the kitchen as she had tended to her needs all her life and could see no good reason for this threat to her independence. After Mrs Davies had again seriously compromised her personal safety a number of times, MP had no alternative but to organize a Mental Health Act section assessment with the GP and approved social worker. Mrs Davies's family was also kept fully informed about this turn of events. The section assessment was carried out and the opinions of the GP and approved social worker gained. Even though the degree of risk was substantial, it was decided not to place Mrs Davies under a section of the Mental Health Act 1983 and take her to hospital against her will.

This situation has proved extremely challenging for the CMHN over a long period of time. The intervention that appears to assist MP the most is the sharing of knowledge and responsibility with other colleagues and access to regular clinical supervision. Strategies for risk management have also been extremely important in this case (see also Chapter 5 in this book by Manthorpe) and access to regular clinical supervision has helped the CMHN to understand and act on her own knowledge of the client and her situation.

Conclusion

The public information brochure *Who Cares* (Health Education Authority 1997), which is aimed at carers of people with confusion, aligns the role of the CMHN in dementia care with the person with dementia and defines their specialist skills as 'an ability to help with the person's emotional and behavioural problems' (Health Education Authority 1997: 30). Whilst adopting a more holistic, family-centred approach, what becomes apparent from the case studies presented in this chapter is that the CMHNs' interpersonal skills and ability to build partnerships and trust helps to inform their decision-making and priority setting. Perhaps where the literature is lacking is in the evaluation of community mental health nursing practice in this arena and how CMHNs then adapt and measure their practice accordingly.

As a starting point, we feel that it is important that CMHNs look at the person with dementia's behaviour through a lens of meaning, building up a picture of what the person is doing and how they are attempting to communicate. Whilst assessment scales can be a useful way of framing this event, their boundaries and constructions are potentially limiting. It would seem more important that the CMHN views the world of the person with dementia through empathetic eyes, whilst also attending to the very real and practical needs of families. Perhaps what is needed is a stream of collaborative research enquiry that takes a fresh look at challenging behaviour and, as Chapman *et al.* (1999) cogently argue, starts from the premise of 'whose problem?'. At present, there are no solutions, only indicators for future actions.

References

Allen-Burge, R., Stevens, A.B. and Burgio, L.D. (1999) Effective behavioural interventions for decreasing dementia: related challenging behaviour in nursing homes, *International Journal of Geriatric Psychiatry*, 14: 213–32.

Alzheimer's Society (1994) *Home Alone: Living Alone with Dementia*. London: Alzheimer's Society.

American Psychiatric Association (1994) *DSM-IV: Diagnostic and Statistical Manual of Mental Disorders*, 4th edn. Washington, DC: American Psychiatric Association.

Beck, C., Heithoff, K., Baldwin, B. *et al.* (1997) Assessing disruptive behaviour in older adults: the Disruptive Behaviour Scale, *Aging and Mental Health*, 1(1): 71–9.

Burns, A., Jacoby, R. and Levy, R. (1990) Psychiatric phenomena in Alzheimer's disease, *British Journal of Psychiatry*, 157: 86–94.

Chapman, A., Jackson, G.A. and McDonald, C. (1999) *What Behaviour? Whose Problem?* Stirling: Dementia Services Development Centre, University of Stirling.

Cohen-Mansfield, J. (1986) Agitated behaviour in the elderly. II: Preliminary results in the cognitively deteriorated, *Journal of American Geriatrics Society*, 34: 722–7.

Emerson, E. (1995) *Challenging Behaviour Analysis and Intervention in People with Learning Difficulties*. Cambridge: Cambridge University Press.

Finkel, S.I., Lyons, J.S. and Anderson, R.L. (1993) A brief agitation rating scale (BARS) for nursing home elderly, *Journal of the American Geriatric Society*, 41: 50–2.

Hawranik, P.G. and Strain, L.A. (2001) Cognitive impairment, disruptive behaviors, and home care utilization, *Western Journal of Nursing Research*, 23(2): 148–62.

Health Education Authority (1997) *Who Cares? Information and Support for the Carers of Confused People*. Information booklet. London: Health Education Authority.

Holm, A., Michel, M., Stern, G.A. *et al.* (1999) The outcomes of an inpatient treatment program for geriatric patients with dementia and dysfunctional behaviors, *The Gerontologist*, 39(6): 668–76.

Innes, A. and Jacques, I. (1998) The construction of challenging behaviour, *Elderly Care*, 10(5): 17–19.

Johnson, J.R. (1996) Risk factors associated with negative interactions between family caregivers and elderly care receivers, *International Journal of Aging and Human Development*, 43: 7–20.

Jones, R.G. (2001) Ethical and legal issues in the care of people with dementia, *Reviews in Clinical Gerontology*, 11: 245–68.

Keady, J. and Nolan, M. (1996) Behavioural and Instrumental Stressers in Dementia (BISID): refocusing the assessment of caregiver need in dementia, *Journal of Psychiatric and Mental Health Nursing*, 3(3): 163–72.

Killick, J. and Allan, K. (2001) *Communication and the Care of People with Dementia*. Buckingham: Open University Press.

Kitwood, T. (1997) *Dementia Reconsidered: The Person Comes First*. Buckingham: Open University Press.

Kuhlman, G.J., Wilson, H.S., Hutchinson, S.A. and Wallhagen, M. (1991) Alzheimer's disease and family caregiving: critical synthesis of the literature and research agenda, *Nursing Research*, 40(6): 331–7.

Maurer, K., Volk, S. and Gerbaldo, H. (1997) Auguste D and Alzheimer's disease, *Lancet*, 349: 1546–9.

Mintzer, J.E., Lewis, L., Pennypaker, L. *et al.* (1993) Behavioral Intensive Care Unit (BICU): a new concept in the management of acute agitated behavior in elderly demented patients, *The Gerontologist*, 33(6): 801–6.

Moniz-Cook, E., Woods, R., Gardiner, E., Silver, M. and Agar, S. (2001) The Challenging Behaviour Scale (CBS): development of a scale for staff caring for older people in residential and nursing homes, *British Journal of Clinical Psychology*, 40: 309–22.

Mungas, D., Weiler, P., Fronzi, C. and Henry, R. (1989) Assessment of disruptive behaviour associated with dementia: the Disruptive Behaviour Rating Scales, *Journal of Geriatric Psychiatry and Neurology*, 2: 196–202.

Palmer, C. (1999) *Evidence Based Briefing: Dementia. A Compilation of Secondary Research Evidence, Guidelines and Consensus Statements.* London: Royal College of Psychiatrists.

Palmsteirna, B. and Wistedt, B. (1987) Staff observation aggression scale: presentation and evaluation, *Acta Psychiatrica Scandinavia*, 76: 657–63.

Patel, V. and Hope, R. (1992) A Rating Scale for Aggressive Behaviour in the Elderly – The RAGE, *Psychological Medicine*, 22: 211–21.

Silver, M. (1998) The challenging behaviour vignettes: assessing the management styles care staff use to deal with challenging behaviour in residential and nursing homes for older people. Unpublished MSc thesis, University of Hull.

Stelzmann, R.A., Schnitzlein, H.N. and Murtagh, R.R. (1995) An English translation of Alzheimer's 1907 paper, 'Über eine eigenartige Erkankung der Hirnrinde', *Clinical Anatomy*, 8: 429–31.

Swearer, J.M., Drachman, D.A., O'Donnell, B.F. and Mitchell, A.C. (1988) Troublesome and disruptive behaviour in dementia: relationships to diagnosis and disease severity, *Journal of the American Geriatrics Society*, 36: 784–90.

PART THREE

**Leading and developing community
mental health nursing in dementia**

16

Clinical supervision and dementia care
Issues for community mental health nursing practice

Angela Carradice, John Keady and Sue Hahn

Introduction

With recent changes in UK health care priorities, treatment provided in the National Health Service (NHS) aims to be guided by evidence based practice and clinical governance (Department of Health 1997). These values emphasize the importance of quality service provision which targets interventions that scientific evaluations propose as the most likely to provide successful outcomes (Gray 1997). Within this climate there is a drive for improving practice and accountability within all professions. The professional body for nursing, the United Kingdom Central Council for Nursing, Midwifery and Health Visiting (UKCC) – now the Nursing and Midwifery Council – advocates the development of a more 'reflective, knowledgeable, accountable and flexible nurse practitioner' (UKCC 1986) and there is a clear expectation that clinical supervision should be integral to accountability and practice development (Department of Health 1994; UKCC 1994, 1996). As yet, the provision and uptake of clinical supervision is in its infancy and this chapter suggests a number of explanations for this. The text then uses a case study to explore the value of clinical supervision to community mental health nursing practice in dementia care by illustrating some beneficial processes in practice. Finally, some implications for practice development are considered.

Development of clinical supervision within nursing: influences and obstacles

The development of clinical supervision within nursing has been directly influenced by the explosion of literature and policy recommendations that support the advancement of practice development through reflective discourse (Graham 1999). However, although there are examples of excellent practice, in reality the growth of provision has been slow and obstacles continue to exist. One factor that causes tension is the meaning of clinical supervision to nurses. Traditional overseeing of practice has been viewed as having a managerial, rather than an educational or clinical function, and this has proven to be a challenge to the effective establishment of clinical supervision (Platt-Koch 1986; Hill 1989). At the root of some of these difficulties is the continued confusion between the meaning of management supervision and that of clinical supervision (Yegdich 1999). The former is focused within an appraisal process on what the professional does, whereas the latter is associated more with developing how the nurse (in this instance) works. Without a clear understanding of this paradigm, clinical supervision will be vulnerable to misinterpretation and to being transformed into managerial supervision (Yegdich 1999). Accordingly, it is not surprising that there is scepticism and resistance within nursing to the adoption of this approach (Cutcliffe and Proctor 1998).

Another reason for clinical supervision not being practised extensively within nursing may be that it is not widely understood by nurses (White *et al.* 1993). However, within psychology, psychotherapy and counselling there are a range of models of clinical supervision which could provide guidance to nursing (Sloan *et al.* 2000). For example, models exist that conceptualize the purposes and processes of supervision (see Scaife 2001 for a detailed summary), and contributions are available from specific therapeutic paradigms such as psychodynamic psychotherapy (Scanlon and Weir 1997) and cognitive therapy (Sloan *et al.* 2000). To complement the models of supervision, there is an abundance of accessible reviews of the processes used, practical descriptions of the complex skills involved in providing clinical supervision and advice about how to make the best use of clinical supervision (see Inskipp and Proctor 1993, 1995).

Despite this vast literature there appears to be little consideration of supervision models within the nursing profession. Most publications that consider supervision issues describe either implementation or subjective evaluation and do not consider the practical application of supervision models. Indeed, it has been observed that most nurses set about clinical supervision 'blindly' with a lack of attention to frameworks (White *et al.* 1998). The few exceptions that exist in the literature, such as those by Fowler (1996a) and van Ooijen (2000), do not provide sufficient conceptualization to meet the needs of the profession. Supervision models may not provide all the answers for nursing, but they are a strong foundation from which to build good practice. Scaife (2001) suggests that the advantages of models is that they can help professionals to organize their ideas about what is happening, thus maintaining their role as participant in the process at the same time as being able to take the position of observer; in other words, thinking about what is happening. There continues to be a need for the development of a clearer conceptualization to increase the likelihood of provision and uptake of clinical supervision (Yegdich 1999).

Despite the demand for clinical supervision to be integral to nursing practice, there has been no central strategy for implementation as recommended by the *Working in Partnership* report (Department of Health 1994). The result has been that local initiatives have attempted to develop the use of clinical supervision largely using cascade models. Indeed, there are a number of reports in the literature describing the successful implementation of this approach within localities (see, for example, Devine and Baxter 1995). However, these initiatives are, by and large, ad hoc, and a central strategy would provide the context for the necessary managerial support and funding to implement large-scale provision of supervision. Such a strategy should also address training, since although recommendations have been made (Department of Health 1994; Coleman and Raffety 1995; Cutcliffe and Proctor 1998), training needs continue to be neglected for both student and experienced nurses (Fowler 1996b).

These factors contribute to a situation whereby the quality of clinical supervision is still unpredictable (Faugier and Butterworth 1995; Scanlon and Weir 1997) and the availability of effective clinical supervision (and/or its uptake) remains patchy (Faugier 1994; Faugier and Butterworth 1995). Whilst these tensions remain, it is likely that nursing culture will continue to struggle to embrace clinical supervision (Bond and Holland 1998; Kelly *et al.* 2001).

Clinical supervision: areas for nursing practice development

Although widespread implementation of clinical supervision has been slow to develop, it provides the potential to enhance the necessary development of nursing practice (UKCC 1996). Few studies have considered the outcomes of mental health nursing treatment approaches, and those published suggest poor outcomes and conclude that they are not efficacious (Sheppard 1991; Adams 1996). Criticisms of nursing approaches that aim to account for poor outcomes (see Gournay *et al.* 1993) include:

- Noticeable discrepancies between the treatment approaches indicated as most efficacious for a clinical problem and the interventions chosen by nurses.
- The use of unfocused assessments.
- A lack of systematic approaches to defining problems.
- Not identifying treatment targets.

In community mental health nursing generally, these factors have been partially linked to a lack of theoretically driven interventions to help counter such poor performance outcomes (Matthew 1990; Sheppard 1991). Furthermore, this absence of an evidence base to practice is not helped by the structure of nurse training that provides little guidance to nurses about how to apply, and evaluate, appropriate theoretical underpinnings to their work (Sheppard 1991; Kenny 1993; Ferguson and Keady 2001). These findings suggest that 'trial and error' experience, rather than theoretical training, is used to develop nurses' work. One concern is that if the theoretical models adopted by nurses are limited and fragmentary, as suggested by Sheppard (1991), then practice may well mirror this deficit.

These areas of disquiet are reflected within dementia care nursing. Adams (1996) explained that there are few empirical studies describing the work of nurses with older people generally, and those published suggest poor outcomes (see, for example, Matthew 1990). As with all nursing practice, theoretical understanding is essential to assessment and treatment in dementia care. Accordingly, nurses need a comprehensive theoretical framework to guide their work with carers of people with dementia (Keady and Nolan 1996; Challenger and Hardy 1998). In this case, theoretical guidance has emerged in the nursing literature (see, for example, Nolan *et al.* 1994, 1996) but little attention has been given to theory–practice links. In her study of community mental health nursing practice with family carers of people with dementia, Carradice *et al.* (2002) used a qualitative methodology to consider whether some theoretical developments have been absorbed by nurses to underpin practice, or not. The findings suggested that nurses do have theoretical knowledge to guide their work with carers, but that the model used is pragmatic and unsophisticated. Moreover, there was a range of gaps in understanding and weaknesses in conceptualization that would directly impact on the nurses' work with carers. For example, the nurses in the study sample did not have a comprehensive framework to guide questions asked during assessment, and to inform development of the hypotheses during the formulation. Such deficits were likely to impact upon the choice of intervention and efficacy of this approach (Carradice *et al.* 2002). In addition, it was also suggested that nurses struggled to reflect on their practice, especially on how to improve their practice when carers were finding their interventions unhelpful (Carradice 1999).

Christopher Johns has emphasized the value of reflective practice in nursing which involves a guided process, and he provides a model that can be used in clinical supervision (Johns 1995a,b). As well as integration of theory into practice and improved reflection skills, it is crucial that nurses are able to understand, recognize and, when appropriate, intervene with the role of the 'self' in clinical work – this includes awareness of attitudes, values, experiences, beliefs, limitations and so on. Self-awareness is an essential nursing skill (Department of Health 1994) and also central to reflective practice.

Clinical supervision: opportunities for development

Clinical supervision can be a useful tool for developing and maintaining the three interdependent skills crucial to the development of effective nursing practice, namely: integration of theory into practice; the use of reflection; and the essential self-awareness. An understanding of these attributes in clinical supervision derives from experiential learning theory (Kolb 1984) which proposes that the construction of new knowledge, development of skills and application in practice follow a learning cycle. Initially, it is suggested that the practitioner has concrete experience followed by reflective observation, then engages in abstract conceptualization and finally active experimentation. Repeating this experiential learning cycle helps to develop practice and reflection during supervision and can enhance learning at each stage. This process can also facilitate the integration of theory into practice, reflection and self awareness leading to what Schön (1983) refers to as knowing-in-action (skilled performance based on procedural knowledge) and reflection-in-action (the ability to reflect, reappraise and improvise practice within a situation). Scaife and Scaife (2001) describe how Binder and Strupp (1997) said that it is the combination of knowledge-in-action and reflection-in-action that reflects therapeutic competence and expertise.

There is a growing number of research studies resulting in an abundance of impressions and anecdotal evidence of positive outcomes that support the usefulness of clinical supervision (see Butterworth *et al.* 1997). On the other hand, the quantity of studies has not been matched by empirical rigour (see Ellis *et al.* 1996 for detailed recommendations of the features of a well-designed clinical supervision study), and few studies have attempted to consider the impact of clinical supervision on performance and client care (Holloway and Neufeldt 1995). Owing to methodological weaknesses, acceptance of the positive findings must always be carefully, and critically, considered (Sloan 1998). Intuitively, however, clinical supervision has the potential to reap a number of benefits for practitioners, and certainly those receiving supervision report beneficial experiences. From the available literature, two main themes emerge. First, the potential benefits for nursing practice, and secondly, the central purpose of clinical supervision is to increase the quality of client care.

Potential benefits for nursing practice

Under this theme the literature can be synthesized into three main areas. First, the integration of theory into practice (see, for example, Severinsson and Kamaker 1999; Arvidsson *et al.* 2000). Secondly, an improved ability to reflect on practice which encompasses the necessary self-awareness (see Hallberg *et al.* 1994; Olsson and Hallberg 1998; Graham 1999). Thirdly, positive additional outcomes including: increased confidence (White *et al.* 1998; Hadfield 2000); greater trust in themselves (Arvidsson *et al.* 2000); strengthened identity (Segesten 1993); feeling valued (Scanlon and Weir 1997); and personal growth (Severinsson and Hallberg 1996).

The central purpose of clinical supervision is to increase the quality of client care

Anecdotal evidence for this theme also exists in the literature. For example, subjectively practitioners report increased quality of client care (White *et al.* 1998) and Severinsson and Borgenhammar (1997) found that experts in clinical supervision believe it is beneficial to client care. Improved creation of a 'good relationship' with clients has been reported (Graham 1999; Arvidsson *et al.* 2000; Hadfield 2000) and, in dementia care, increased nurse–patient cooperation (Edberg *et al.* 1996) and confirmed uniqueness of people with dementia to aid the provision of more person-orientated care (Berg and Hansson 2000). In residential settings, Berg *et al.* (1994) also reported a decreased level of burnout and increased creativity in caring for people with dementia. In addition, a number of studies report increased satisfaction at work (Berg *et al.* 1994; Hallberg *et al.* 1994; Arvidsson *et al.* 2000) which is thought to influence the quality of nursing care (Edberg *et al.* 1996; Begat *et al.* 1997).

Although the research findings are positive, there is a long way to go before the efficacy of clinical supervision can be demonstrated (Sloan 1998) and, as suggested earlier, methodological rigour needs to be further considered.

Clinical supervision specific to dementia care nursing

The aforementioned difficulties surrounding the provision and uptake of clinical supervision for mental health nursing in general are magnified in dementia care nursing as it has largely been neglected in the literature. Of the literature that does exist, interesting dynamics emerge, including the inherent challenge posed by working with someone with dementia: this challenge may cause the nurse to contribute towards the loss of value and dignity experienced by the person with dementia themself (Edberg *et al.* 1996; Graham 1999). For example, Miller (1985) suggested that nurses could 'push' the patient into greater dependence by doing for the person, rather than allowing the person to do for themself. It also appears important for nurses to understand the loss of personhood associated with having dementia (Henry and Tuxill 1987).

It has been noticed that nurses can lack the knowledge of 'patients as people' (Hallberg *et al.* 1994) that can help them react to the person and their changing sense of self. As Graham (1999) noted, this directly influences the provision of high-quality individualized care that can maintain the person's dignity and value. It is also reported that working with people with dementia in residential care settings can result in negative emotional experiences for the nurses involved, including: a sense of meaninglessness in the care provided (Norberg and Asplund 1990); an insufficiency of emotional investment (Hallberg and Norberg 1990); and feelings of emptiness (Hallberg and Norberg 1995). Supervision focused on the expression of feelings can help to reduce such emotional strain and improve relationships with people with dementia (Olsson *et al.* 1998). The dementia care literature also stresses the value of clinical supervision using a framework for reflection on client work from competing angles. For example, Graham (1999) outlines five perspectives: the patient; the significant other; co-workers; the NHS trust; and society. He reports that structuring clinical supervision around these perspectives helps to synthesize thinking, reflection and awareness on experiences, and can help to stimulate debate about the meaning and purpose of the work.

This literature is of undoubted interest, but the reported studies do not comprehensively address nursing practice issues, and attention should be given to the specific needs of nurses working in dementia care. This addition to knowledge includes the need to raise the profile of clinical supervision, develop appropriate frameworks for supervision and provide descriptions about how to facilitate effective supervision in order to address practice development. The next section describes a case study which aims to illustrate in practice the principles outlined above and introduce specific examples of processes that can be used to enhance the success of clinical supervision.

Clinical supervision in dementia care: putting principles into practice

The following case study is taken from a 15-month intervention study conducted in North Wales where two of the authors (JK and SH) had an integral role (see

Wenger *et al.* 2000; Keady *et al.* 2001). The project was entitled Dementia Action Research and Education (DARE) and its central aim was to 'evaluate whether early interventions would be associated with better outcomes over a 15-month period for caregivers and people with dementia, when considered separately and together' (Wenger *et al.* 2000: 4). Whereas a detailed description of the research methodology underpinning the project is beyond the scope of this chapter, some of the main tenets of the project are outlined in order to provide a context for the case study that follows.

The DARE project: a brief project outline

The DARE project employed two part-time dementia care specialists to deliver tailored interventions to people with dementia and their families; SH acted as one dementia care specialist and a social worker as the other. Joint two-hour clinical supervision sessions were provided fortnightly by JK and Professor Bob Woods (a renowned clinical psychologist in the field of dementia care) at the University of Wales, Bangor. The intervention group comprised 27 older people with dementia and their families, whereas the control group numbered 23. In most cases the dementia had not been previously diagnosed, and there was no current contact with specialist dementia services. Over both groups the mean age of participants was 84 years and the majority of carers were either spouses or adult children, a characteristic representative of other studies in the field (see Levin *et al.* 1989; Nolan and Keady 2001). Ethical approval to conduct the study was gained through the North West Wales Health Authority Local Research Ethics Committee.

The role of the dementia care specialist was to provide early information, education and support to the person with dementia and their family using psychosocial techniques as a basis for treatment. To operationalize this process, the dementia care specialists were able to draw on a number of interventions and organizational tasks, including: organizing family meetings; one-to-one direct work with the person with dementia; broaching the sharing of the diagnosis; liaison with other service providers; and supportive counselling for the carer. This approach built upon an earlier (carer-only) study by Pollitt *et al.* (1989) where elements of an early psychosocial intervention for carers of people with mild dementia provided a rationale and context for care.

The interventions were evaluated independently by the projects' research fellow at 8- and 15-month intervals using a range of clinical and health-related measures (for further information see White *et al.* 2000).

Clinical supervision: developing a contract and the use of ecomaps

The key predictor of success of clinical supervision is thought to be the quality of the supervisory alliance (Scaife 2001). This 'good enough' relationship is essential to provide the necessary 'holding environment' (Winnicott 1965) with which the supervisees can feel safe enough to explore their practice. Within supervision, the use of contracting is helpful to developing a trusting alliance (Scaife 2001). In this study contracting began with shared values built upon the guidance given in the *Working in Partnership* report (Department of Health 1994: 21), namely that:

- skills should be constantly redefined throughout professional life;

- critical discussion about clinical practice is a means to professional development;

- introduction to the process of clinical supervision should begin in professional training and continue thereafter as an integral aspect of professional development;

- clinical supervision requires time, energy and commitment; it is not an incidental activity and must be planned and effectively resourced.

In order to operationalize these standards, guiding principles for clinical supervision sessions (see Figures 16.1 and 16.2) were agreed by the four stakeholders during the first clinical supervision meeting in March 1998.

A description of the interventions, the tape recordings of sessions (with the informed consent of participants) and notes of the practitioner's thoughts and feelings about their work were used as the basis of clinical supervision. One of the aims of clinical supervision is to enhance reflection on practice and holistic conceptualization of the work. It was decided that to help facilitate meaningful discussion, ecomaps would be compiled on each client/family situation.

Social workers began using graphic aids, such as social network maps, genograms and ecomaps, in the early 1970s as a means of recording their interventions

---

Clinical supervision is to be:

- informal in its nature
- conducted in a group setting
- supportive
- educative
- undertaken with honesty and in an environment of trust
- routinely provided at an agreed time and venue
- protected from external commitments, barring an emergency
- provided by all members of the group

Figure 16.1 Guiding principles for the nature of clinical supervision

---

The content of clinical supervision is to be:

- flexible in approach
- case by case
- Incorporate a case review process
- Intervention based introducing:
  - practice example(s)
  - tape recording/transcript of interventions
  - discussion
  - peer support and clinical guidance
  - reflective practice to inform decision making

Figure 16.2 Guiding principles for the content of clinical supervision

in complex cases and in seeking supervisory support (Meyer 1976). Ecomaps are a simple simulation that can be used as an assessment, planning and intervention tool. They depict the major ecological and interactive systems of the person in the community and the 'energy flow' between the relationships. The final product presents clear information regarding relationship, support system possibilities and needs. They are particularly useful in helping stimulate different or more complete perspectives on the work.

The case study that follows is taken directly from the caseload of SH and summarizes elements of clinical supervision and use of ecomaps to help support practice development. In this case, a move into a supportive care environment for the person with dementia had a demonstrable impact on raising quality of life for all parties involved in the situation. The case was discussed at each of the two-week clinical supervision sessions using the guiding principles outlined in Figures 16.1 and 16.2 as an agreed framework. Space does not permit a detailed review of each session, so, instead, the intervention milestones are described to provide a flavour of the value of clinical supervision on the understanding of the clinical picture, decision making, and the temporal nature of the changing family dynamics. A key to interpreting the diagrams portrayed in the ecomaps is as follows:

- A circle contains the name of the key personnel in the family/domestic situation.

- The perimeter of the box is used to symbolize distance to/from key personnel in the family/domestic situation.

- The thickness of the line linking the key personnel details the strength of that relationship (actual and/or perceived). As a rule, the thicker the line the stronger the relationship.

Case study

July 1998: Point of first contact – constructing a picture of the domestic situation

Clare is the primary carer for her mother, Joan, who has been diagnosed as being in the early stages of dementia and experiences symptoms of depression. Joan lives in a small village in the Conwy Valley in North Wales and has lived alone since her husband died seven years ago. Joan is an independent woman, 79 years of age and has had three children, the youngest of whom died at the age of 12 in a drowning accident. Clare lives some distance away in Cheshire and travels to see her mother as much as it is practicable to do so.

The referral to SH was made following Joan's augmented over-75s assessment screen when areas of cognitive deficit were uncovered. As guided by the DARE study protocol, this triggered a referral to the project officer and further diagnostic tests, all undertaken with Joan's consent, that confirmed the existence of a dementia. Once the referral to the DARE project was made and Joan had consented to take part in the study, SH organized an initial meeting in Joan's home with both Clare and Joan. This meeting was undertaken in order to gather a detailed history and explore their understanding of the diagnostic process and meaning of recent events. As in clinical supervision, the aim of this early phase of the work was to build a trusting relationship with Clare and Joan in order to ensure continuity of contact.

September 1998: Building on the relationship

Three months after referral, a more complete picture of the family and domestic situation emerged. Specifically, SH was experiencing difficulties in identifying and meeting the needs of Joan and Clare, both individually and jointly. The reasons behind this were complex, but in brief Joan was highly dependent on both her daughter and her neighbour to enable her to continue with her day-to-day life; Joan was also reluctant to trust anyone else outside her home situation. At the same time, Clare was experiencing difficulty in accepting any offers of help from SH and it had become evident that the relationship between Clare and Joan was highly interdependent. From Joan's perspective, SH, as well as most other members of the family and social network (excluding her daughter and neighbour), were not seen as particularly important and were therefore 'pushed out' of the picture. Drawn by SH, the two ecomaps shown in Figures 16.3 and 16.4 were used in clinical supervision at the time to capture this value system.

The ecomap in Figure 16.3 reveals the dependence Joan has upon Clare. Although Joan recognizes that she needs her neighbour, the neighbour feels less 'attached' to Joan and to meeting her needs – hence the dotted lines. Joan's relationship with her son was also lacking in reciprocity; again, this is shown by the broken narrow line from son to mother.

The ecomap in Figure 16.4 demonstrates the way in which Clare feels that all the people in her life are dependent upon her in some way; however, this dependency is not fully reciprocated by other family members. The relationship between Clare and her husband is complicated further by the fact that Clare does not trust her husband owing to previous adverse life experiences.

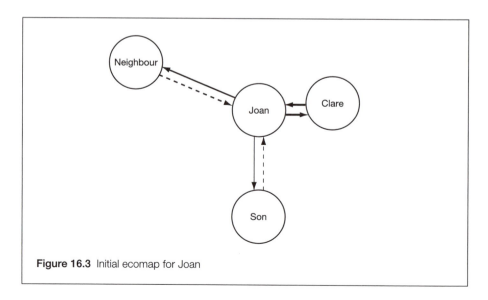

Figure 16.3 Initial ecomap for Joan

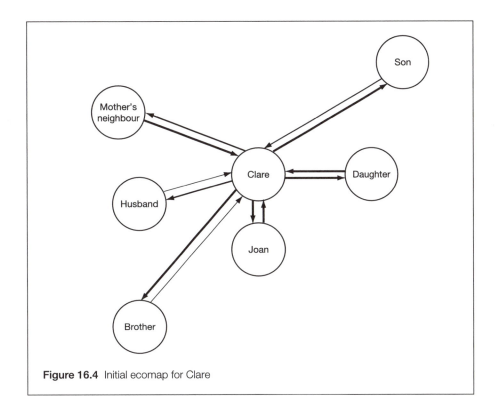

Figure 16.4 Initial ecomap for Clare

Clinical supervision: facilitating decision making

For Joan

During presentation of the two initial ecomaps in clinical supervision, the real and potential risks to Joan and the way in which her needs could be met were considered. It had to be remembered at all times that it was Joan's priority to remain in her own home. On a practical level it was identified that one of the greatest risks for Joan was in omitting her medication as this resulted in a relapse of her physical and emotional health and, as a consequence, a greater stress on her family, particularly Clare. To overcome this anxiety it was agreed between Joan and SH that a trained home care worker would visit to support her medication compliance. It was vital that this decision was explored with Joan in a way that gave her a sense of ownership in the decision making and resultant action.

For Clare

Clare was experiencing distressing feelings of guilt, anger and resentment. She believed she carried the full weight of caring, a strain she identified as 'not being able to do right for doing wrong'. On the one hand, Clare wanted to be in a position to provide love and support for her mother in the best possible way. On the other hand, she was cognizant of her mother's need to live her own life. Unfortunately, it seemed to Clare that this latter aspiration could not be achieved as she felt her mother was unsafe to be left alone. Clare also felt guilty about 'not being there' to support her mother and help to 'sort things out' in her day-to-day life. No matter which way Clare turned she felt a sense of failure or frustration, and this was having a detrimental impact upon her emotional health.

It was decided that SH should begin by exploring the areas in which Clare felt the greatest anxiety, and this became the focus of the intervention and the reporting in subsequent clinical supervision sessions. Over time, it became apparent that Clare's priorities were twofold. First, her mother's unreliability at taking her medication and her inability to 'check' to see if she had done this appropriately. Secondly, the frequent telephone calls to Clare's home when her mother expressed her feelings of emptiness and loneliness for which Clare felt guilty.

As well as the practical aim of organizing a home care worker to monitor medication compliance, in prioritizing the intervention plan for Clare it was decided that SH would explore Clare's heightened sense of failure and frustration. In the one-to-one counselling sessions that ensued, Clare revealed that she felt a sense of 'wanting to please everyone'. Clare attributed this feeling to emotional insecurity experienced in childhood, and fears that if she did not do what others wanted, she would be left alone. To positively influence this emotional state, the necessity of offering Clare additional counselling was raised in clinical supervision and a treatment plan was developed. Through these additional counselling sessions it became evident that the problems that Clare experienced with her caring role were largely tied up with her own 'need to be needed' whilst fearing the loss (both physically and emotionally) of her mother. This was illustrated by the way that Clare usually colluded with her mother in the breakdown of services that were either offered or put in place to alleviate the situation at home. Indeed, Clare viewed herself as the 'rock' around which all care revolved, no matter how 'emotionally battered' she became as a result of this responsibility.

November 1998: Moving on

With negotiation and full involvement, home support services were eventually arranged for Joan and accepted as necessary by Clare. However, Joan still telephoned Clare to say that she felt lonely and Clare had real difficulty in minimizing the experiences of her guilt about being a distant carer.

In counselling, Clare continued to explore her feelings of guilt and 'inadequacy', but found it impossible to withdraw from her mother and the role of carer. The counselling enabled Clare to consider what she wanted for herself and her life. Throughout these sessions she was keen to talk, and often became tearful and distressed. Through reflecting on this emotional material in clinical supervision, it became clear that Clare had lost her sense of identity and saw herself as only being available to meet the needs of others. The counselling process enabled Clare to realize that an additional motivation for caring for her mother was linked to protection in that she wanted to shield her mother from feelings of emotional pain, a pain she had seen her mother endure over the loss of her 12-year-old son. Ultimately, Clare was overcompensating for this tragic event and felt responsible for her mother's happiness. Only through expressing and then accepting these feelings could Clare begin to move on and become more aware of her own needs.

Gradually, through this acceptance, Clare began to realize that improvements in the family situation would necessarily involve compromise and that she was not responsible for the pain that may result. Towards the end of this period, it transpired that Clare was keen for her mother to move nearer to her in Cheshire in order to provide support closer to home. Clare viewed this as a potential solution that would benefit all concerned, although her mother, at this time, was unwilling to consider such a move.

January 1999: Next intervention milestone

At a clinical supervision session some two months later, the caring and domestic situation had changed, as the ecomaps in Figures 16.5 and 16.6 reveal.

Figure 16.5 shows that the relationship between Joan and Clare remained strong, but there had been a subtle shift in importance in the relationship for the neighbour. The neighbour now felt more responsible for Joan's welfare, although this was not reciprocated fully by Joan. With the introduction of the home care worker, Clare was able to withdraw from this 'monitoring' responsibility. Joan accepted that Clare felt supported by the home carer, although Joan refused to consider that she gained anything from their input.

The ecomap in Figure 16.6 demonstrates the way in which Clare is feeling well supported by her own daughter and the home carer. The relationship between Clare and the neighbour is now more balanced, as it is between Clare and her brother. Joan still has the greatest impact on Clare's life, although Clare is now able to put her altruistic motivation to care in context and be realistic about the demands of providing care. The relationship between Clare and her husband is a little more distant, but Clare feels comfortable with this outcome.

May 1999: Introducing a new dynamic

This new supportive routine broke down when Joan stopped the visits of the home carer, a move that restimulated Clare's anxieties about her mother's condition and

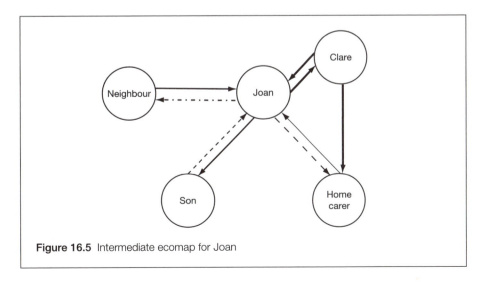

Figure 16.5 Intermediate ecomap for Joan

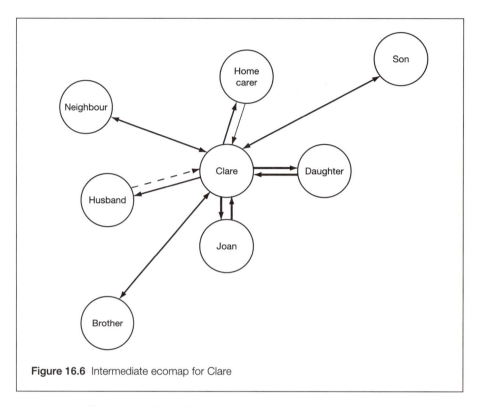

Figure 16.6 Intermediate ecomap for Clare

her responsibility for it. In her clinical supervision notes at the time, SH recorded her feelings of concern about being unable to develop a workable package of care. This frustration was heightened as SH identified with the way in which Clare responded to the demands of her mother. Ultimately, there remained a conflict of interest, and whatever system was put into place failed due to a lack of continuity and, as Clare saw it, her mother's decision making.

Taking the situation as a whole, three issues were apparent:

1   Joan's wish to remain in her own home with support only from Clare.
2   Clare's need to support her mother.
3   The difficulties presented by the geographical distance.

Given that Joan was having increased difficulty in managing independently and that Clare could not carry on the way she had been, the compromise seemed to be that Joan could live closer to her daughter. Arranging for her mother to move to a small residential home in Cheshire on a trial basis was seen by Clare to be a solution to the dilemma. Following intensive discussion and reflection, it became clear that Clare was hoping for an idealized conclusion. SH had internalized this view and with the support received from clinical supervision, she was able to see and accept that this was unrealistic, an awareness SH then took back to her clinical work. The revised aim was for a clearer understanding to be developed by both Clare and Joan of the necessity of compromise to move forward. This illustrated the parallel process whereby SH mirrored the feelings of Clare in the supervision and the supervisors were able to intervene with SH in such a way that she was able to have new understanding to inform her work (see Inskipp and Proctor 1993, 1995 for further explanation of parallel process).

Outcome

As SH thought that all alternatives had been explored, a reasonable compromise was considered to be that Joan needed to accept that her quality of life would be improved if she moved closer to her daughter. It was important that Joan felt fully involved in this decision-making process and ideally that she could suggest this as a solution herself. A meeting was arranged in which SH's role was to ensure that Joan was not pressurized to accept a change to her lifestyle, whilst Joan and Clare discussed potential options. During the discussion Joan decided to give the trial 'a go' based on her wish to be closer to her granddaughter.

July 1999: Nearing the end

The final ecomaps (Figures 16.7 and 16.8) were put together by SH and the family, including Joan, and were drawn towards the end of the intervention period.

Treatment outcomes combined with interpretation of final ecomaps

At a six-month follow-up Clare reported that Joan 'had settled well' into the residential home. As Figure 16.7 reveals, Clare's situation had altered considerably.

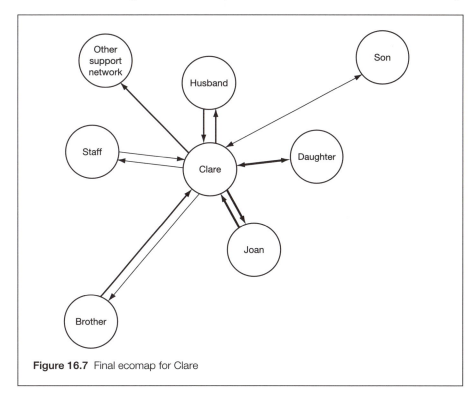

Figure 16.7 Final ecomap for Clare

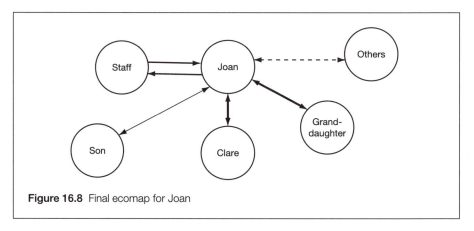

Figure 16.8 Final ecomap for Joan

Clare felt less guilty about the situation, felt more relaxed and was now able to enjoy the relationship with her mother and her daughter. Clare describes how this final ecomap highlights the relationships that are important to her, but not in terms of need and dependency. Acknowledging this perspective added to her new-found sense of personal choice and freedom. She no longer felt totally responsible for her mother's happiness and had greater insight into her motivation and commitment to her mother's care. Clare remarked that this eased the burden of caring and reported that she was able to follow her own interests and felt less 'torn' between members of her family. Clare's daughter took on some of the caring role and was keen to support her own mother through this experience.

As Joan's ecomap illustrates (Figure 16.8), there was a shift in Joan's relationships, notably in that she was less dependent on Clare. Joan now relied far more on the staff for meeting her physical needs and company. Her granddaughter is, for the first time, significant, and there is no sense of burden or codependency. Now that Joan lived closer to her family, particularly her granddaughter, she had more visitors and was regularly invited for lunch and taken out on social occasions. Joan no longer experienced depression, was less anxious (assessed via the project worker through independent measures) and her physical health stabilized. There was a significant improvement in her quality of life.

The impact of clinical supervision on negotiated care: a personal reflection

Throughout the 15-month intervention period, SH was encouraged to share her own feelings about the work. The aim of clinical supervision was to provide the sense of emotional 'containment' (Hinshelwood 1991) to tolerate the feelings associated with the work, to be able to 'reflect-in-action' (Schön 1983) and develop what Casement (1985, 1990) terms the 'internal supervisor' where skills from supervision are internalized and transferred into the clinical situation. Over time it emerged that SH struggled with the difficulty of supporting Clare within the context of her mother's experience of Alzheimer's disease, and the way in which it would have been easier to make decisions for Joan without consulting her fully. Becoming aware of and articulating this dilemma helped SH intervene in her approach to the work. This self-awareness helped SH to monitor and prevent herself from acting to disempower Joan. Without this insight the intervention may have become 'stuck', with SH being unsure how to proceed.

In this case study, clinical supervision played a vital role in understanding and determining the needs of Joan and Clare, both individually and jointly. It enabled SH to reflect upon the situation and the effect it was having on her, which led to a more objective and professional relationship. Reflection and clarification were therefore important elements in the process of the supervisory relationship. Ecomaps were a useful visual aid that reinforced the process of clarification; they provided a way in which to describe a situation and to explore the complexities of relationships. They also supported the process of conceptualization and planning and provided a useful point of reference for all parties in the process. In addition, the ongoing nature of clinical supervision and the use of ecomaps facilitated a shift in perspective for the dementia care specialist that enabled SH to become more person-centred and self-aware. This process allowed the whole picture to emerge, thus creating an environment in which SH could remain objective and focused in supporting Clare and Joan to reach a satisfactory compromise. Finally, a reflective and client-centred approach was used in clinical supervision, which was then paralleled in the counselling sessions.

Conclusion

It is crucial within dementia care nursing that more attention is paid to clinical supervision since it has been a neglected area. This chapter suggests that clinical supervision is an essential element of practice development within nursing, and specifically for dementia care nursing. Essential components of practice development include improved use of theory–practice links, reflective practice and the essential self-awareness. The case study was used to demonstrate practical examples of helpful processes that enhance practice and illustrate the value of clinical supervision for dementia care nursing.

The development of clinical supervision has been slow and obstacles hinder its widespread quality provision and uptake. The chapter suggests that lack of central strategy, the confusion between management supervision and clinical supervision, a continued lack of conceptual clarity and the neglect of training needs all contribute to this situation. It is vital that some progress is made to address these factors in order to ensure that clinical supervision appropriately contributes to the maintenance and enhancement of quality community mental health nursing practice.

Acknowledgements

JK and SH would like to acknowledge the Department of Health for funding the DARE study and to the other project grantholders: Professor G.C. Wenger,

Professor R.T. Woods, Dr M. Devakumar and Ms A. Scott. We would also like to acknowledge Joan and Clare (not their real names) for allowing us access to their lives and permission to record their experiences.

References

Adams, T. (1996) Informal family caregiving to older people with dementia: research priorities for community psychiatric nursing, *Journal of Advanced Nursing*, 24: 703–10.

Arvidsson, B., Löfgren, H. and Fridlund, B. (2000) Psychiatric nurses' conceptions of how group supervision in nursing care influences their professional competence, *Journal of Nursing Management*, 8: 175–85.

Begat, I., Severinsson, E. and Berggren, I. (1997) Implementation of clinical supervision in a medical department: nurses' views of the effects, *Journal of Clinical Nursing*, 6: 389–94.

Berg, A. and Hansson, U.W. (2000) Dementia care nurses' experiences of systematic clinical group supervision and supervised planned nursing care, *Journal of Nursing Management*, 8(3): 357–68.

Berg, A., Welander Hansson, U. and Hallberg, I.R. (1994) Nurses' creativity, tedium and burnout during one year of clinical supervision and implementation of individually planned nursing care. Comparison between a ward for severely demented patients and a similar control ward, *Journal of Advanced Nursing*, 20: 742–9.

Binder, J.L. and Strupp, H.H. (1997) Supervision of psychodynamic psychotherapies, in C.E. Watkins Jr (ed.) *Handbook of Psychotherapy Supervision*. New York: Wiley.

Bond, M. and Holland, S. (1998) The surface picture: the development and value of clinical supervision, in *Skills of Clinical Supervision for Nurses*. Buckingham: Open University Press.

Butterworth, A., Carson, J., White, E. *et al.* (1997) *It is Good to Talk: An Evaluation of Clinical Supervision and Mentorship in England and Scotland*. Manchester: Manchester University Press.

Carradice, A. (1999) A qualitative study of the theoretical models used by mental health nurses to guide their assessments with carers of people with dementia. Unpublished D.Clin.Psy. thesis, University of Sheffield.

Carradice, A., Shankland, M. and Beail, N. (2002) A qualitative study of the theoretical models used by UK mental health nurses to guide their assessments with family caregivers of people with dementia, *International Journal of Nursing Studies*, 39(1): 17–26.

Casement, P. (1985) *Learning from the Patient*. London: Routledge.

Casement, P. (1990) *Further Learning from the Patient*. London: Routledge.

Challenger, J. and Hardy, B. (1998) Dementia: the difficulties experienced by carers, *British Journal of Community Nursing*, 3(4): 166–71.

Coleman, M. and Raffety, M. (1995) Using workshops to implement supervision, *Nursing Standard*, 9(50): 27–9.

Cutcliffe, J.R. and Proctor, B. (1998) An alternative training approach to clinical supervision, *British Journal of Nursing*, 7(5): 280–5.

Department of Health (1994) *Working in Partnership: A Collaborative Approach to Care*. London: The Stationery Office.

Department of Health (1997) *The New NHS: Modern, Dependable*. London: The Stationery Office.

Devine, A. and Baxter, T.D. (1995) Introducing clinical supervision: a guide, *Nursing Standard*, June 289(40): 32–4.

Edberg, A., Hallberg, I.R. and Gustafson, L. (1996) Effects of clinical supervision on nurse–patient cooperation quality, *Clinical Nursing Research*, 5(2): 127–49.

Ellis, M.V., Ladany, N., Krengel, M. and Schult, D. (1996) Clinical supervision research from 1981 to 1993: a methodological critique, *Journal of Counselling Psychology*, 43: 35–50.

Faugier, J. (1994) Thin on the ground, *Nursing Times*, May 18: 90(20).

Faugier, J. and Butterworth, T. (1995) Clinical supervision: a positional paper, in *Clinical supervision: A Resource Pack*. London: NHS Management Executive.

Ferguson, C. and Keady, J. (2001). The mental health needs of older people and their carers: exploring tensions and new directions, in M. Nolan, G. Grant and S. Davies (eds) *Working with Older People and their Families: Key Issues in Policy and Practice*. Buckingham: Open University Press.

Fowler, J. (1996a) How to use models of clinical supervision in practice, *Nursing Standard*, 10(29): 42–7.

Fowler, J. (1996b) The organisation of clinical supervision within the nursing profession: a review of the literature, *Journal of Advanced Nursing*, 23(3): 471–8.

Gournay, K., Devilly, G. and Brooker, C. (1993) The CPN in primary care: a pilot study of the process of assessment, in C. Brooker and E. White (eds) *Community Psychiatric Nursing: A Research Perspective*. London: Chapman & Hall.

Graham, I.W. (1999) Reflective narrative and dementia care, *Journal of Clinical Nursing*, 8: 675–83.

Gray, R. (1997) *Evidence-based Practice*. London: Churchill Livingstone.

Hadfield, D. (2000) Clinical supervision: user's perspectives, *Journal of Child Health Care*, 4(1): 30–40.

Hallberg, I.R. and Norberg, A. (1990) Staff's interpretation of the experiences behind vocally disruptive behaviour in severely demented patients and their feelings about is. An exploratory study, *International Journal of Aging and Human Development*, 31: 297–307.

Hallberg, I.R. and Norberg, A. (1995) Nurses' experience of strain and their reactions in the care of severely demented patients, *International Journal of Geriatric Psychiatry*, 10: 757–66.

Hallberg, I.R., Hansson, U.W. and Axelsson, K. (1994) Satisfaction with nursing care and work during a year of clinical supervision and individualised care: comparison between two wards for the care of severely demented patients, *Journal of Nursing Management*, 1: 297–307.

Henry, C. and Tuxill, A.C. (1987) Persons and humans, *Journal of Advanced Nursing*, 12: 383–8.

Hill, J. (1989) Supervision in the caring profession: a literature review, *Community Psychiatric Nursing Association Journal*, 5: 9–11.

Hinshelwood, R.D. (1991) *A Dictionary of Kleinian Thought*. London: Free Association Press.

Holloway, E.L. and Neufeldt, S.A. (1995) Supervision: its contribution to treatment efficacy, *Journal of Consulting and Clinical Psychology*, 63: 207–13.

Inskipp, I. and Proctor, B. (1993) *The Art, Craft and Tasks of Counselling Supervision. Part 1: Making the Most of Supervision*. London: Cascade.

Inskipp, I. and Proctor, B. (1995) *The Art, Craft and Tasks of Counselling Supervision. Part 2: Becoming a Supervisor*. London: Cascade.

Johns, C. (1995a) The value of reflective practice for nursing, *Journal of Clinical Nursing*, 4(1): 23–30.

Johns, C. (1995b) Time to care? Time for reflection, *International Journal of Nursing Practice*, 1: 37–42.

Keady, J. and Nolan, M. (1996) Behavioural and Instrumental Stressers in Dementia (BISID): refocusing the assessment of caregiver need in dementia, *Journal of Psychiatric and Mental Health Nursing*, 3(3): 163–72.

Keady, J., Hahn, S. and Woods, R.T. (2001) Sharing a diagnosis of dementia: exploring the nursing role. Paper presented to the Royal College of Nursing of the United Kingdomto the Research Society Triennial International Nursing Research Conference, Glasgow, 4 April.

Kelly, B., Long, A. and McKenna, H. (2001) A survey of community mental health nurses' perceptions of clinical supervision in Northern Ireland, *Journal of Psychiatric and Mental Health Nursing*, 8: 33–44.

Kenny, T. (1993) Nursing models fail in practice, *British Journal of Nursing*, 2(2): 133–6.

Kolb, D.A. (1984) *Experiential Learning: Experience as the Source of Learning and Development*. Englewood Cliffs, NJ: Prentice Hall.

Levin, E., Sinclair, I. and Gorbach, P. (1989) *Families, Services and Confusion in Old Age*. Aldershot: Avebury.

Matthew, L. (1990) A role for the CPN in supporting the carer of clients with dementia, in C. Brooker (ed.) *Community Psychiatric Nursing: A Research Perspective*. London: Chapman & Hall.

Meyer, C.H. (1976) *Social Work Practice: The Changing Landscape*. New York: Free Press.

Miller, A. (1985) A study of the dependency of elderly patients in wards using different methods of nursing care, *Age and Ageing*, 14: 132–8.

Nolan, M. and Keady, J. (2001) Working with carers, in C. Cantley (ed.) *A Handbook of Dementia Care*. Buckingham: Open University Press.

Nolan, M., Grant, G., Caldock, K. and Keady, J. (1994) *A Framework for Assessing the Needs of Family Caregivers: A Multi-disciplinary Guide*. Bangor: Base Publications.

Nolan, M., Grant, G. and Keady, J. (1996) *Understanding Family Care*. Buckingham: Open University Press.

Norberg, A. and Asplund, K. (1990) Caregivers' experiences of caring for severely demented patients in the terminal phase of life, *Western Journal of Nursing Research*, 12: 75–84.

Olsson, A. and Hallberg, I.R. (1998) Caring for demented people in their homes or in sheltered accommodation as reflected on by home-care staff during clinical supervision sessions, *Journal of Advanced Nursing*, 27: 241–52.

Olsson, A., Bjorkheim, K. and Hallberg, I.R. (1998) Systematic clinical supervision of home carers working in the care of demented people who are at home: structure, content and effect as experienced by participants, *Journal of Nursing Management*, 6(4): 239–42.

Platt-Koch, L.M. (1986) Clinical supervision for psychiatric nurses, *Journal of Psychological Nursing*, 26(1): 7–15.

Pollitt, P.A., O'Connor, D.W. and Anderson, I. (1989) Mild dementia: perceptions and problems, *Ageing and Society*, 9: 261–75.

Scaife, J. (2001) *Supervision in the Mental Health Professions: A Practitioner's Guide*. Sussex: Brunner–Routledge.

Scaife, J. and Scaife, J. (2001) Supervision and learning, in J. Scaife (ed.) *Supervision in the Mental Health Professions: A Practitioner's Guide*. Sussex: Brunner–Routledge.

Scanlon, C. and Weir, W.S. (1997) Learning from practice? Mental health nurses' perceptions and experiences of clinical supervision, *Journal of Advanced Nursing*, 26(2): 295–303.

Schön, D.A. (1983) *The Reflective Practitioner: How Professionals Think in Action*. London: Temple Smith.

Segesten, K. (1993) The effects of professional group supervision of nurses, *Scandinavian Journal of Caring Sciences*, 7: 101–4.

Severinsson, E.I. and Borgenhammar, E.V. (1997) Expert views on clinical supervision, *Journal of Nursing Management*, 5: 175–83.

Severinsson, E.I. and Hallberg, I.R. (1996) Systematic clinical supervision, working milieu and influence over duties: the psychiatric nurse's viewpoint – a pilot study, *International Journal of Nursing Studies*, 33(4): 394–406.

Severinsson, E.I. and Kamaker, D. (1999) Clinical nursing supervision in the workplace: effects on morale, stress and job satisfaction, *Journal of Nursing Management*, 7: 81–90.

Sheppard, M. (1991) *Mental Health Work in the Community: Theory and Practice in Social Work and Community Psychiatric Nursing*. London: Falmer Press.

Sloan, G. (1998) Clinical supervision: characteristics of a good supervisor, *Nursing Standard*, 12(40): 24–30.

Sloan, G., White, C. and Coit, F. (2000) Cognitive therapy supervision as a framework for clinical supervision in nursing: using structure to guide discovery, *Journal of Advanced Nursing*, 32(3): 515–24.

UKCC (1986) *Report on the Reorganisation of Basic Nurse Education*. London: United Kingdom Central Council for Nursing, Midwifery and Health Visiting.

UKCC (1994) *Draft Guide to Arrangements for Inter-agency Working for the Care and Protection of Severely Mentally Ill People*. London: United Kingdom Central Council for Nursing, Midwifery and Health Visiting.

UKCC (1996) *Position Statement on Clinical Supervision for Nursing and Health Visiting*. London: United Kingdom Central Council for Nursing, Midwifery and Health Visiting.

van Ooijen, E. (2000) *Clinical Supervision: A Practical Guide*. Edinburgh: Churchill Livingstone.

Wenger, G.C., Woods, B., Keady, J., Scott, A., Devakumar, M. and White, N. (2000) *Dementia Action Research and Education*, Final Report to the Department of Health. Bangor: Institute of Medical and Social Care Research, University of Wales.

White, E., Riley, E., Davies, S. and Twinn, S. (1993) *A Detailed Study of the Relationships between Teaching, Support, Supervision and Role Modelling in Clinical Areas, Within the Context of Project 2000 Courses*. London: English National Board for Nursing, Midwifery and Health Visiting.

White, E., Butterworth, T., Bishop, V. *et al.* (1998) Clinical supervision: insider reports of a private world, *Journal of Advanced Nursing*, 28(1): 185–92.

White, N., Keady, J., Woods, R.T. *et al.* (2000) *Screening for Dementia in the Community*, CSPRD Research Summary, Series No. 2. Bangor: CSPRD, University of Wales.

Winnicott, D.W. (1965) *Maturation Processes and the Facilitating Environment*. London: Hogarth Press.

Yegdich, T. (1999) Clinical supervision and managerial supervision: some historical and conceptual considerations, *Journal of Advanced Nursing*, 30(5): 1195–204.

17

Multi-agency and inter-agency working
Issues in managing a community mental health nursing service in dementia

Cathy Mawhinney, Paul McCloskey and Assumpta Ryan

Introduction

Historically, services for older people have been under-resourced, understaffed, underdeveloped and have lacked recognition by the professions (McCormack 2001). For most of the twentieth century, older people with dementia who could not be managed by family and friends were cared for in large psychiatric hospitals. This strategy changed with the realization that an ever-increasing ageing population required a more dynamic approach and the government's decision to retract long-stay hospital beds, both of which culminated in the development of a community care policy and the NHS and Community Care Act 1990. In addition to these changes, there was also a growing impetus to move away from a purely medical model of intervention towards an holistic, person-centred psychotherapeutic model of treatment (Kitwood 1993; Holden and Woods 1995). The person-valuing paradigm was born. The shift towards community care was further reflected in the Carers (Recognition and Services) Act 1995, which entitles family carers to a separate assessment of their ability to care. More recently, this position has been consolidated in standards set by the *National Service Framework for Older People* (Department of Health 2001) which states that 'older people who have mental health problems should have access to integrated mental health services, provided by the NHS and councils to ensure effective diagnosis, treatment and support for them and their carers' (p. 90).

All these divergent factors have come together to form a relatively new environment in which community mental health nurses (CMHNs) now practise. There is a new service to manage and CMHNs are key players in a multi-agency structure charged with the task of providing a service for people with dementia and their carers. Dementia is a disorder that transcends traditional health and social services boundaries and therefore an integrated care pathway that reflects a multi-agency and inter-agency approach is mandatory. This new approach provides great opportunities for CMHNs to make use of their therapeutic selves and develop interventions to help dementia sufferers and their carers. It is crucial that all health and social care professionals work collaboratively and collectively to compile essential health and social data in order to promote the overall health of their community (Long 2001). However, there are issues relating to role definition, teamwork, multi-agency and inter-agency workings and resource limitations, all of which render the management of a community mental health nursing service in dementia a complex and challenging task.

Role definition

The role of the CMHN in dementia care is relatively new, previously uncharted territory and consequently has not been clearly defined. It seems to depend on where one works and who one asks. In Northern Ireland, as in other regions, it is not unusual for two CMHNs working in different trusts, often less than 20 miles apart, to have completely different roles and functions. In some areas, CMHNs appear to have emerged as interchangeable beings. Practice boundaries have become blurred and consequently, without an epistemology for practice, the profession is left vulnerable and open to misinterpretation both from within its own boundaries and by other professional groups. Thus, inadequate or inappropriate role definition can lead to role conflict, which then becomes a disabling influence on the profession, the individual, the team and the service. This is not a personal issue. Role conflict occurs where there is inadequate or inappropriate role definition and is distinct from personality clashes.

Few will disagree that the role of the CMHN working in dementia care should be based upon the principles of good community mental health nursing practice. These have been defined by Long (2001) and include: the search for recognized and unrecognized mental health needs; the prevention of disequilibrium in mental health; the facilitation of mental-health-enhancing activities; therapeutic approaches to mental health care and influencing policies affecting mental health. However, the work of the CMHN in dementia care cannot be reduced to categories or tasks as this only serves to dilute the philosophy and the way in which interventions are delivered. In their everyday practice, CMHNs use an armoury of skills for the benefit of the client and carer. According to Gunstone (1999), these interventions are delivered with love, which is a very powerful tool and the quintessential element in the helping process. However, immense difficulties arise for the manager in measuring this invisible work and consequently it is in danger of not being acknowledged.

Leadership and management

It is now recognized that harmonious working relationships and good teamwork result in a high level of work performance (Heller 1997). In fact, it would seem that 'making teamworking work is the new, indispensable skill' (Heller 1997: XIV). However, it is often the case that managers are appointed because of their knowledge, skills and expertise in community mental health nursing with very little emphasis on their team-building skills. Yet, Mullins (1999) argues that the quality of management is one of the most important factors in the success of any organization, and Heller (1999) stresses that an effective manager must be a well-organized administrator who is highly adept in understanding people's basic needs and behaviour in the workplace. Honesty and enthusiasm are recurrent themes in nurses' descriptions of popular and effective managers (Legge 2001), and good management is central to delivering patient-centred care (Department of Health 1997). Despite this, management within the NHS continues to suffer from particularly bad press, with complacency and mismanagement the 'order of the day' (Morris 2000).

Managing a community mental health nursing service in dementia requires both management and leadership skills. Peter Drucker, who is widely regarded as an expert in management theory, suggests management is a practice, a discipline and a task but it is also about people. Every achievement of management is the achievement of a manager. Every failure is a failure of the manager (Drucker 1979). Stewart (1994) offers a somewhat different perspective in that he defines a manager as someone who achieves results through other people, whilst Levine and Crom (1994) consider management a complex challenge involving functions such as planning, organizing, directing and controlling the activities of subordinate staff. Leadership, on the other hand, is personal (Handy 1993). It is concerned with motivating, encouraging, communicating and involving people (Belbin 2001). Although there is a wealth of literature debating the essence of leadership (Yuki 1994; Heller 1997; Mullins 1999), there is a general consensus that leadership transforms. Jarvis and Manley (2001) support this view and suggest that transformational leadership combined with expertise in practice, research and education, helps develop a workplace culture where quality improvement and staff empowerment is the norm.

Leading and managing a community mental health nursing service in dementia is a complex task with multi-faceted roles and dimensions. Managers are also charged with the task of fighting for increased manpower and demanding more resources for practice development and research. An effective manager must have a vision for the development of the role of the CMHN in dementia care. They must also be proactive in ensuring that the team is prepared to respond appropriately to challenges, not least those presented by changing demographic trends, nurse prescribing guidelines, information technology and the emergence of specialist nurse consultant posts. The nurse manager must also ensure that the expertise of CMHNs and their unique and dynamic combination of therapeutic skills and psychotherapeutic approaches to care are utilized to maximum effect at micro, median and macro levels (Long 2001). At a more strategic level, the nurse manager or team leader has a responsibility for developing specialist practice in dementia care and consequently must be proactive in forging links with educational institutions in order to carry this initiative forward.

Team building and teamwork

People with dementia are a unique client group in so far as their needs are sometimes met by health and social care professionals with a remit for the care of older people whereas in other situations their needs are met by mental health service providers. Different localities have particular demographic, geographic, historic and legislative influences, as well as social work and health care traditions, which must be taken into account when developing a comprehensive, cohesive dementia service. As it is clearly impossible for any one profession to possess all the knowledge, skills and resources required to meet the total health care needs of society, good care should be the product of a good team (UKCC 1996). Good teamwork requires individual team members to recognize and respect the role and function of other team members whilst at the same time ensuring that the interest of the client remains paramount.

Setting up a multi-disciplinary team is a challenge. Placing a number of people from different disciplines in the same building is not teamwork. People have not been brought together merely to engage in social relationships but are there to perform a body of work: hence Belbin's assertion that teamwork should cover the components of the composite word – team and work (Belbin 2000). The UKCC (1998) suggests that hard work and negotiation between all health care professions is required if good teamwork is to be achieved. Gaining commitment, nurturing talent and ensuring people are motivated and productive require open communication and trust between managers and staff.

West (1994) describes a team as having the following attributes: a common purpose, team identity, interdependent functions and agreed values that regulate behaviour. Adair (1986) believes a team is a group of individuals who share a common aim and where the job and skills of each member fit with those of the others. Ønyett (1997) refers to empowerment, flexibility, good staff morale and good communication as characteristics of teamwork. This is supported by the UKCC (1998) which acknowledges that 'providing care is an inter-professional and inter-agency activity which in order to be effective, must be based on co-operation, shared understanding and respect' (p. 8). Clearly, the common denominator among all definitions of teamwork is the emphasis on shared aims and objectives. Hartlebury (1990) believes that clear aims and objectives, arrived at in a democratic way, lead to greater motivation, greater creativity and initiative, less conflict, fewer demands on management and better use of time and energy.

In order to lead and manage a team effectively, it is essential for CMHN managers to have a working knowledge and understanding of the dynamics that exist and drive the development of a team (Belbin 1998). Working together has positive connotations, but in practice carries threats of loss of identity, redistribution of power and loss of autonomy (Biggs 1997). There is clearly a need for more research on the negative and positive consequences of inter-agency working, not only to test effectiveness and efficiency but particularly to explore the preferences of the service users (Cox 1998). A useful team-building exercise used by the authors has been a training tool devised by Pearpoint *et al.* (1991) known as PATH. All team members attend a once-off PATH training day and the session provides a forum in which to highlight core values, identify and discuss roles, and examine processes and relationships. Team members are involved in establishing mutually agreed aims and objectives and have an opportunity to share fears, concerns and aspirations. At the end of the session, an action plan is formulated, objectives set and a review date agreed.

Team-building exercises such as PATH help to focus a team's attention on common goals, which in turn may be used to inform a mission statement and guide the development of organizational policies. In this way all team members have a sense of ownership and have contributed to the development of the team's aims and objectives. This is crucial to the success of any team, as it is well documented that clear aims and objectives lead to a more effective team (Heller 1999; Mullins 1999; Belbin 2000). Good teamwork leads to effective, efficient working relationships and empowerment for staff. It also promotes cooperation, shared understanding and is central for effective inter-agency and inter-professional activity. However, once-off days like those used in PATH are not likely to change or improve team dynamics unless there is also the infrastructure in place for continuous and integrated team building.

A successful team never stands still, and the team leader will never finish building the team. Such is the ambiguity of the times we live in that it is not the goalposts that keep moving but the playing field itself (Underwood 2001). Dementia care has been described as a developing landscape, but living in this evolving world brings with it high degrees of uncertainty and ambiguity. The nurse manager or team leader must develop skills to continue to operate the service effectively and support staff through changing times whilst ensuring the core values and mission of the team remains constant. The team leader must also strive to include all the necessary ingredients in the infrastructure of the team. This promotes job satisfaction and good staff morale, which results in improved staff performance and a strong, supportive collegial environment. An appropriate infrastructure should include regular staff meetings, as consultation is important in helping team members to feel valued. Other important initiatives include the establishment of effective information and communication systems, clinical and peer supervision; mentorship; regular staff appraisals; multi-disciplinary recordkeeping and case reviews; reflective dialogue; significant incident debriefing; journal clubs and social interaction outside the work environment.

Clinical supervision must be acknowledged as the cornerstone of clinical practice (Tingle 1995). As seen in Chapter 16, the value of clinical supervision lies in the relationship between the maintenance of high standards of patient care whilst at the same time developing a system of formal collegial support. The UKCC (1995) believes that clinical supervision is a multi-faceted task and provides a safeguard for standards of practice, the delivery of quality care and the development of expertise. Nurses are the greatest resource in health care and it is imperative to move forward with knowledgeable practice and quality patient care (Butterworth *et al.* 1996). CMHNs work on a daily basis with cognitively impaired clients whose challenging behaviour is often a source of great distress to family and friends. Because of the emotional trauma associated with this type of work, collegial support is vital and should exist alongside clinical supervision if burnout is to be avoided. In the absence of existing protocols, the team leader is responsible for researching and identifying an appropriate model of clinical supervision (Kohner 1994; Farrington 1995) and motivating team members to embrace the challenges therein.

Promoting cooperation and collaboration

Only when roles and responsibilities within the team are operationalized can the CMHN manager begin to consider relationships outside of the team. Good external relationships depend on communication, understanding, mutual support, flexibility and acceptance of help (Marson *et al.* 1990). The person with dementia, in their journey through their illness, can potentially come in contact with a range of health and social care providers. These may include general practitioners (GPs), social workers, occupational therapists, district nurses, health visitors, care managers, psychiatrists and many more depending on the individual circumstances of the person. Many of these professionals may not be members of a specialist multi-disciplinary team and their role and that of the CMHN may have the potential to complement or conflict with each other. It is therefore essential that all individuals and agencies with a remit for dementia care have an awareness of each other's role and function, both uni-professionally and as part of a specialist multi-disciplinary team.

Perhaps the most important contact is the GP, who often initiates referrals to the CMHN or team. The authors' own experience reflects the necessity of developing referral pathways so that referrals are appropriate and preliminary health care screening has been undertaken prior to referral to the CMHN specializing in dementia care. This will have the dual benefit of directing resources to clients in greatest need whilst raising GP awareness of the services available for clients who, following screening, present with memory impairment. Whilst, on paper, this approach would appear to be of benefit both to the client and to the referring GP, a study by Renshaw *et al.* (2001) concluded that almost half of the GPs questioned ($n = 500$) felt that it would be of little benefit to make an early diagnosis, with comments such as 'dementia is untreatable, so why diagnose?'. Comments like this suggest that an alarming degree of clinical nihilism continues to exist among some GPs. However, on a more positive note, the study's findings also indicated that where measures had been undertaken to heighten awareness of interventions, both pharmacological and psychological, GPs were more likely to believe in the benefits of early diagnosis.

Clearly, CMHNs need to work collaboratively with their GP colleagues to raise the index of suspicion about the insidious onset of dementia and to move towards a more enlightened approach to the management of the disorder. The work of Naidoo and Bullock (2001) has proved to be invaluable in providing a framework by which GPs, after carrying out relatively simple screening, can then refer cognitively impaired clients to specialist teams and memory clinics. The authors are currently involved in developing local referral pathways aimed at increasing the number of early referrals from GPs, thus initiating contact with the specialist dementia team at a much earlier point in the trajectory of the dementia process than has been the case heretofore. The ultimate aim of this initiative is to maximize the effectiveness of interventions through the initiation of early cognitive rehabilitation and to move from a reactive model to a proactive model of management.

Whilst GPs are often the first point of contact for a person with cognitive impairment, other health and social care professionals also have extensive contact with the older population and as a result are ideally placed to observe cognitive or behavioural changes. District nurses frequently visit clients in the community for a myriad of physical health needs. This regular contact with older people affords an opportunity for early intervention in situations where a client's cognitive impairment is a source of concern to the nurse or the family. However, in order for this concern to result in practical action, lines of communication must be established between district nurses and specialist community mental health nursing teams for older people. It is useful from the outset if roles and responsibilities are clearly defined so that each professional involved in a client's care is aware what others are doing. Often misunderstandings can develop, particularly when nurses from different areas of practice are working with the same client. Regular meetings and shared learning opportunities should be encouraged as a means of improving knowledge and understanding of each other's role. Procedures for referrals should also be established between teams, with referral criteria and trigger points agreed, documented and discussed with all staff involved. The specialist skills of different teams will then be understood thus reducing the risk of professional hegemony.

Having undertaken this process, the authors can verify that it works and has led to increased referral rates and to improved communication between community mental health nursing staff and district nurses. In fact, both teams now view each other as a resource and frequently co-work cases and complete joint visits. Of course, one can, as Belbin (2000: 56) suggests, 'encroach often innocently into some incumbent's closely guarded territory', and if lines of communication have not been established between and within professions, an atmosphere of 'them and us' can easily develop. However, if holistic person-centred care is to be established then it will require all professionals involved to act in a manner which rises above petty parochialism and embraces a true multi-dimensional response to the person's needs. This form of close cooperation and co-working should also be established with other professions allied to medicine. Indeed, the *National Service Framework for Older People* (Department of Health 2001: 103) states that 'the Specialist Mental Health Service for Older People should also have agreed working and referral arrangements with speech and language therapists, physiotherapists, dieticians, chiropodist/podiatrists, community dental services, pharmacists, district nurses, health visitors, trained bi or multi lingual co-workers and housing workers'. One could add to this list, the Alzheimer's Society and the range of other private and voluntary sectors involved in the delivery of care to people with dementia and their carers.

Inter-agency communication

Perhaps the greatest challenge in multi-agency and inter-agency working for a CMHN manager is the relationship with local social services departments. Dementia in its progression will have a profound effect on the person and their family, and the requirement for a multi-agency response is self-evident. The historical separation of health and social care provision in Britain has meant that care provision has often been patchy and uncoordinated, and the need for greater understanding and cooperation between health and social services is well documented in the literature (Campbell and McLoughlin 2000; Vernon *et al.* 2000). Failure to work within a cooperative coordinated approach, which promotes the sharing of information and joined-up working can lead not only to a poor service but also to increased risk to vulnerable adults living in the community. This is supported by Alaszewski *et al.* (2000: 118) who state that 'the effective care and support of vulnerable individuals in the community depends on the effective co-ordination of all services which are intended to provide them with care and support'. However, division between agencies providing this support, which have been reinforced by traditional professional rivalries, have meant that some vulnerable clients have fallen into the gaps between agencies, with disastrous consequences both for themselves and for others (Alaszewski *et al.* 2000).

Within a Northern Ireland context, a review of services and standards of care of people with dementia and their carers was conducted in 1994. The Dementia Policy Scrutiny report (Department of Health and Social Services (Northern Ireland) 1995) highlighted the diversity of services throughout the province, ranging from centres of excellence to almost non-existent in some parts. The report also recognized that dementia as an illness requires a multi-professional response across the range of health and social care agencies, and advocated a multi-disciplinary approach as the best method of responding to this challenge. The report therefore recommended the establishment of specialist dementia teams within Trusts to include a representative from community mental health nursing, social work, psychogeriatric medicine and occupational therapy. As noted earlier, health and social services have been integrated in Northern Ireland since 1972, and the implementation of this report's recommendations may not prove as difficult as in other parts of the UK. However, as Campbell and McLoughlin (2000) have suggested, this integration may be more apparent at a strategic rather than at an operational level. Even within systems that are integrated on paper, there are often misunderstandings among health and social care professionals leading to fear of loss of autonomy and professional recognition.

Within a system of multi-agency and inter-agency service provision, it is essential that roles and lines of communications are clearly established. These principles will also be relevant when the CMHN interfaces with other agencies involved in the provision of social services, including voluntary and independent organizations. Some of the difficulties which inhibit closer collaboration between health and social services have been outlined by Hudson (1999a,b). These include: different patterns of employment and accountability in health and social services; different approaches to, and structures for, making decisions; different models of distributing resources; different professional cultures. These differences are highlighted when a CMHN specializing in dementia care has to access resources from an agency which facilitates a much broader client group. The latter organization's perception of dementia, and the priority it places in meeting the needs of people with dementia and their carers, will have an influence on how it responds to the resource issue. One example of the tragic consequences that can result from poor communication and co-ordination between agencies has been demonstrated in the report into the circumstances surrounding the death of Mr Frederick McLernon (Department of Health and Social Services (Northern Ireland) 1998). This report recommended that in situations where the referring individual or agency has requested specific services and these are found to be inappropriate to the client's need, the outcome of the assessment should be discussed (with the client's consent) with the person who has made the referral to ensure that all relevant information has been taken into account.

CMHNs working in these types of situation are faced with the challenge of changing the culture of the organization in which they work. The very nature of dementia in its clinical presentation often makes it difficult for the individual to make their needs known. In addition, relatives, often older people themselves, consider their role as carer as part of their family duty. They can often perceive requests for help and assistance, in whatever form, as a failure on their part. The end result is that potentially many individuals are not receiving the community support they need. This places a huge responsibility on the CMHN manager to access timely and effective resources from local social services. Tunmore and Thomas (1992), who argue that one of the major components of CMHN role is to identify, challenge and attempt to change those factors that adversely affect the mental health of the present and future population, support this view. In essence, the CMHN manager must act as an advocate to promote a change of culture. This culture change will involve the promotion of the ideals of equality and citizenship which look beyond the label of 'demented', a term which in itself is poorly understood and serves only to perpetuate the notion of incapacity and paternalistic attitudes.

The work of the late Professor Tom Kitwood (1997) has been influential in recognizing that people with dementia have the ability to make choices and that health and social care providers have a duty to 'hear the voices within' (Goldsmith 1996: 5). This type of intervention is in itself not easy because it is intensive and time consuming. The concept of person-centred dementia care planning advocated by Kitwood and others does not always sit easily in the wider health and social care arena. In essence it challenges many of the nihilistic perceptions held by those charged with providing health and social care to people with dementia and their carers. There is, however, evidence in the literature which clearly demonstrates good practice in terms of the delivery of health and social care for people with dementia (Tuppen 1998; Cameron 1999; Hammond 2000).

What is common in all these reports is the level of coordination, the concept of a shared philosophy and common aims and objectives regardless of the professional backgrounds of the people involved. The creation of specialist dementia teams with their multi-agency membership recognizes the need for holistic client-centred care. Furthermore, such teams can provide clients and carers with a resource whereby an identified key worker can access the specialist skills and knowledge of other team members as and when required.

As with other agencies, it is necessary for the CMHN manager to devise protocols for the acceptance and receipt of referrals from local social services and district nursing teams. Issues around the key worker role and the process of transferring and co-working cases need to be operationalized. Once the wider health and social services organization realizes that they have within their trust a valuable resource, then relationships can and should improve. It is the authors' experience that whilst policies, procedures and protocols are essential, true collaboration exists only when successful outcomes are apparent. The authors also believe that experiential working is the single most effective way of promoting better relationships between agencies. This brings with it a realization that the specialist team does not present a threat to generic services but rather is a resource which, when used appropriately, can improve outcomes for clients, carers and professionals alike. The authors' experience of helping to develop the Northern Ireland Dementia Forum, a multi-agency, regional forum for health and social care professionals working in the field of dementia care, has been a useful learning exercise. The forum provides an opportunity for regular meetings so that ideas of best practice, service developments and new initiatives are shared. It is envisaged that the forum will help to ensure high standards of practice and care throughout the region and beyond.

Towards the future

Many older people have complex needs and, as such, a single intervention approach to management is inappropriate. Much of the work undertaken by nurses is hidden and its effectiveness is contingent upon the nature of the interpersonal relationship between the CMHN and the older person (Gunstone 1999). The nurse's therapeutic presence and the effectiveness of the 'Being' model (Long 1995) are inherently difficult to measure. However challenging the task, it is crucial that nurses develop ways of measuring their interventions and benefits to the health status of clients and their carers. Kitson (1997) believed that clinical effectiveness in the context of work with older people is that of being able to do the right thing whilst doing the right thing, and this is dependent on the effectiveness of teams and teamwork.

Services for clients and their carers will not improve until the perceived gap between acute and community care has been bridged. Unplanned, inappropriate discharges must rapidly be consigned to the history books. The relationship between primary care providers and specialist dementia teams needs to be developed and sustained. GP fundholding will cease to exist from 1 April 2002 and will be replaced with local health and social care groups. These groups are designed as a mechanism to facilitate partnerships and better cooperation between primary care professionals and others, as well as promote the involvement of local communities and other agencies in the planning and delivery of services (Department of Health, Social Services and Public Safety (Northern Ireland) 2001). CMHNs working in dementia care must be represented on this group. If mental health practitioners are to feel safe and secure in today's working environment, they must be given a platform in which to highlight the grey areas in this black and white world, particularly to the people who set the psychiatric care agenda (Pratt 2001). It is also important that CMHNs specializing in dementia care continue to lobby for dementia to be classified under the umbrella of serious and enduring mental illnesses as this would be hugely significant in addressing the needs of people with dementia and their families (Adams 1996).

The scope of professional practice is ever changing in response to client need, and CMHNs must be prepared to accept statutory responsibilities if their role is to expand. The issue of nurse prescribing is in a consultation period and it remains to be seen what recommendations will emerge. However, the use of cholinesterase inhibitors in clinical practice is exciting and it may well be that CMHNs working in this field will be involved in supplementary prescribing in the not too distant future. Clearly, the development of new pharmacological treatments for people with dementia will have important implications for the development of dementia care nursing (Adams and Page 2000). However, nurse managers will have a key role to play in supporting and guiding nurses to achieve the required level of confidence and competence in their prescribing role whilst at the same time ensuring that such an initiative is brought forward with the full support of other members of the multi-disciplinary team, particularly medical colleagues.

Research is essential to the maintenance of good practice and, as the field expands, the more that research becomes necessary. This is supported by Perrin (1996: 128) who states that 'it is research and evaluation which will develop and extend this specialism to the point where it has efficacy, expertise and authority and a voice of potency in health care today'. Few will deny that there is a paucity of research about the role of the CMHN in dementia care and this needs to be addressed. CMHNs specializing in dementia need to develop a sound understanding of research and be able to critically appraise research in the field of dementia. Knowledge of research methodologies, statistics and good presentation skills will be essential requirements of tomorrow's nurse managers. As education and research are inextricably linked, new educational initiatives are necessary if specialist programmes in dementia nursing are to be developed and recognized. In the absence of specialist skills and knowledge, nurses will have great difficulty in achieving recognition for their contribution to the care of people with dementia and their carers (Carr *et al.* 1980). Recognition of the need to provide therapeutic interventions, education, training and supportive counselling whilst ensuring evidence-based practice, has increased the demand on practitioners in collaboration with nurse educationalists to develop appropriate post-registration specialist education in this area. In Northern Ireland, CMHNs and other health and social care representatives are collaborating with the University of Ulster to develop an MSc in dementia studies. This programme of study, the first of its kind in Northern Ireland, is designed to appeal to a range of health and social care professionals who are interested in specializing in dementia care and addresses a dearth of educational development in this area.

With the implementation of devolution in Wales, Scotland and Northern Ireland there is an opportunity for CMHNs to be more influential in deciding how, when and where dementia services are provided. The nurse as a political animal, whilst not a new concept, is one which the authors believe will take on greater significance as regional government becomes a reality. The ability to lobby effectively at regional health committee meetings and increased awareness of how decisions are made is now a necessity. The future planning, resourcing and direction of dementia care will be decided at local assembly level, but in order to respond to changing health and social care demands, it is necessary for nurses to become more political.

Conclusion

Collaboration in the planning and delivery of care for people with dementia between health, social services, voluntary and private sectors is now a major drive in government policy. The extent to which nurses develop and sustain good working relationships with other agencies will have an impact on the quality of the service received by clients. Clearly, multi-agency/inter-agency working brings with it great opportunities to develop the care and service provision for people with dementia and their carers. However, it is essential that the core values of effective multi-agency/inter-agency working are fully implemented at a strategic level and not left to individual trusts or local authorities to implement at their discretion. It is incumbent on CMHNs specializing in dementia to raise their profile so that other agencies within the health and social care arena have an understanding of the specialist skills, knowledge and practice available to them. Equally, CMHNs must recognize the unique contribution of other individuals and agencies involved in dementia care provision and in doing so embrace the concept of holistic care.

References

Adair, J. (1986) *Effective Teambuilding: How to Make a Winning Team*. London: Pan.

Adams, T. (1996) Informal family caregiving to older people with dementia: research priorities for community psychiatric nursing, *Journal of Advanced Nursing*, 24: 703–10.

Adams, T. and Page, S. (2000) New pharmacological treatments for Alzheimer's disease: implications for dementia care nursing, *Journal of Advanced Nursing*, 31(5): 1183–8.

Alaszewski, A., Alaszewski, H., Ayer, S. and Manthorpe, J.M. (2000) *Managing Risk in Community Practice: Nursing, Risk and Decision Making*. London: Baillière Tindall/ Royal College of Nursing.

Belbin, R.M. (1998) *Team Roles at Work*. Oxford: Butterworth-Heinemann.

Belbin, R.M. (2000) *Beyond the Team*. Oxford: Butterworth-Heinemann.

Belbin, R.M. (2001) *Managing Without Power*. Oxford: Butterworth-Heinemann.

Biggs, S. (1997) Inter-professional collaboration: problems and prospects, in J. Øvretveit, P. Mathias and T. Thompson (eds) *Interprofessional Working for Health and Social Care*. London: Macmillan.

Butterworth, T., Bishop, V. and Carson, J. (1996) First step towards evaluating clinical supervision in nursing and health visiting: theory, policy and practice development, a review, *Journal of Clinical Nursing*, 5(2): 127–32.

Cameron, K. (1999) Dementia care in the community: an opportunity for collaboration, *Nursing Times*, 31: 44–5.

Campbell, J. and McLoughlin, J. (2000) The 'joined up' management of adult health and social care services in Northern Ireland: lessons for the rest of the UK, *Managing Community Care*, 8: 6–13.

Carr, P.J., Butterworth, C.A. and Hodges, B.E. (1980) *Community Psychiatric Nursing*. London: Churchill Livingstone.

Cox, S. (1998) Multidisciplinary and interprofessional working: the dementia context, in D. Sheard and S. Cox (eds) *Teams, Multidisciplinary Teams and Interprofessional Working and Dementia*. Stirling: University of Stirling.

Department of Health (1990) *The NHS and Community Care Act*. London: The Stationery Office.

Department of Health (2001) *National Service Framework for Older People*. London: The Stationery Office.

Department of Health (1997) *The New NHS: Modern, Dependable*. London: The Stationery Office.

Department of Health and Social Services (Northern Ireland) (1995) *Dementia in Northern Ireland*. Report of the Dementia Policy Scrutiny. Belfast: The Stationery Office.

Department of Health and Social Services (Northern Ireland) (1998) *From Policy to Practice: The Care of Mr Frederick Joseph McLernon (Deceased)*. Belfast: The Stationery Office.

Department of Health, Social Services and Public Safety (Northern Ireland) (2001) *Minister Announces the Way Forward for Primary Care*. Press statement. Belfast: Castle Buildings, Stormont.

Drucker, P.F. (1979) *Management*. London: Pan.

Farrington, A. (1995) Models of clinical supervision, *British Journal of Nursing*, 4(15): 876–8.

Goldsmith, M. (1996) *Hearing the Voice of People with Dementia: Opportunities and Obstacles*. London: Jessica Kingsley.

Gunstone, S. (1999) Expert practice: the interventions used by a community mental health nurse with carers of dementia sufferers, *Journal of Psychiatric and Mental Health Nursing*, 6: 21–7.

Hammond, B. (2000) Joint working success, *Journal of Dementia Care*, July/August: 12–13.

Handy, C.B. (1993) *Understanding Organisations*, 4th edn. London: Penguin.

Hartlebury, M. (1990) Teambuilding: a practical approach, in S. Marsdon, M. Hartlebury, R. Johnston and B. Scammell (eds) *Managing People*. London: Macmillan Education.

Heller, T. (1997) *In Search of European Success*. London: HarperCollins.

Heller, R. (1999) *Managing People*. London: Dorling Kindersley.

Holden, U.P. and Woods, R.T. (1995) *Positive Approaches to Dementia Care*. Edinburgh: Churchill Livingstone.

Hudson, B. (1999a) Primary health care and social care: working across professional boundaries. Part One: The changing context of inter-professional relationships, *Managing Community Care*, 7(1): 15–22.

Hudson B. (1999b) Primary health care and social care: working across professional boundaries. Part Two: Models of inter-professional collaboration, *Managing Community Care*, 7(2): 15–20.

Jarvis, J. and Manley, K. (2001) *Leading the Way*, Royal College of Nursing Bulletin, 19/01/02–3/02/02 issue no. 19.

Kitson, A.L. (1997) Using evidence to demonstrate the value of nursing, *Nursing Standard*, 11(28): 34–9.

Kitwood, T. (1993) Person and process in dementia, *International Journal of Geriatric Psychiatry*, 8: 541–5.

Kitwood, T. (1997) *The New Culture of Dementia Care*. Buckingham: Open University Press.

Kohner, N. (1994) *Clinical Supervision in Practice*. London: King's Fund Centre.

Legge, A. (2001) Have you got the right stuff?, *Nursing Times*, 97(25): 24.

Levine, S. and Crom, M. (1994) *The Leader in You*. Edinburgh: Simon & Schuster.

Long, A. (1995) Community mental health nursing, in D. Sines, F. Appleby and E. Raymond (eds) *Community Health Care Nursing*. London: Blackwell Science.

Long, A. (2001) Community mental health nursing, in D. Sines, F. Appleby and E. Raymond (eds) *Community Health Care Nursing*, 2nd edn. London: Blackwell Science.

Marson, S., Hartlebury, M., Johnston, R. and Scammel, B. (1990) *Managing People*. London: Macmillan Education.

McCormack, B. (2001) Clinical effectiveness and clinical teams: effective practice with older people, *Nursing Older People*, 13(5): 14.

Morris, C. (2000) Management matters? *Interchange News*, no. 15. London: The NHS Confederation.

Mullins, L.J. (1999) *Management and Organisational Behaviour*, 5th edn. London: Pitman.

Naidoo, N. and Bullock, R. (2001) *An Integrated Care Pathway for Dementia: Best Practice for Dementia Care*. Swindon: Kingshill Research Centre.

Ønyett, S. (1997) The challenge of managing community mental health teams, *Health and Social Care in the Community*, 5(1): 40–7.

Pearpoint, J., O'Brien, J. and Forest, M. (1991) *PATH: A Workbook for Planning Positive Possible Futures*. Canada: Toronto Inclusion Press.

Perrin, T. (1996) *Problem Behaviour and the Care of Elderly People*. Oxfordshire: Winslow Press.

Pratt, D. (2001) Risk management in mental health, *Nursing Times*, 97(25): 38.

Renshaw, J., Surfield, P., Cloke, L. and Orrell, M. (2001) General practitioners' views on the early diagnosis of dementia, *British Journal of General Practice*, 51(462): 37–8.

Stewart, R. (1994) *Managing Today and Tomorrow*. London: Macmillan.

Tingle, J. (1995) Clinical supervision is an effective risk management tool, *British Journal of Nursing*, 4(14): 794–5.

Tunmore, R. and Thomas, B. (1992) Models of psychiatric consultation liaison in nursing, *British Journal of Nursing*, 1(9): 447–51.

Tuppen, J. (1998) Working together: a model for co-ordinating community care, *Journal of Dementia Care*, March/April: 10–11.

UKCC (1995) *Clinical Supervision for Nursing and Health Visiting*, Registrar's Letter, 24 January. London: United Kingdom Central Council.

UKCC (1996) *Guidelines for Professional Practice*. London: United Kingdom Central Council.

UKCC (1998) *Guidelines for Mental Health and Learning Disabilities Nursing*. London: United Kingdom Central Council.

Underwood, C. (2001) Changing times, *Modern Management*, 15: 2.

Vernon, S., Ross, F. and Gould, M.A. (2000) Assessment of older people: politics and practice in primary care, *Journal of Advanced Nursing*, 31(2): 282–7.

West, M.A. (1994) *Effective Teamwork*. Leicester: BPS Books (The British Psychological Society).

Yuki, G. (1994) *Leadership in Organisations*, 3rd edn. Harlow: Prentice Hall International.

18

Higher-level practice
Addressing the learning needs for community mental health nursing practice in dementia care

Jan Dewing and Vicki Traynor

Introduction

In this chapter our aims are twofold: first, we describe the development of the higher-level practice (HLP) standard (UKCC 2002). We look at why HLP is an issue for specialist nurses such as community mental health nurses (CMHNs). Then we consider issues of practice-based competence and show how a competency-based approach combined with evidence of learning in, and from, everyday practice can be used to help demonstrate achievement of HLP. Secondly, we seek to show the kinds of learning experience CMHNs working in dementia care can acquire when aspiring to attain HLP registration. We make reference to an action research project with Admiral Nurses as this was centred on the development of competencies and work-based learning (see also Chapter 13). At the time of writing, the new Nursing and Midwifery Council has not yet added to HLP so we refer to the United Kingdom Central Council (UKCC) as the developer and author of the HLP standard. We also refer throughout this chapter 'to those of us with dementia' instead of people with dementia to emphasize that there is no divide; no 'us and them'.

Higher level of practice

There are two main sets of professionally driven arguments related to nursing competency that seem relevant to CMHNs working with those of us who have dementia. First, there is a gathering broad-based professional agenda towards demonstrating competency in nursing and other health and social care professions. This is in part internally driven: for example, work undertaken by the Royal College of Nursing (RCN) in developing faculties of nursing each with a competency and career progression framework. It is also in part influenced by the growing calls from a variety of sources for greater public protection (Lenburg 1999; UKCC

1999a; Department of Health 2001a; Royal College of Nursing 2001). Secondly, proliferation of nursing roles, such as advanced practitioners and specialist nurses with huge variation in grades, remit and skills, led to some degree of concern about the competence required for such jobs as well as confusion over what nurses with such unusual titles actually do in and for nursing practice. Thus the UKCC sought to review the situation and suggested that the way forward lay in recognizing that a higher level of practitioner should be encouraged and standardization of what competence could be expected was needed for greater public protection. After all, pre-registration nursing students were required to achieve competencies in order to register (Norman *et al.* 2000), yet registered nurses, including those claiming to be most skilled in clinical or patient care, were not required to do this.

The UKCC has been driving work on HLP because its primary role is to ensure the safety of the public. Recently, it examined how the public could be assured about the standard of practice provided by nurses carrying out diverse and specialist roles (UKCC 1999a). A report by the UKCC (1995) identified two levels of practice beyond the entry point of registration: advanced and specialist. However, it was not long before the UKCC began to rethink its framework in response to rapid changes in health care provision (UKCC 2002) and confusion over the two levels from within the profession. It was not until 1999 that the UKCC publicized its intentions in relation to developing HLP (UKCC 1999b). The final report (UKCC 2002) sets out a standard for HLP with seven elements:

1   Providing effective health care.

2   Leading and developing practice.

3   Improving quality and health outcomes.

4   Innovation and changing practice.

5   Evaluation and research.

6   Developing self and others.

7   Working across professional and organizational boundaries.

Current policy and politics are also a driver for increased and better quality nursing. For example, the NHS modernization programme is intended to set out investment and reform for a twenty-first-century health and welfare service (Department of Health 1998). Clinical governance agendas and commission for health improvement (CHI) will all contribute towards the need to be clearer about competence and competencies in all professions. In England, national service frameworks (NSFs) (Department of Health 2001b) were established as part of the modernization agenda to improve services through the setting of national standards to drive up quality and to try to reduce existing variations in care (Dewing and Ford 2001). The *National Service Framework for Older People* focuses on four themes with eight standards in total:

1   *Respecting the individual.* The standards applied to this theme are rooting out age discrimination and providing person-centred care.

2   *Intermediate care.* The standards applied to this theme are the provision of intermediate care.

3   *Providing evidence-based specialist care.* The standards covered in this theme are general hospital care, stroke, falls, promoting older people's mental health.

4   *Promoting an active healthy life.* The standards in this theme are about the promotion of health and active life in older age.

There are some natural links to be made between the NSF standards and elements of the UKCC's standard for HLP. CMHNs in England could use the four themes as part of a framework for gathering evidence of attainment. Integration of national policy themes from the other countries could work equally well.

Dementia and HLP?

The field of dementia care is becoming more complex regardless of the policy and political agenda. Not only is multi-disciplinary screening, assessment and medical pharmacological treatment growing in possibility and potential, but humanistic caring and associated therapeutic opportunities are constantly expanding (Dewing 2000; Cantley 2001; Traynor and Dewing 2001). Achieving the standards set out in the NSF is proving challenging for many teams. Each standard has milestones for progress with target dates for achievement. Further milestones and dates will be rolled out as the NSF develops. The themes all require contribution from a registered nurse. If the final theme of promoting an active, healthy life is to be achieved and health gain is to be met, then skilled CMHNs are needed as part of the overall care that an older person with dementia receives. Maintaining health, let alone promoting health in an older person with dementia, and in supporters/carers, is not a simple matter. The older person with a dementia process has a variety of health needs, some age related, some due to physical illness and some related to dementia that mean they will be neither stable nor predictable for long periods of time. Equally, we have for a long time underestimated the health care needs of supporters/ carers. The work of Admiral Nurses (see Chapter 13) has, for example, demonstrated how complex achieving quality of health with carers can be.

Accumulating research in many fields indicates that much can be done for those of us with dementia and that there is still more to be achieved. Nursing has a major role to play in promoting and maintaining subjective quality of health as a contribution to social well-being and social inclusion. The debates about the contribution that skilled nursing and skilled CMHN can make to the quality of life for those of us with dementia and our families have been covered in other chapters and will not be expanded upon here.

However, we believe that those of us with a dementia deserve practitioners who have knowledge and skills in both the condition of dementia (in its broadest sense) and ways of knowing about the subjective experience of the person that enables both clinically effective evidence-based and person-centred interventions. Subjective experience in this instance is related to life cycle, biography and ultimately with ageing processes. Therefore, we would argue that all nurses working in dementia care wanting to progress to HLP should have accumulating expertise in both mental health and biopsychosocial aspects of ageing. CMHNs generally regard themselves to be specialist nurses. We would see that in the future, as the move towards competency-based health and social care professions continues, specialist nurses in all fields of practice will be expected to provide evidence of what this means through attaining HLP registration.

Understanding competency

A competency is a statement about a level or type of competence. There has been, and probably still is, no overall agreement as to what constitutes competence. Certainly incompetence is probably easier to recognize and describe, although it still carries value assumptions. As a minimum, newly registered practitioners must be competent to assess the need for care, provide care, monitor and evaluate and to do this in institutional and non-institutional settings (UKCC 1986). Following registration the practitioner is required to maintain and develop their professional knowledge and competence (UKCC 1990). In the case of HLP, defining competence becomes more ambitious and perhaps also more ambiguous. This is indeed the case where competency is taken entirely as measurable or observable behaviours.

Like Lankshear *et al.* (1996) in an English National Board study, we adopt the definition of competence (set out by Eraut and Cole 1993: ii) as 'the ability to perform to an agreed standard, a specified set of tasks, processes and functions over an agreed range of contexts and situations'. This definition encapsulates a broad perspective on competencies as suggested by both the occupational standards and outcomes-based approach and the generic attributes model of competency. It is linking competence to standards and thus suggesting that competence can be achieved in different dimensions and at differing levels.

Within the nursing literature, there is disagreement about the appropriateness of a competency-based approach to the education and development of nurses and nursing practice. In addition, there is confusion about which of several approaches should be adopted. Approaches will naturally reflect how competency is defined by proponents of particular models. One approach is described as the American, generic or holistic approach. In the generic model, competency refers to a person's overall capacity and tends to be used about characteristics of a person rather than a statement about range of competence (Eraut 1994). Thus a CMHN, for example, could be observed to carry out a nursing activity in a way that is behaviourally competent but attitudinally unprofessional or ethically unacceptable.

In contrast, O'Hagan (1996) suggests that competency means to be 'fit, proper, or qualified'. This is probably the meaning the UKCC drew on when it referred to a competent nurse as one who is 'safe to practise with minimal supervision'. Competency-based education approved by the UKCC aimed to provide nurses who are 'fit for purpose'. In this way, a registered practitioner is one who has demonstrated their competence for performing a set of predefined competency statements that the UKCC deemed necessary to be a competent practitioner.

Another influential development of the word 'competent' is presented by Benner (1984). Interpretations of her work have suggested that a competent nurse is one who is no longer a novice and not yet an expert – as if competent was a stage a nurse passed through comparable to being good enough, average or satisfactory. A competent nurse's practice is distinguished by the nurse's ability to integrate theory and knowledge to deliver effective nursing care and is what we would expect of a newly qualified practitioner. This is in direct contrast to a novice nurse who cannot easily transfer knowledge and skills learnt in one setting to another, unknown setting. Benner's (1984) work is derived from Dreyfus's skills acquisition model of work and has been influential in the UK for structuring pre-registration curricula (Norman *et al.* 2000). Benner's work says that beginning nurses learn how to perform a certain set of tasks, in certain situations, and as they develop their practice they learn to integrate theory and practice and are able to perform these tasks on different practice settings. In this model, there is no overall concept of a competent nurse who is 'fit for purpose'. Rather, a competent nurse is one who can integrate theory and practice to deliver effective nursing care in a wide range of settings. This nurse then moves on to become more expert.

Benner (1984) suggests that an expert nurse is one who uses intuition and is able to draw on lifelong experiences to deliver effective nursing care in complex situations or in situations not previously experienced. In this case the concept of competencies may become unhelpful or redundant and the expert nurse may seek to use attributes instead (see later in this chapter). The enthusiastic adoption of Benner's work by UK educationalists has partially contributed to the current confusion about which model of competence is appropriate. In our opinion, Benner (1984) confuses us by suggesting that competence is a descriptor for a nurse with an ability to integrate theory and practice across a range of settings and that an expert nurse is one who can draw on lifelong experience to deliver effective nursing care regardless of the context in which the care is delivered. Benner (1984) then adopts a literal meaning of competence to mean fit, proper or qualified. She does not consider the importance of 'fitness for purpose'. She ignores the need to find out what level of competence is expected of, say, a senior nurse with senior responsibilities. In contrast, we argue that nurses at all levels of skill need to be competent within what is expected at that level. So, to prepare nurses to be experts and ensure they are 'fit for purpose' we can develop a set of competencies which, when demonstrated, reflect expert nursing practice.

The 'fit for purpose' model of competency is derived from what is known as outcomes-based competency education. The focus in the competency statements, and the way in which nurses demonstrate their competence, centre on the outcomes of the fulfilling the competencies. Thus, clients' and services' needs are the focus and the competency statements are structured around developing nurses' practice in order to improve the way they carry out their nursing practice.

Benner's (1984) work is presented as distinct from the UKCC's model of competency which is around the concept of 'fit for purpose'. Some educationalists have critiqued the 'fit for purpose' approach as reductionist and behaviouristic. They suggest that nursing practice is a sophisticated profession which cannot be described through a set of discrete set of tasks which is suggested by the 'fit for purpose' approach to competency. This criticism can be challenged by suggesting that as long as the 'fit for purpose' includes an ability to integrate theory and knowledge into practice there is no reason why it cannot be useful to even a very sophisticated profession such as nursing. It does, however, mean that standards and competency statements must not only reflect the professional artistry but also be achievable and measurable in some way.

The fitness for practice and purpose approach taken by the UKCC challenged Benner's (1984) conception of competence. The UKCC suggested that it is important to educate nurses to be 'fit for purpose' and it set about developing this model to apply to nurses regardless of the grades or roles. Project 2000 was put in place to prepare undergraduate nurses. Then, in the mid-1990s, Post-Registration Education and Practice (PREP) was launched into the nursing profession. Whilst PREP was never intended to be a guarantee of competence, it contributed to registered nurses entering into lifelong learning and continuous skills updating in order to stay on the effective nursing register.

The UKCC has more recently developed a standard for HLP (UKCC 2002) to be achieved rather than setting out actual competencies. The standard is, however, reasonably detailed. Nurses are left with the problem of deciding whether the standard can be used alone or whether and how they can be related to competencies. Using the 'fit for purpose' model of competency it is possible to draw up competency statements which could be used to help nurses to demonstrate their HLP or expert practice.

There are three main points for CMHNs to reflect on:

1   Other developments over and above UKCC agenda including the NHS pay modernization report (Department of Health 2001c) mean that the move towards a competency-based profession is growing.

2   HLP will be regulated and practice-based evidence of attainment will be required. Applicants such as CMHNs will be assessed on a portfolio of evidence, a visit by a member of the assessment panel and appearing before an assessment panel (UKCC 2002). It will be for the Nursing and Midwifery Council to determine further developments on regulating a higher level of practice.

3   Regardless of how (or when) the above happens, CMHNs who regard themselves as specialist or expert practitioners have a responsibility, over and above PREP, to demonstrate their fitness for purpose to the public and the profession. Evidence relating to attainment of the HLP standard (and competencies) must come from day-to-day practice. Demonstrating attendance at academic courses and study days will not be sufficient, neither will descriptive accounts of applying knowledge in practice.

Attributes

Benner (1984) describes domains of nursing in a similar way to how Manley and McCormack (1997) describe attributes of the expert nurse. Attributes can be thought of as a desirable characteristic of practice. In effect an attribute is a statement about a personal quality nurses must possess if they are to be effective practitioners. For example, five key attributes have been developed by the RCN Gerontological Nursing Programme as part of the BSc(Hons) in gerontological nursing (Royal College of Nursing Institute 2001: 4–5). They are:

1   *Holistic knowledge: synthesis of different types of knowledge about older people.*

2   *Saliency: seeing and acting on the most pertinent issues in a situation.*

3   *Knowing the patient: getting to know the patient as a person and working with them in an individualized way; developing partnership with the older person to achieve health and maximize potential.*

4   *Moral agency: responds to needs of older person in an holistic way both at a personal and social level; respects dignity and protects personhood at times of vulnerability; enables person to feel safe and valued and works to support integrity in personal relationships with them and between the older person and others.*

5   *Skilled know-how: performance is fluid, seamless and highly proficient.*

It can be seen from this that the notion of attributes sits more comfortably with Benner's picture of the skilled nurse working in an holistic way. This approach seems well suited to HLP and gives CMHNs another option for organizing the UKCC standard with a broader professional framework. But it must be said that determining higher-level competence in practice in terms of describing attributes and gathering evidence is a challenging, although extremely interesting and engaging, process. The attributes above offer another way in which CMHNs can structure their development and gather evidence for HLP registration.

Assessing competence

Accepted definitions of competence and competency have been influenced by ways of assessing, demonstrating and testing competency, often led by educationalists. As has already been said, traditional means of demonstrating competence was through direct observation of behaviours. Given that the UKCC recognizes HLP is also about values, attitudes and decision making as well as the seen components of behaviours, assessment must be directed at finding evidence of these. This means a range of assessment methods are needed over and above direct observation as set out by the UKCC (2002) following the pilot project of the proposed HLP standard and assessment process.

The approach we are adopting is described as an outcomes-based approach and is rooted in a belief that work-based learning is one way of developing a professional workforce of nurses delivering relevant and high-quality nursing care (Flanagan *et al.* 2000). The traditional approach to practice was to see it as work. Learning was something that took place through education routes such as formal courses or study days and usually away from the workplace. This approach meant that learning took place in episodic chunks. So, for example, nurses would read academic journals only when they were on a formal course. For newly registered nurses there is clearly a need to acquire formal knowledge about how to undertake a range of activities and tasks. Newly registered practitioners need this sort of knowledge to develop in confidence and competence. The same is often true for practitioners moving into a new care setting or into a new speciality as in both cases the culture and way of doing things may differ.

With lifelong learning in nursing, there are two important principles. First, it is acknowledged that learning is taking place continuously within practice, and secondly, that education provides supplemented rather than constituted learning. For learning to be said to have taken place it must be synthesized, evaluated and used in practice for the benefit of patients and service delivery. One way of utilizing the competency-based approach is to use work-based learning to demonstrate competency (Flanagan *et al.* 2000). Again we draw on Benner's (1984) work to show that competency does not have to take a linear or simplistic task approach. Benner outlined how the critical incident technique, reflective practice and nursing narratives can be used to illustrate how a practitioner is delivering their nursing care. Benner (1984) suggests using this model to help nurses articulate what they are doing. She would suggest that the different levels of nursing practice that a nurse is delivering can be demonstrated using any one of these techniques.

To take a broader view, we suggest CMHNs can use these and similar techniques to demonstrate how they are delivering their nursing care at a higher level of practice. We would suggest that these techniques can be used by nurses to demonstrate their competency at whatever level of practice is expected of them. For example, a newly qualified nurse can demonstrate their competency to integrate theory and practice across various settings through a critical incident, a reflective practice account, or a nursing narrative. A CMHN working for HLP will demonstrate their expert competence through an in depth critical analysis and synthesis. At HLP the nurse will be expected to be analytical and to synthesize knowledge in relation to practice. Undoubtedly there will be academic implications to this level of practice as the following case vignette illustrates.

Case vignette

Jane, a CMHN, is working towards HLP registration. She has identified and agreed the structure of her portfolio with a mentor. Jane has an experience where an older person with altered capacity is asked to make a decision about where they want to live (at home or in residential care) in a brief space of time and in a communal hospital setting. She decides to use this in her portfolio. She identifies several key issues that she can influence in order to provide improved care:

* Confidentiality.
* Decision making and capacity issues.
* Multi-disciplinary team attitudes and skills.
* Life's transitions and older persons' abilities to adapt, and how well this is recognized or facilitated.

Jane's foundation was to describe what happened, but this is not her evidence. Her evidence is the summary of the types of knowledge she considered in relation to each of the above. She presented this in a diagram like a mind map and related it to the attributes described earlier in the chapter. In relation to the issue of capacity she summarized for herself organic changes affecting decision making, national and local policies on consent and capacity, and relevant knowledge from key writers in this area. Her learning from this was twofold. First, that capacity and decision making is situation specific. So the evidence she put into her portfolio was the outcomes from how she went about working with the team to learn about this and change their policy and methods when an older person with altered capacity was making life-changing decisions. This was her second learning point. Jane would be able to attach to her portfolio the new policy and results from a questionnaire the team completed on their feelings about the change in their practice.

Whilst we differ from Benner (1984) in that we suggest that all levels of nurses can demonstrate that they are competent to practise, we accept that an interpretative qualitative approach is a more useful way of demonstrating nursing competence than assessing that specific sets of tasks have been performed. We would suggest that, for the novice nurse or the nurse new to a client group or setting, it might be acceptable to assess certain discrete tasks, but a more experienced nurse will need a more in-depth approach to demonstrate their competence to practice and that they are 'fit for purpose'. Observation of behaviours or actions as part of a nursing activity is not as straightforward as it seems. It is possible that a naive observer (such as an inexperienced practitioner) and an expert practitioner could be observed to undertake the same behaviours. Whereas, to an expert observer, the overall behaviours are the same, the artistry and fluidity of the expert stands out from the inexperienced practitioner (Benner 1984). Furthermore, in structured conversation the expert would be able to break down the situation into more parts, demonstrate better use of language to describe and explain both the situation and their own feelings, thoughts and decisions.

There are two main points here. First, that competence, when thought of as values, attitudes knowledge and skill (not just behaviour), can be captured by another person. In this way competence is more about attributes. Secondly, the observer must know what expert or HLP looks like when they come across it – it takes a practitioner with expertise to recognize it in another person. More fundamentally there is a need for practitioners to consider a range of ways in which they can collect evidence of achieving competencies and development to HLP. This may include, for example, analysis and summaries of reflections, accounts from service users, peer and colleagues, teaching plans and evaluations.

In summary, the approach we advocate for demonstrating HLP is derived from the 'fitness for purpose' approach which the UKCC has adopted for assuring that nurses are competent to practise at whatever level they expect to practise at. The way in which competence should be demonstrated also needs to be 'fit for purpose'. That is, adopting the qualitative interpretative approaches described by Benner (1984) seems most appropriate. Assessment must then be criterion focused and consensus agreement between assessors reached that it is appropriate for a particular level. Whilst this may be open to extremes of interpretation, reducing nursing practice to a set of discrete tasks is not helpful. Benner (1984) suggests that job analysis of nursing results in a reductionism within nursing with more and more competencies and sub-competencies in a fruitless attempt to try to define nursing by the tasks that practitioners perform. A much quoted extract from her work suggests that nursing competency is defined by a practitioner's ability to perform nursing tasks under varied circumstances in the real world (see, for example, Bartlett *et al.* 1998; Norman *et al.* 2000). She suggests an alternative 'interpretative' approach to competence in nursing (Benner 1982). Further she suggests that nurses describe, in qualitative terms, what they are doing rather than relying on objective mechanistic attempts to describe a complex profession dependent on interpersonal relationships. Objectively testing the performance of tasks does not reveal whether a practitioner is competent to deliver the quality of nursing care. Rejection of this reductionist approach does not have to be a rejection of a competency-based approach to demonstrate certain levels of practice. By using interpretative qualitative techniques nurses can demonstrate the competent delivery of care.

An example of competencies and HLP: the Admiral Nurses' Competency Project

The RCN Gerontological Nursing Programme has completed a project adopting a participatory action research approach to facilitate a structured process towards the development of higher-level competencies for the Admiral Nurse service in England (Traynor and Dewing 2002). The project was funded by the Dementia Relief Trust. Admiral Nurses are usually CMHNs who combine a client case-load with a teaching and consultancy role to work in the field of dementia with a focus on carers' need (see Chapter 13 for more details).

Methodology

An action research approach using qualitative data collection and analysis was adopted to carry out this project. An action research approach was adopted because the aim of action research is to enable practitioners to engage in the research process and have an effect on the outcome of the findings (Hart and Bond 1995). That is, action research has an educative and learning focus. By being involved in an action research project, practitioners have the opportunity to use their participation to develop their practice. In addition, by engaging the practitioners in the research process, the applicability and ownership of the findings is enhanced because the practitioners' input can be used to ensure the findings are relevant.

There are variations to action research. In this project, emancipatory action research was adopted. The main aim of adopting an emancipatory action research approach is to facilitate clinicians to challenge taken-for-granted assumptions about their ways of working and to develop more effective ways of working (Manley 2000a,b, 2001). This in itself is a necessary part of moving towards HLP. In this way, Admiral Nurses actively took part in the research process. The project resulted in the development of a competency framework which was relevant and the Admiral Nurses were provided with numerous opportunities to review their current ways of working and develop their practice towards the model of practice and practitioner envisaged by the UKCC in their HLP model.

Methods

There were three distinct phases to this project: a 'scoping exercise'; development of the competency framework; and piloting the competency framework. It began with a scoping exercise. The project facilitators observed all aspects of the Admiral Nurses' work by spending time with each Admiral Nurse team. This included carer visits and observing teaching and consultancy sessions. In addition, Admiral Nurses and other stakeholders (service managers and Dementia Relief Trust staff and trustees) took part in detailed interviews to describe what the Admiral Nurse service does and their vision for the future.

The project facilitators and Admiral Nurses analysed transcriptions of the observation visits and the interviews to draw out the core competencies for the Admiral Nurse service. Monthly focus groups were held with the Admiral Nurses to develop the competencies into themes and items and to discuss ongoing issues arising from participation in action research. Reference groups were held with carers to ensure the core competencies were relevant to the main client group. Finally, the competencies were built into a resource pack that would guide the nurses through their use. The pack included ideas around how to self-assess, what counted as evidence, and achieving peer and collegiate validation of evidence. The final framework was piloted by the majority of Admiral Nurses and amended according to their experiences.

Outcomes

The outcome of this project has been the development of a competency-based framework for enabling Admiral Nurses to move towards HLP as befits a specialist nursing service. The participatory approach enabled Admiral Nurses to raise issues about several aspects of their practice, supervision, management, learning and support systems and to begin to question how these are enabling (or otherwise) movement towards HLP. The core competencies are:

1 Therapeutic work (interventions).
2 Sharing knowledge about dementia and carer issues.
3 Advanced assessment skills.
4 Prioritizing work.
5 Prevention and health promotion.
6 Person-centred and ethical practice.
7 Balancing needs of the person with dementia and the carer.
8 Promoting 'best' practice.

The competencies cover the range of client, teaching and consultancy practice which the Admiral Nurses carry out. Each competency is related to a UKCC HLP standard and includes statements about how the Admiral Nurse could demonstrate their competence within each of the HLP standards described by the UKCC (2002).

One of the action cycles involved reviewing other competency frameworks. As a result of this, the Admiral Nurses decided they wanted to include different levels of competency for themselves. Three levels were agreed. It might be that not all Admiral Nurses will want to work towards HLP, but by structuring the competency statements around the HLP standard the competency framework can be used to facilitate this process by those who do. The minimum level of competence is set at that expected of an Admiral Nurse in a post for between one and two years and thus it is developmental. Two examples are provided. Within the theme 'Prioritizing work', the competencies to cover HLP element 6 'Developing self and others', at the three levels are set out in Table 18.1, whilst Table 18.2 sets out the competencies required at the three levels within the theme 'Sharing knowledge about dementia care and carer issues', element 4 'Innovation and changing practice'.

Tables 18.1 and 18.2 demonstrate how the nurses can have a structure against which to self-assess the best fit of their own competence with both specific role competencies and UKCC HLP standard. The competency framework will be used by Admiral Nurses to structure how they demonstrate that their practice as a specialist nurse is competent and remains well above that which is expected of a newly registered practitioner. The competency framework includes resources and tools which can be used to structure how Admiral Nurses gather work-based evidence to demonstrate their competence.

Table 18.1 Competency framework for prioritizing work

Theme 4: Prioritizing work	*Intermediate*	*Advanced – in addition to Intermediate*	*Expert – in addition to Intermediate and Advanced*
HLP element 6: Developing self and others	Keeps reflective diary and participates in supervision to see how clients' involvement in care planning and prioritization is successfully facilitated Teaching sessions carried out on care planning and prioritization of clients' care	Actively engages in lifelong learning in the area of prioritizing work Facilitates others to critically review impact of supervision on prioritizing work Provides supervision to others trying out ways to facilitate clients' involvement in care planning and prioritization Undertakes postgraduate studies which include strategic ways to approach prioritizing work, for example, management courses Involved in developing undergraduate courses, for example management courses Teaches on postgraduate courses, for example management courses	Actively engages self and others in lifelong learning in the area of prioritizing work Takes on a leading role in innovative approaches to reflecting on practice and learning from experience and others' practice to prioritize work Contributes to evaluation of supervision system and its impact on how work is prioritized Involved in developing curriculum for postgraduate courses, for example management courses

Table 18.2 Competency framework for sharing knowledge about dementia care and carer issues

Theme 2: Sharing knowledge about dementia care and carer issues	Intermediate	Advanced – in addition to Intermediate	Expert – in addition to Intermediate and Advanced
HLP element 4: Innovation and changing practice	Critically reflects on information provided and ways of sharing information Disseminates information resources information to colleagues locally through newsletters and non-peer-reviewed journals Presents work at local forums	Develops innovative ways of sharing information Publishes work through peer-reviewed journals Presents work at national conferences	Takes on a leading role on national developments for information sharing with colleagues Presents work at international conferences Facilitates others to publish work in peer-reviewed journals and present work at national conferences

Conclusion

Underpinned by the philosophy and practice of lifelong learning, professional development for specialist nurses that is structured around the HLP standard fits with professional agendas and the government's vision for the contribution that nursing should make to improved health for older persons with a dementia (Department of Health 1999), the agenda for change (Department of Health 2001c), and the agenda of the Nursing and Midwifery Council. Thus, even though all CMHNs may not be actively seeking to register as a higher-level practitioner, the standard and approaches to demonstrating practice at this level should be something all CMHNs are actively seeking to work towards. Accumulating evidence of achievement in a portfolio through the means of broad-based competencies is a way in which CMHNs can demonstrate HLP and thus openly account to the public and peers that they are practising and achieving outcomes commensurate with specialist practice.

References

Bartlett, H., Westcott, L., Hind, P. and Taylor, H. (1998) *An Evaluation of Pre-registration Nursing Education: A literature review and comparative study of graduate outcomes.* Oxford: Oxford Centre for Health Care Research and Development, Oxford Brookes University.

Benner, P. (1982) Issues in competency-based testing, *Nursing Outlook*, May, 303–9.

Benner, P. (1984) *From Novice to Expert*. California: Addison-Wesley.

Cantley, C. (ed.) (2001) *A Handbook of Dementia Care*. Buckingham: Open University Press.

Department of Health (1998) *Modernising Health and Social Services: National Priorities Guidance*. London: The Stationery Office.

Department of Health (1999) *Making a Difference: Strengthening the nursing, midwifery, and health visiting contribution to health and healthcare*. London: The Stationery Office.

Department of Health (2001a) *Report of the Public Inquiry into Children Having Heart Surgery at the Bristol Royal Infirmary 1984–1995: Learning from the Bristol Inquiry*. London: The Stationery Office.

Department of Health (2001b) *Modern Standards and Service Models: National Service Framework for Older People*. London: The Stationery Office.

Department of Health (2001c) *Pay Modernisation: Agenda for Change in the NHS*. London: The Stationery Office.

Dewing, J. (2000) Promoting well being in older people with cognitive impairment. *Elderly Care*. 12(4): 19–24.

Dewing, J. and Ford, P. (2001) Mental health and the NSF, *Mental Health Practice*. 14(9): 24–6.

Eraut, M. (1994) *Developing Professional Competence: Knowledge and Competence*. London: Falmer Press.

Eraut, M. and Cole, G. (1993) *Assessing Competence in the Professions*, Research and Development Series Report No. 14. Sheffield: Department of Employment.

Flanagan, J., Baldwin, S. and Clarke, D. (2000) Work-based learning as a means of developing and assessing nursing competency, *Journal of Clinical Nursing*. 9: 360-8.

Hart, E. and Bond, M. (1995) *Action Research for Health and Social Care: A Guide to Practice*. Buckingham: Open University Press.

Lankshear, A., Brown, J. and Thompson, C. (1996) *Mapping the Nursing Competencies Required in Institutional and Community Settings in the Context of Multi-disciplinary Health Care Provision: An Exploratory Study*. London: ENB for Nursing, Midwifery and Health Visiting.

Lenburg, C.B. (1999) Redesigning expectations for initial and continuing competence for contemporary nursing practice, *Online Journal of Issues in Nursing*, published 30 September at http://www.nursingworld.org/ojin/topic10/tpc101.htm (accessed October 2001).

Manley, K. (2000a) Organisational culture and consultant nurse outcomes. Part 1: Organisational culture, *Nursing Standard*, 14(36): 34–8.

Manley, K. (2000b) Organisational culture and consultant nurse outcomes. Part 2: Nurse outcomes, *Nursing Standard*, 14(37): 34–9.

Manley, K. (2001) Consultant nurse: concept, processes, outcome. Unpublished Doctoral Study, University of Manchester/Royal College of Nursing Institute: London.

Manley, K. and McCormack, B. (1997) Exploring expert practice. MSc Module, Royal College of Nursing Institute, London.

Norman, I., Watson, R., Calman, L., Redfern, S. and Murrells, T. (2000) *Evaluation of the Validity and Reliability of Methods to Assess the Competence to Practise of Pre-registration Nursing and Midwifery Students in Scotland*. Edinburgh: National Board for Nursing, Midwifery and Health Visiting for Scotland.

O'Hagan, K. (1996) Social work competence: an historical perspective, in K. O'Hagan (ed.) *Competence in Social Work Practice: A Practical Guide for Professionals*. London: Jessica Kingsley.

Royal College of Nursing (2001) *Learning the Lessons: A Summary of the RCN's Response to the Bristol Inquiry*. London: Royal College of Nursing.

Royal College of Nursing Institute (2001) *Values through the Ages: Ageing in Society*. London: Royal College of Nursing Institute.

Traynor, V. and Dewing, J. (2002) The development of a HLP competency framework for the Admiral Nurse service: a participatory action research approach. Unpublished Report, Dementia Relief Trust, London.

Traynor, V. and Dewing, J. (2001) Admiral Nurses' Competency Project, *Journal of Dementia Care*, 9(4): 38.

UKCC (1986) *Project 2000: A New Preparation for Practice*. London: United Kingdom Central Council.

UKCC (1990) *The Post-registration and Education and Practice Project*. London: United Kingdom Central Council.

UKCC (1995) *PREP and You: Maintaining your Registration Standards for Education following Registration*. London: United Kingdom Central Council.

UKCC (1999a) *A Higher Level of Practice: Report of the Consultation on the UKCC's Proposals for a Revised Regulatory Framework for Post-Registration Clinical Practice*. London: United Kingdom Central Council.

UKCC (1999b) *A Higher Level of Practice: A Pilot Standard*. London: United Kingdom Central Council.

UKCC (2002) *Report of the Higher Level of Practice Pilot and Project: Executive Summary*. London: United Kingdom Central Council.

Index

abuse
  historic perspective 11–12
  risk of 67–9
access to services 58–9, 173–4
activity 27–8
activity group 156
Activity Monitoring Admiral Nurse
    Database (AMANDA) 177–8
Adams, T. 45, 51, 55, 56, 57, 59, 65,
    77, 78, 80–1, 83, 84, 130, 161,
    165, 168, 178, 189, 217, 245
  and Page, S.C. 130, 246
Admiral Nurse Assessment Schedule
    (ANAS) 171–2, 175–8
Admiral Nurse Competency Project
    259–62
Admiral Nurse service 161–2
  assessing practice efficacy 181–2
  case studies 177–8, 179–81
  consultancy 172
  evidence base 173–7
  future challenges 182–3
  interventions 174–9
  origins and philosophy 171–3
Adults with Incapacity Act
    (Scotland) (2000) 45, 47, 49,
    54, 55, 58, 197
advocacy role 54–5
ageism 14
agenda setting (CBT) 96–7
Alaszewski, A. 24
  et al. 63, 64, 66, 71, 243
  and Manthorpe, J. 64, 68
Allen, D. 21–2
Alzheimer, A. 7, 199, 200
Alzheimer's disease 199, 200
  pharmacological treatments
    127–8, 129–30
Alzheimer's Scotland – Action on
    Dementia 188–9
Alzheimer's Society 88, 89, 104, 105,
    199, 242
  carer support 150, 151, 152
  living alone 208

AMANDA (Activity Monitoring
    Admiral Nurse Database)
    177–8
American Nurses Association
    (ANA) 48, 201
AMPS UK Ltd, see Assessment of
    Motor and Process Skills
ANAS, see Admiral Nurse
    Assessment Schedule
anxiety 89
Armstrong, M. 178
Ashley, P. 107–8, 115
  and Schofield, J. 107–8, 115
assertive outreach 40–1
Assessing Older People with
    Dementia Living in the
    Community 134
assessment
  Admiral Nurse service 161–2
    practice efficacy 181–2
  of carers 138–9
  CMHN role 78–81
  cognitive function 123–4
  early 135–6
  memory 123–4, 130–1
  physical health 123
  of professional competency 256–9
  risk 70–1
  teamwork 41–2
Assessment of Motor and Process
    Skills (AMPS UK Ltd) 41
assumptions 91
  cultural 108–10
asylums (mental hospitals) 7–8,
    12–13, 33–4
attributes, expert nurse 255–6
Audit Commission 40, 78, 127, 134,
    136
automatic thoughts 91
autonomy 46–7, 50–1, 52, 54, 106
  CMHN 70
  legal (Scotland) 47–8
  and risk 71
  threats to 54–6

Barrowclough, C. and Tarrier, N.
    165, 166
Beck, A.T. 90, 166
  et al. 89, 91–2, 94–5, 99
  and Young, J.E. 95
Beech House Inquiry 68–9
Behavioural Assessment Scale of
    Later Life 42
Belbin, R.M. 238, 239, 240, 242
Benner, P. 19, 253–5, 256, 257, 258–9
bereavement issues 84–5
Berrios, G.E. 3, 5
  and Freeman, H. 7
biographical approaches 26, 79–80,
    82, 114–16, 123
biomedical vs psychosocial
    interventions 14, 24, 189–90
Bond, J. 79
Bradford Dementia Group 108
Brief Assessment Schedule
    Depression Cards 42
brokering services (care
    coordination) 29, 40
Brooker, C. et al. 162
Buber, M. 106
Building Bridges 34
Burns, A. et al. 79, 128, 129, 130, 201

Camberwell Family Interview (CFI)
    163–4
Camden and Islington Community
    Health Services NHS Trust
    68–9
CAMI, see Carers' Assessment of
    Management Index
Care Coordination (Department of
    Health) 40
care coordinator 29, 40
Care Programme Approach (CPA)
    (Department of Health) 34–5
CarenapD 80
care-planning 116
Carer (Recognition and Services)
    Act (1995) 136, 149, 236

carer–patient dyad 110, 114
carer-led assessment process
    (CLASP) 80
carer(s)
    assessment 138–9
    autonomy issues 51–2
    CMHN Dementia Team,
        Scotland 190–3
    crisis 84
    depression 89
    distress, *see* stress
    Early Intervention in Dementia
        (EID) study 137–9, 143–4
    education 53–4, 167
    heterogeneity 174
    information 109–10, 178
    vs patients 80, 82
    vs professional perspectives 21–2,
        24–5, 65–7
    see also Admiral Nurse service;
        Dementia Action Research
        and Education (DARE)
Carers' Assessment of Management
    Index (CAMI) 138–9
Carers' Checklist 178
Caring for Carers 135
Carradice, A. 160, 161, 218
'case finding' 40
CBS, *see* Challenging Behaviour
    Scale
CBT, *see* cognitive-behavioural
    therapy
CFI, *see* Camberwell Family
    Interview
challenging behaviour
    case studies 202–4, 206–7, 208–9
    CMHN practice 202–7
    inner meaning and observed
        reality 200–1
    living alone 208–9
    rating scales 201, 205
    residential care 204–7
Challenging Behaviour Scale (CBS)
    201
Charcot, J.M. 7
Charter Mark 120
Cheston, R. 83, 194–5
    and Bender, M. 79, 80, 107–8, 110
cholinergic deficit 127–8, 129
cholinesterase inhibitors (ChEI) 127,
    128, 129–30

Clarke, C.L. 20, 22, 24, 25, 29, 65–6,
    186–7, 192, 193, 194, 197
    and Gardner, A. 23
    and Heyman, B. 21
    and Wilcockson, J. 23, 24
Clarkson, P. 190
CLASP, *see* carer-led assessment
    process
client pathways 39–40
Clifton Assessment Procedure for
    the Elderly (CAPE) 79
Clinical Board of Nursing Studies
    12
clinical supervision 196–7, 240
    case study 223–31
    DARE project 221–32
    in dementia care 220–3
    impact on negotiated care 230–1
    in nursing
        influences and obstacles 215–17
        opportunities 218–19
        potential benefits 219
        practice development 217–18
    vs managerial 38, 216
CMHN Dementia Team, Scotland
    187, 188
    clinical practice 193–4
    early diagnosis, implications for
        practice 194–6
    reflections 196–7
    roles 188–9
    theoretical base 189–90
co-therapists 157
cognitive assessment 123–4
cognitive model 90–2, 97–8
cognitive-behavioural therapy (CBT)
    88, 89–90
    agenda setting 96–7
    carers 93, 94, 96–9, 149–54, 166–8
    commencement 97
    developing a therapeutic
        relationship 94–5
    group 93–4, 149–54
    guided discovery 95–6
    preparation 93–4
    principles to practice 90–2
    process 92–3
    Socratic dialogue 95–6, 97–8
    termination and relapse
        prevention 99–100
    using the techniques 97–9

collaborative work 58–9, 241–2
    see also multi-disciplinary
        teamwork; partnership
communication
    inter-agency 242–5
    teamwork 42
    in therapeutic relationship 56
competency 253–6
    Admiral Nurse Project 259–62
    assessing 256–9
    core competencies 260
compliance 130
computer technology 106, 107
consent to treatment 201
constraints in exchanging knowledge
    24–5
consultancy roles 137, 172
contract development 221–3
coping strategies 165, 167–8, 174
core beliefs 91
core elements, in positive person
    work 110, 111–14
core and periphery teamwork 36
counselling 50–2, 83, 189
    loss and bereavement 192–3
    post-diagnostic 128–9
critical incidents 58
cultural assumptions 108–10

decision-making 50–2
    facilitating, case study 225–6
    see also autonomy
defensive practice 22
Dementia Action Research and
    Education (DARE) 221–32
Dementia Policy Scrutiny report
    (Northern Ireland) 243
dementia praecox (schizophrenia)
    8, 9
denial *vs* acceptance of diagnosis
    139
Department of Health
    *Assessing Older People with
        Dementia Living in the
        Community* 134
    Building Bridges 34
    Care Coordination 40
    Care Programme Approach (CPA)
        34–5
    Caring for Carers 135
    No Secrets 67–8

Working in Partnership 216–17, 221–2
   see also National Services Framework for Older People
Department of Health and Social Services (N. Ireland) 243–4, 245
depression 89, 124, 127
Derwentside Practice Development Unit 37, 40, 41–2
diagnosis
   disclosure of 135, 136, 139, 193
   early 135–6, 194–6
   in memory clinics 124–5
   nurses' role 136–7
   patient perspectives 193
diagnostic support 52–4
Drickamer, M.A. and Lachs, M.S. 135, 136, 145

early diagnosis 135–6, 194–6
early intervention 135–6
   EID study
      carers 137–9, 143–4
      case examples 139–43
      design 137–9
      findings 139, 145
   group CBT for carers 153–4
ecomaps 222–3, 231
   case study 224–5, 227–8, 229–30
Edberg, A. *et al.* 219, 220
education
   carer 53–4, 167
   patient 53–4
   see also nurse education
EE, *see* expressed emotion
effectiveness of interventions 161–3
   Admiral Nurse service 181–2
ELTOS (Enhanced Lifestyle Through Optimal Stimulus) model 28–9
emotional support 50–2
   see also expressed emotion (EE)
English National Board 12, 64, 252
Enright, S.J. 166, 167
ethical issues, *see* moral/ethical knowledge; negotiated care, study
evidence 18–29
   Admiral Nurse service 173–7
   carer distress 150

case study (Jones) 17–18, 20, 29–30
   early intervention and diagnostic sharing 135–6
   psychosocial interventions with carers 163–4
   see also research; scientific approaches
evidence-based practice 22, 23, 24
expert nurse, attributes 255–6
expertise, lay *vs* professional perspectives 21–2, 24–5, 65–7
expressed emotion (EE) 165
   see also emotional support

Falloon, I. 83–4
   et al. 164, 165, 166–8
family
   responses to diagnosis 135
   therapy 27, 28, 51–2, 83–4, 156–7
   see also carer(s)
Fearnley, K. *et al.* 135, 137, 193
first contact
   case study 223–4
   in memory clinics 122–3
'fitness for purpose' model of competence 253, 254–5, 258
Flanagan, J. *et al.* 256, 257
Forchuk, C. 45, 46, 54, 59
fragmentation of care and knowledge 25
fragmented teamwork 36

Garratt, S. and Hamilton-Smith, E. 28
General Health Questionnaire (GHQ) 138, 143, 162, 163, 166
general practitioners (GPs) 40, 109, 130
   early diagnosis 134, 135, 136
   early intervention study 138, 139
   teamwork 241–2
George, E. *et al.* 178–9
Geriatric Depression Scale 124
Gibson, F. 27, 82
Gilhooly, M.L.M. 89, 149, 167
   and Whittick, J.E. 165
goal setting, stress management 167–8

Goldberg, D.P. and Hillier, V.F. 138, 143, 166
Gournay, K. *et al.* 161, 168, 217
Graham, I.W. 215, 219, 220
Greenhalgh, T. 18–19, 22, 23
group therapy 148–9
   for carers (CBT) 93–4, 149–54
   for younger people with dementia 154–7
   see also self-help group
guided discovery 95–6
Gunstone, S. 45, 51, 57, 58, 60, 136, 237, 245

Health Education Authority 209
Heyman 25, 63, 66
higher-level practice (HLP) 250–3, 260–2
   see also competency
historic perspectives
   involvement of nurses in dementia care 12–13
   multi-disciplinary teamworking 33–5
   responses to dementia 7–10
   science of old age 6–7
   treating disorders of older people 10–12
Ho, D. 51, 60, 77, 136
Holden, U. 78, 79, 80
   and Woods, R.T. 180
home day care 117
homesharing 117
Hospital Anxiety and Depression Scale 89
hospitals
   mental hospitals 7–8, 12–13, 33–4
   'scandals' 11–12
housing 116–17
Hull and East Riding Community Health NHS Trust project 40–1

'I–Thou' meeting 106
individuality 26
   see also biographical approaches
inequalities
   of knowledges 24
   social 25
information giving 109–10, 178
information processing 90–1

inner meaning, of challenging
    behaviour 200–1
institutional care, *see* hospitals
integrated teamwork 35–6
integration, theory–practice 26–8,
    218, 220–3
inter-agency communication 242–5
'interpretative' approach to
    competence 258–9
interventions, *see* early intervention;
    post-diagnostic interventions
intuitive/experiential knowledge 19

Jarvis, J. *et al.* 172
Johns, C. 218
Jones, K. *et al.* 148, 149

Kapp, M. 56
Keady, J. 107, 173
    and Adams, T. 48, 51, 60, 77, 81,
        85, 182
    et al. 220–1
    and Gilliard, J. 122
    and Nolan, M. 52, 60, 80, 107,
        174, 217–18
Kitwood, T. 4, 10, 27, 79, 81–2,
        104–5, 106, 107, 108, 114–15,
        117, 123, 190, 196, 199, 236,
        244
    and Benson, S. 105
    and Bredin, K. 25, 105, 154,
        189–90
'knowing the patient' 21, 22
knowledge
    chains 23–5
    types 18–22
Kraepelin, E. 7, 8, 9

Law Commission 136
lay *vs* professional perspectives 21–2,
    24–5, 65–7
leadership (management) 38–9,
    237–8, 240, 246
legal autonomy (Scotland) 47–8
Levi, B. 46, 55
Liaschenko, J. and Fisher, A. 19, 20,
    21, 28, 29
life histories, *see* biographical
    approaches; reminiscence
    work
lifelong learning 257

lifestyle profile 115
living alone 208–9
Long, A. 236–7, 238, 245
loss issues 84–5
Luker, K.A. *et al.* 21, 28

McCormack, B. 50, 51, 52, 56, 57,
    59, 60, 236
McFadyen, J. *et al.* 45, 55, 59, 60
McGowin, D.F. 107
McWalter, G. *et al.* 78, 79, 80
malignant social psychology (MSP)
    108–10
management, *see* leadership
    (management)
managerial *vs* clinical supervision 38,
    216
Manchester memory clinic 121–31
Manchester support groups 155–7
Marriott, A. 155, 156–7, 166, 167
    et al. 90, 151, 163, 164, 166, 167,
        179
Martin, P.J. 9–10, 12, 22, 23
Mason, A. and Wilkinson, H. 45,
    49
Matthew, L. 57, 60, 161, 217
memory clinics 120–1
    assessment 123–4, 130–1
    case study 125–7
    diagnosis 124–5
    first contact 122–3
    Manchester model 121–31
    nurses' roles 121
    post-diagnostic interventions 127
    treatments 127–31
memory problems 116
Mental Health Acts 11, 136
*Mental Health Framework for
    Scotland* (1997) 58, 60
mental hospitals (asylums) 7–8,
    12–13, 33–4
Miller, A. 220
Miller, C. *et al.* 35, 36
Mini-Mental State Exam (MMSE)
    41, 79
Mishler, E.G. 49
monastic community 5–6
monitoring role 57, 129–31
moral/ethical knowledge 19–20
MSP, *see* malignant social
    psychology

multi-agency working, *see* multi-
    disciplinary teamwork
multi-disciplinary teamwork
    characteristics 35–6
    collaboration 58–9, 241–2
    Derwentside Practice
        Development Unit 37, 40,
        41–2
    development 33–5
    inter-agency communication
        242–5
    key areas 38–42
    leadership (management) 38–9,
        237–8, 240, 246
    risk 69–71
    team building and 238–40
    towards the future 245–6

National Health Service Executive
    67
National Institute for Clinical
    Excellence (NICE) 130
*National Services Framework for
    Older People* 13, 236
    Charter Mark 120
    early intervention 136
    multi-disciplinary working 34, 41,
        242
    risk taking 64
    standards 251–2
    tenets 14
needs
    articulation of 173–4
    care-planning 116
    carers *vs* patients 80
    in dementia 88–9
    perceived 50–9
negative thoughts 99
negotiated care
    impact of clinical supervision
        230–1
    study 49–60
Newcastle carers group CBT 151–3
NHS and Community Care Act
    (1990) 236
NICE, *see* National Institute for
    Clinical Excellence
No Secrets 67–8
Nolan, M.
    et al. 14, 46, 51, 110–14, 143, 144,
        173, 174, 218

and Grant, G. 56
and Keady, J. 221
Nolan, P. 10
normalization 186–7
  see also CMHN Dementia Team,
    Scotland
normalizing strategies 192, 194
norms 26–7
Northern Ireland 243–4
  Dementia Forum 245
nurse consultants 137, 172
nurse education
  higher-level practice (HLP) 250–3,
    260–2
  historic perspective 9, 12–13
  research-based 246
nurse prescribing 245–6
nursing roles, *see* role(s)

Overholser, J.C. 95–6
Øvretveit, J. 35, 38, 39

Packer, T. 137
Padesky, C.M. 96
partnership 195–6
PATH, team building exercises
    239–40
patients
  client pathways 39–40
  education 53–4
  experience of illness 22
  'knowing the patient' 21, 22
  responses to diagnosis 193
  vs carers 80, 82
Payne, M. 35
Peplau, H. 45, 46, 47, 48, 189
Perrin, T. 246
person-centred approaches 81,
    105–8, 244
  challenging behaviour 201
  housing 116–17
  malignant social psychology
    108–10
  positive person work 110–14
  and risk 66
  vs 'relationship-centred care'
    14
  see also biographical approaches
personal autonomy, *see* autonomy
personhood
  definition 107

'rementia' 108
  vs scientific method 10
'personhood club' 115
pharmacological treatments 127–8,
    201, 245–6
phenomenological focus 48, 56
physical health screening 123
*Planning Signposts for Dementia
    Care Services* (Scotland)
    188–9
policy development 13–14
  see also Department of Health
Pollock, L. 46, 60
positive person work 110–14
post-diagnostic interventions 127
  counselling 128–9
Pratt, R. and Wilkinson, H. 52, 60,
    136
prescribing 127–8, 201
  nurse 245–6
problem solving 168, 174–5, 178–9
professional accountability 66–7
professional *vs* lay perspectives 21–2,
    24–5, 65–7
proximal *vs* distal knowledge 23–4
psychosis 161
psychosocial interventions 28, 84,
    160–8
  vs biomedical approaches 14, 24,
    189–90

qualitative approach to competence
    258–9
quality of client care 219
Quinton, A. 105–6

Raines, M.L. 20
rationality 106
  and risk 71
RCN, *see* Royal College of Nursing
reality orientation 26–7
Reed, J.
  and Clarke, C. 26
  and Ground, I. 20
referrals 39–40, 124, 188, 241, 242
reflective practice 215, 218, 230–1
relapse prevention (CBT) 99–100
Relative Assessment Interview 166
'rementia' 108
reminiscence work 27, 82
  see also biographical approaches

research
  importance of 246
  vs service-driven model 120–1
  see also evidence; scientific
    approaches
residential care, challenging
    behaviour in 204–7
resolution therapy 83
respite care 56
Reynolds, W. 45, 46, 48, 50, 52, 56,
    59, 60
right to know (diagnosis) 135, 136,
    139, 193
risk
  assessment 70–1
  and autonomy 71
  definitions and concepts 63–5
  lay *vs* expert views 65–7
  multi-disciplinary teamwork
    69–71
  and normalization 197
  policy at agency level: proactive
    and reactive 67–9
  positive aspects of risk taking 64
  and rationality 71
Rogers, C. 105
role(s)
  advocacy 54–5
  assessment 78–81
  challenging behaviour 202–4
  definition 237
  diagnosis 136–7
  in memory clinics 121
  monitoring 57, 129–31
  research 49
  social 57
  support 50–4
  therapeutic 81–5, 161–3
Rosenfeld, R. 49
Ross, F. and Meerabeau, L. 25
Royal College of Nursing (RCN)
    10–11, 46, 250–1, 255–6,
    259
Royal College of Psychiatrists
    201
Rule of St Benedict 5, 7

Sabatino, C. 47
Sackett, D.L. *et al.* 22
Sailors, P.R. 47, 52
Scaife, J. 216, 218, 221

schizophrenia 164
  dementia praecox (historic
      perspective) 8, 9
scientific approaches
  biomedical *vs* psychosocial
      interventions 14, 24, 189–90
  historic perspective 6–7
  knowledge 18–19
      consequences of dominance 21
  see also evidence; research
Scotland
  Adults with Incapacity Act (2000)
      45, 47, 49, 54, 55, 58, 197
  legal autonomy 47–8
  *Mental Health Framework for
      Scotland* (1997) 58, 60
  see also CMHN Dementia Team,
      Scotland
screening, *see* assessment
Seedhouse, D. 20
self-awareness 218, 231
self-help group 194–5
  see also group therapy
senile dementia 7, 8
senile haemorrhage 7
'senile insanity' 9
senium praecox 7
service context knowledge 20
service *vs* research-driven model of
      care 120–1
Shaw, A. and Shaw, I. 65
Silvester, S. and McCarthy, M.
      171–2, 176, 177
Sloan, G. 95, 219
  et al. 216
social connectedness, *see* social
      relationships
social inequalities 25
'social knowledge' 20, 21
social model of care 46–7, 123, 127
social norms, *see* norms
social relationships 27, 57, 106–7

Social Services Inspectorate 70
social workers 222–3
Socratic dialogue 95–6, 97–8
solution-focused brief therapy 178–9
Standing Medical Advisory
      Committee 130
Stanley, D. and Cantley, C. 80
Stelzmann, R.A. *et al.* 199, 200
Sterin, G. 107, 116
Stevenson, O. 70, 71
stress 143, 150, 152–4, 160, 163–4,
      173, 174
  management 167, 189
      models 84, 174–5
  vulnerability model 164–5
supervision, *see* clinical supervision
support groups 154–7, 194–5
support roles 50–4
systems (family) therapy 27, 28,
      51–2, 83–4, 156–7

Taylor, William and Keith (inquiry)
      69
team management *see* leadership
      (management)
teamwork, *see* multi-disciplinary
      teamwork
termination of therapy (CBT)
      99–100
theory–practice integration 26–8,
      218, 220–3
therapeutic relationship 28–9
  Admiral Nurses 178
  assessment 81
  challenging behaviour 202
  CMHN Dementia Team,
      Scotland 190–3
  communication skills 56
  development in CBT 94–5
  historic perspective 10
  lifestyle profile 115
  in memory clinics 122, 129, 130–1

36 Hour Day 150
Thompson, L.W. *et al.* 94
Thorne, S.E. *et al.* 20, 21, 28
time
  caregiving changes over 173
  pacing strategy 192, 194
triadic approach 121–2
Trinder, L. 20, 23

United Kingdom Central Council
      for Nursing, Midwifery and
      Health Visiting (UKCC)
  clinical supervision 215, 217
  'fitness for purpose' 253, 254–5,
      258
  higher-level practice (HLP)
      standards 250–1, 252, 255,
      256, 260–1
  Post-Registration Education and
      Practice (PREP) 255
  teamwork 239, 240

validation therapy 83

Watkins, P. 79, 80
Wilford, S. 83–4
Wilkinson, H. 25, 47
  Mason, A. and 45, 49
  Pratt, R. and 52, 60, 136
Woods, B. *et al.* 162, 182
Woods, Bob 221
Working in Partnership (Department
      of Health) 216–17, 221–2

Yale, R. 154, 155
Yegdich, T. 216
younger people with dementia,
      group CBT 154–7

Zarit, S.H. *et al.* 84, 150, 161, 167,
      173, 174–5, 178, 189
Zubin, J. and Spring, B. 164

COMMUNICATION AND THE CARE OF PEOPLE WITH DEMENTIA

John Killick and Kate Allan

The combination of creativity and critical analysis which the joint authors as poet and psychologist bring to this book is especially productive . . . The interweaving of substantial practice examples based on conversations with people with dementia give persuasive authority to the careful exposition and detailed analysis. The book is much more than an exhortation to carers about how they should communicate. It challenges them to understand themselves and shows how they might use themselves to engage with people with dementia.

Faith Gibson, Emeritus Professor of Social Work

This book argues that communication is at the heart of all approaches to dementia care, and is an in-depth exploration of ways of establishing and developing communication with people with dementia. It examines both the nature of dementia as a condition and the subjective experience of those affected. The authors consider in detail how communication between people with dementia and those who care for them changes, and how it can be maintained and enhanced. They include a significant amount of material quoted from people with dementia, and suggest ways of interpreting their words and actions. We learn about what it might be like to have dementia, and what sort of help is needed by people in this situation. Throughout the book the authors address the ethical issues and the implications for practice.

Communication and the Care of People with Dementia is a key resource for students and professionals in health and social care work, including those in such fields as social work, nursing, occupational therapy, speech therapy, physiotherapy, clinical psychology, geriatric medicine, and the management of services.

Contents

Introduction – Part one: Basics – Conversations with Alice: 'A far fetch' – Personhood: 'The truth is mine, not yours' – Nonverbal communication: 'I just want to hold you and hold you one minute' – Language: 'Words can make or break you' – Memory: 'Playing in the House of Ages' – Interpretation: 'After all, what is this lump of matter if you can't make sense of it?' – Part two: Practicalities – Making contact: 'Getting in a normal situation' – Developing the interaction: 'With you I am putting things together' – Endings: 'With regard to silence, I think it should be observed' – Writing: 'It's a good idea, this writing it down' – Part three: Themes – Narrative: 'I want to make up my story for myself' – Relationships: 'I like us being with us' – Awareness: 'I'm thinking when I'm not saying anything' – Part four: Implications – Implications for care: 'I need help, yes. But it's the way that it's done' – Ethical implications: 'What I want to know is, what is this doing for you?' – Part five: Conclusion – Conversations with Jane: 'My mind, my whole sphere of life is full' – References – Index.

352pp   0 335 20774 X (Paperback)   0 335 20775 8 (Hardback)

A HANDBOOK OF DEMENTIA CARE

Caroline Cantley (ed.)

Recently, professional understanding of dementia has broadened and has opened up new thinking about how we can provide more imaginative, responsive and 'person-centred' services for people with dementia. Against this background *A Handbook of Dementia Care* provides a wide-ranging, up-to-date overview of the current state of knowledge in the field. It is comprehensive, authoritative, accessible and thought-provoking. It asks:

- How do different theoretical perspectives help us to understand dementia?
- What do we know about what constitutes good practice in dementia care?
- How can we improve practice and service delivery in dementia care?
- How do policy, organizational issues and research impact on dementia care?

This handbook provides a unique, multidisciplinary and critical guide to what we know about dementia and dementia care. It is written by leading academics, practitioners and managers involved in the development of dementia care. It demonstrates the value of a wide range of perspectives in understanding dementia care, reviews the latest thinking about good practice, and examines key ethical issues. It explores the way organizations, policy and research shape dementia care, and introduces a range of approaches to practice and service development.

A Handbook of Dementia Care is an essential resource for students and professionals in such fields as gerontology, social work, nursing, occupational therapy, geriatric medicine, psychiatry, mental health, psychology, social services and health services management, social policy and health policy.

Contents

Introduction – Part one: Understanding dementia – Bio-medical and clinical perspectives – Psychological perspectives – Sociological perspectives – Philosophical and spiritual perspectives – The perspectives of people with dementia, their families and their carers – Part two: Practice knowledge and development – Understanding practice development – Assessment, care planning and care management – Living at home – Communication and personhood – Therapeutic activity – Working with carers – Care settings and the care environment – Ethical ideals and practice – Part three: Policy, organizations and research – Understanding the policy context – Understanding people in organizations – Developing service organizations – Developing quality in services – Involving people with dementia and their carers in developing services – Research, policy and practice in dementia care – Conclusion: The future development of dementia care – Glossary – References – Index.

400pp   0 335 20383 3 (Paperback)   0 335 20384 1 (Hardback)

DEMENTIA RECONSIDERED
THE PERSON COMES FIRST

Tom Kitwood

For some years now, Tom Kitwood's work on dementia care has stood out as the most important, innovative and creative development in a field that has for too long been neglected. This book is a landmark in dementia care; it brings together, and elaborates on, Kitwood's theory of dementia and of person-centred care in an accessible fashion, that will make this an essential source for all working and researching in the field of dementia care.

Robert Woods, Professor of Clinical Psychology, University of Wales

Over the last ten years or so Tom Kitwood has made a truly remarkable contribution to our understanding of dementia, and to raising expectations of what can be achieved with empathy and skill. This lucid account of his thinking and work will communicate his approach to a yet wider audience. It is to be warmly welcomed.

Mary Marshall, Director of the Dementia Services Development Centre, University of Stirling

- What is the *real* nature of the dementing process?
- What might we reasonably expect when dementia care is of very high quality?
- What is required of organizations and individuals involved in dementia care?

Tom Kitwood breaks new ground in this book. Many of the older ideas about dementia are subjected to critical scrutiny and reappraisal, drawing on research evidence, logical analysis and the author's own experience. The unifying theme is the personhood of men and women who have dementia – an issue that was grossly neglected for many years both in psychiatry and care practice.

Each chapter provides a definitive statement on a major topic related to dementia, for example: the nature of 'organic mental impairment', the experience of dementia, the agenda for care practice, and the transformation of the culture of care.

While recognizing the enormous difficulties of the present day, the book clearly demonstrates the possibility of a better life for people who have dementia, and comes to a cautiously optimistic conclusion. It will be of interest to all professionals involved in dementia care or provision, students on courses involving psychogeriatrics or social work with older people, and family carers of people with dementia.

Key features:

- One of the few attempts to present the whole picture.
- Very readable – many real-life illustrations.
- Offers a major alternative to the 'medical model' of dementia.
- Tom Kitwood's work on dementia is very well known.

Contents
Series editor's preface – Brian Gearing – Acknowledgements – Introduction – On being a person – Dementia as a psychiatric category – How personhood is undermined – Personhood maintained – The experiences of dementia – Improving care: the next step forward – The caring organization – Requirements of a caregiver – The task of cultural transformation – References – Index.

176pp   0 335 19855 4 (Paperback)   0 335 19856 2 (Hardback)

WORKING WITH OLDER PEOPLE AND THEIR FAMILIES
KEY ISSUES IN POLICY AND PRACTICE

Mike Nolan, Sue Davies and Gordon Grant (eds)

Addressing the needs of older people and their carers is an essential element of both policy and practice in the fields of health and social care. Recent developments promote a partnership and empowerment model, in which the notion of 'person-centred' care figures prominently. However, what 'person-centred' care means and how it can be achieved is far from clear.

Working with Older People and their Families combines extensive reviews of specialist literatures with new empirical data in an attempt at a synthesis of themes about making a reality of 'person-centred' care. Uniquely, it seeks to unite the perspectives of older people, family and professional carers in promoting a genuinely holistic approach to the challenges of an ageing society.

Working with Older People and their Families is recommended reading for students on health related courses such as nursing, medicine and the therapies. It is also of relevance to students of social work and social gerontology, researchers, managers and policy makers.

Contents
The changing face of health and social care – Quality of life, quality of care – Who's the expert: redefining lay and professional relationships – Acute and rehabilitative care for older people – Community care – The care needs of older people and family care-givers in continuing care settings – Palliative care and older people – The mental health needs of older people and their carers: exploring tensions and new directions – Older people with learning disabilities, health, community inclusion and family caregiving – Integrating perspectives – Appendix 1: Literature review: Methodology – Bibliography – Index.

224pp   0 335 20560 7 (Paperback)   0 335 20561 5 (Hardback)

RESEARCHING AGEING AND LATER LIFE
THE PRACTICE OF SOCIAL GERONTOLOGY

Anne Jamieson and Christina Victor (eds)

The changing demographic profiles of modern societies have led to a growing interest in understanding ageing and later life among those working within the social sciences and humanities. This edited volume addresses the methodological challenges entailed in studying the process of ageing and life course changes, as well as the experience of being old. The book focuses on the theory and practice of doing research, using a wide range of examples and case studies. The contributors, who are prominent researchers in the field, review the range of practices in the use of different methodologies and give in-depth examples, based on their own research experience. The book covers a variety of disciplines and methodologies, both quantitative and qualitative, and a diversity of sources, including fiction, photographs, as well as the traditional social science sources. *Researching Ageing and Later Life* will be essential reading for those wishing for an insight into the realities of doing research in this area.

Contents

Introduction – Part 1: The who, what and how of social gerontology – Theory and practice in social gerontology – Strategies and methods in the study of ageing and later life – Part 2: Using existing sources – Using documentary material: Researching the past – Using existing research and statistical data: Secondary data analysis – Using the Mass Observation Archive – Using 'cultural products' in researching images of ageing – Part 3: Creating new data – Doing longitudinal research – Doing life history research – Doing case study research in psychology – Doing diary based research – Doing evaluation of health and social care interventions – Part 4: The roles and responsibilities of the researcher – Researching ageing in different cultures – Ethical issues in researching later life – The role of older people in research – The use of gerontological research in policy and practice – References – Appendix: Web resources – Index.

288pp   0 335 20820 7 (Paperback)   0 335 20821 5 (Hardback)